Next-Generation Mobile and Pervasive Healthcare Solutions

Jose Machado
University of Minho, Portugal

António Abelha
University of Minho, Portugal

Manuel Filipe Santos
University of Minho, Portugal

Filipe Portela
University of Minho, Portugal

A volume in the Advances in Medical Technologies and Clinical Practice (AMTCP) Book Series

IGI Global
DISSEMINATOR OF KNOWLEDGE

Published in the United States of America by
IGI Global
Medical Information Science Reference (an imprint of IGI Global)
701 E. Chocolate Avenue
Hershey PA, USA 17033
Tel: 717-533-8845
Fax: 717-533-8661
E-mail: cust@igi-global.com
Web site: http://www.igi-global.com

Library of Congress Cataloging-in-Publication Data

Names: Machado, Jose Manuel, editor. | Abelha, Antonio, 1964- editor. | Santos, Manuel Filipe, editor. | Portela, Filipe, editor.
Title: Next-generation mobile and pervasive healthcare solutions / Jose Machado, Antonio Abelha, Manuel Filipe Santos, and Filipe Portela, editors.
Description: Hershey, PA : Medical Information Science Reference, [2018] | Includes bibliographical references.
Identifiers: LCCN 2017010732| ISBN 9781522528517 (hardcover) | ISBN 9781522528524 (ebook)
Subjects: | MESH: Medical Informatics Applications | Telemedicine | Mobile Applications | Global Health
Classification: LCC R855.3 | NLM W 26.5 | DDC 610.285--dc23 LC record available at https://lccn.loc.gov/2017010732

This book is published in the IGI Global book series Advances in Medical Technologies and Clinical Practice (AMTCP) (ISSN: 2327-9354; eISSN: 2327-9370)

British Cataloguing in Publication Data
A Cataloguing in Publication record for this book is available from the British Library.

Advances in Medical Technologies and Clinical Practice (AMTCP) Book Series

Srikanta Patnaik
SOA University, India
Priti Das
S.C.B. Medical College, India

ISSN:2327-9354
EISSN:2327-9370

Mission

Medical technological innovation continues to provide avenues of research for faster and safer diagnosis and treatments for patients. Practitioners must stay up to date with these latest advancements to provide the best care for nursing and clinical practices.

The **Advances in Medical Technologies and Clinical Practice (AMTCP) Book Series** brings together the most recent research on the latest technology used in areas of nursing informatics, clinical technology, biomedicine, diagnostic technologies, and more. Researchers, students, and practitioners in this field will benefit from this fundamental coverage on the use of technology in clinical practices.

Coverage

- Telemedicine
- Nursing Informatics
- E-health
- Biomedical Applications
- Clinical Studies
- Neural Engineering
- Medical Imaging
- Clinical Nutrition
- Clinical High-Performance Computing
- Diagnostic Technologies

IGI Global is currently accepting manuscripts for publication within this series. To submit a proposal for a volume in this series, please contact our Acquisition Editors at Acquisitions@igi-global.com or visit: http://www.igi-global.com/publish/.

The Advances in Medical Technologies and Clinical Practice (AMTCP) Book Series (ISSN 2327-9354) is published by IGI Global, 701 E. Chocolate Avenue, Hershey, PA 17033-1240, USA, www.igi-global.com. This series is composed of titles available for purchase individually; each title is edited to be contextually exclusive from any other title within the series. For pricing and ordering information please visit http://www.igi-global.com/book-series/advances-medical-technologies-clinical-practice/73682. Postmaster: Send all address changes to above address.

Titles in this Series

For a list of additional titles in this series, please visit: www.igi-global.com/book-series

Innovative Research in Thermal Imaging for Biology and Medicine
Ricardo Vardasca (University of Porto, Portugal) and Joaquim Gabriel Mendes (University of Porto, Portugal)
Medical Information Science Reference • copyright 2017 • 340pp • H/C (ISBN: 9781522520726) • US $210.00 (our price)

Internet of Things and Advanced Application in Healthcare
Catarina I. Reis (Polytechnic Institute of Leiria, Portugal) and Marisa da Silva Maximiano (Polytechnic Institute of Leiria, Portugal)
Medical Information Science Reference • copyright 2017 • 349pp • H/C (ISBN: 9781522518204) • US $210.00 (our price)

Integrating Biologically-Inspired Nanotechnology into Medical Practice
B.K. Nayak (K.M. Centre for Post Graduate Studies, India) Anima Nanda (Sathyabama University, India) and M. Amin Bhat (Sathyabama University, India)
Medical Information Science Reference • copyright 2017 • 394pp • H/C (ISBN: 9781522506102) • US $190.00 (our price)

Recent Advances in Drug Delivery Technology
Raj K. Keservani (Rajiv Gandhi Proudyogiki Vishwavidyalaya, India) Anil K. Sharma (Delhi Institute of Pharmaceutical Sciences and Research, India) and Rajesh Kumar Kesharwani (National Institute of Technology, Warangal, India)
Medical Information Science Reference • copyright 2017 • 510pp • H/C (ISBN: 9781522507543) • US $215.00 (our price)

Advancing Medicine through Nanotechnology and Nanomechanics Applications
Keka Talukdar (Nadiha High School, India) Mayank Bhushan (Pondicherry University, India) and Anil Shantappa Malipatil (Guru Nanak Dev Engineering College – Bidar, India)
Medical Information Science Reference • copyright 2017 • 359pp • H/C (ISBN: 9781522510437) • US $195.00 (our price)

Pattern and Data Analysis in Healthcare Settings
Vivek Tiwari (Maulana Azad National Institute of Technology, India) Basant Tiwari (Devi Ahilya University, India) Ramjeevan Singh Thakur (Maulana Azad National Institute of Technology, India) and Shailendra Gupta (AISECT University, India)
Medical Information Science Reference • copyright 2017 • 358pp • H/C (ISBN: 9781522505365) • US $215.00 (our price)

IGI Global
DISSEMINATOR OF KNOWLEDGE

701 East Chocolate Avenue, Hershey, PA 17033, USA
Tel: 717-533-8845 x100 • Fax: 717-533-8661
E-Mail: cust@igi-global.com • www.igi-global.com

Table of Contents

Preface xiv

Chapter 1
Promoting Better Healthcare for Patients in Critical Condition: An IoT-Based Solution to Integrate Patients, Physicians, and Ambulance Services 1
Itamir Barroca, UFRN, Brazil
Gibeon Aquino, UFRN, Brazil
Maria Alzete Lima, UFRN, Brazil

Chapter 2
Internet of Things in Pervasive Healthcare Systems 22
Teresa Guarda, Universidad Peninsula de Santa Elena (UPSE), Ecuador
Maria Fernanda Augusto, Universidad Peninsula de Santa Elena (UPSE), Ecuador
Oscar Barrionuevo, Universidad de las Fuerzas Armadas (ESPE), Ecuador
Filipe Mota Pinto, Polytechnic Institute of Leiria, Portugal

Chapter 3
Benefits of Bring Your Own Device in Healthcare 32
Filipe Portela, University of Minho, Portugal
Ailton Moreira da Veiga, University of Minho, Portugal
Manuel Filipe Santos, University of Minho, Portugal

Chapter 4
Big Data and mHealth: Increasing the Usability of Healthcare Through the Customization of Pinterest – Literary Perspective 46
Nancy Shipley, Towson University, USA
Joyram Chakraborty, Towson University, USA

Chapter 5
Mobile Health Systems and Electronic Health Record: Applications and Implications 67
Kijpokin Kasemsap, Suan Sunandha Rajabhat University, Thailand

Chapter 6
Pervasive Computing in Supporting Pediatric and Neonatology Care Unit Decision Process............ 86
Bia Martins, University of Minho, Portugal
Tiago André Saraiva Guimarães, University of Minho, Portugal
Mariana Santos, Unidade Local de Saúde do Alto Minho, Portugal
Simão Frutuoso, Centro Materno Infantil do Norte, Portugal
Filipe Portela, University of Minho, Portugal
Manuel Filipe Santos, University of Minho, Portugal

Chapter 7
Augmented Reality in Surgery: A New Approach to Enhance the Surgeon's Experience 96
José Inácio, University of Minho, Portugal
João Ribeiro, Peek Health S.A., Portugal
Jaime Campos, Peek Health S.A., Portugal
Sara Silva, Peek Health S.A., Portugal
Victor Alves, University of Minho, Portugal

Chapter 8
Recommendation System: A Potential Tool for Achieving Pervasive Health Care 111
Shashi Kant Srivastava, Indian Institute of Management Indore, India
Sudipendra Nath Roy, Indian Institute of Management Indore, India

Chapter 9
Real-Time Healthcare Intelligence in Organ Transplantation: Real-Time Intelligence in Organ Transplantation 128
Bruno Fernandes, University of Minho, Portugal
Cecília Coimbra, University of Minho, Portugal
António Abelha, University of Minho, Portugal

Chapter 10
Advanced Issues of Health Informatics and Clinical Decision Support System in Global Health Care 153
Kijpokin Kasemsap, Suan Sunandha Rajabhat University, Thailand

Chapter 11
Applied Business Intelligence in Surgery Waiting Lists Management... 171
Cristiana Neto, University of Minho, Portugal
Inês Dias, University of Minho, Portugal
Maria Santos, University of Minho, Portugal
Hugo Peixoto, University of Minho, Portugal
José Machado, University of Minho, Portugal

Chapter 12
Pervasive Business Intelligence Platform to Support the Decision-Making Process in Waiting Lists 186
Marisa Esteves, University of Minho, Portugal
Filipe Miranda, University of Minho, Portugal
António Abelha, University of Minho, Portugal

Chapter 13
Business Intelligence for Nutrition Therapy 203
Rita Reis, University of Minho, Portugal
Ana Mendonça, University of Minho, Portugal
Diana Lisandra Azevedo Ferreira, University of Minho, Portugal
Hugo Peixoto, University of Minho, Portugal
José Machado, University of Minho, Portugal

Chapter 14
Indian Healthcare Service Management Through Data Mining: Datamining for Healthcare Services 219
Manaswini Pradhan, Fakir Mohan University, India

Compilation of References 234

About the Contributors 279

Index 284

Detailed Table of Contents

Preface xiv

Chapter 1
Promoting Better Healthcare for Patients in Critical Condition: An IoT-Based Solution to Integrate Patients, Physicians, and Ambulance Services 1
Itamir Barroca, UFRN, Brazil
Gibeon Aquino, UFRN, Brazil
Maria Alzete Lima, UFRN, Brazil

The high cost of healthcare services, the aging population and the increase of chronic disease is becoming a global concern. Several studies have indicated the need to minimize the process of hospitalization and the high cost of patient care. A promising trend in healthcare is to move the routines of medical checks from a hospital to the patient's home. Moreover, recent advances in microelectronics have boosted the advent of a revolutionary model involving systems and communication technology. This new paradigm, the Internet of Things (IoT), has a broad applicability in several areas, including healthcare. Based on this context, this chapter aims to describe a computer platform based on IoT for the remote monitoring of patients in critical condition. Furthermore, it is planned to approach the current advances and challenges of conceiving and developing a set of technology-centric, targeting issues relevant to underdeveloped countries, particularly in regards to Brazil's health infrastructure.

Chapter 2
Internet of Things in Pervasive Healthcare Systems 22
Teresa Guarda, Universidad Peninsula de Santa Elena (UPSE), Ecuador
Maria Fernanda Augusto, Universidad Peninsula de Santa Elena (UPSE), Ecuador
Oscar Barrionuevo, Universidad de las Fuerzas Armadas (ESPE), Ecuador
Filipe Mota Pinto, Polytechnic Institute of Leiria, Portugal

Throughout the stunning development of wireless communication technologies, sensors and wireless sensor networks (WSN) are being used in almost every area, such as in healthcare field. The ubiquitous sensing enabled by WSN technologies, in particularly the wireless medical sensor network (WMSN), might be one important key success factor in the modern medical system. The recent advances, and wireless devices proliferation, had proved the technical feasibility of the pervasive health care systems. The data collected by sensors are very sensitive and important, and the leakage of them could compromise security and privacy. This work presents the pervasive health care systems (PHCS) focusing on security and privacy of pervasive environments.

Chapter 3
Benefits of Bring Your Own Device in Healthcare 32
Filipe Portela, University of Minho, Portugal
Ailton Moreira da Veiga, University of Minho, Portugal
Manuel Filipe Santos, University of Minho, Portugal

Bring Your Own Device (BYOD) has become very popular topic in information technology because this approach allows the employees to bring their personal devices into organization and they want to use them to access the organization information. This trend has some benefits both for organization and to employees. This paper aims to identify those benefits as well the advantages and disadvantages of BYOD usage in organization. Also, it is present a SWOT analysis of BYOD usage. It is introduced an approach about BYOD in healthcare also. Utilizing personal devices at work is beneficial to organizational employees because they are in some way satisfies, and they have more freedom and choice to use their devices. This freedom and choice can easily lead the employees to be more productivity, flexibility. The organization who embraces BYOD policies found their employees happier, more productive, and more collaborative.

Chapter 4
Big Data and mHealth: Increasing the Usability of Healthcare Through the Customization of Pinterest – Literary Perspective 46
Nancy Shipley, Towson University, USA
Joyram Chakraborty, Towson University, USA

Technology has greatly improved healthcare. Research has shown that improved user experience can vastly increase the volume and quality of knowledge gained from the accessible resources. Electronic medical records have been mandated by the U.S. government transitioning the medical field to computer based applications with the goal of efficiency and meaningful use. From this vast data, the end user could potentially increase their healthcare understanding through a centralized mobile-platform that brings the expertise from medical professionals, smart health and well-being best practices, alternative medicine and social media such as crowd-sourcing materials. In this chapter, we present a mHealth solution incorporating the features of Pinterest in order to provide a single portal for the dissemination of healthcare information.

Chapter 5
Mobile Health Systems and Electronic Health Record: Applications and Implications 67
Kijpokin Kasemsap, Suan Sunandha Rajabhat University, Thailand

This chapter reveals the overview of mobile health systems; the adoption of mobile health systems; mobile health systems and patient monitoring; the overview of mobile health technology; the advanced issues of Electronic Health Record (EHR); and the challenges of EHR in global health care. Mobile health helps deliver the health care services with quality care, improved workflow, and increased patient interaction while minimizing complexity and cost to achieve the desired goals in health care settings. EHR systems are the real-time and patient-centered records that make information available instantly and securely to authorized users. The chapter argues that applying mobile health systems and EHR has the potential to improve health care efficiency and gain sustainable competitive advantage in global health care.

Chapter 6
Pervasive Computing in Supporting Pediatric and Neonatology Care Unit Decision Process............ 86
Bia Martins, University of Minho, Portugal
Tiago André Saraiva Guimarães, University of Minho, Portugal
Mariana Santos, Unidade Local de Saúde do Alto Minho, Portugal
Simão Frutuoso, Centro Materno Infantil do Norte, Portugal
Filipe Portela, University of Minho, Portugal
Manuel Filipe Santos, University of Minho, Portugal

Neonatal units, and especially the sections devoted to intensive care require an individualized medical prescription, based on body weight and gestational age making them among the hospital settings where treatment errors are most likely to occur. These errors may harm patients and their families, as well as increase the duration of hospital stay and its costs. Tools such as Sabichão have sought, over the last years, to aid clinical decision-making to reduce clinical error. However, with the increased use and dissemination of mobile platforms, it's now possible and essential to bring the available assistance closer to the health providers and their practice. This paper describes a Framework that seeks to present itself as a more efficient and ubiquitous alternative to an existing Clinical decision support system.

Chapter 7
Augmented Reality in Surgery: A New Approach to Enhance the Surgeon's Experience.................. 96
José Inácio, University of Minho, Portugal
João Ribeiro, Peek Health S.A., Portugal
Jaime Campos, Peek Health S.A., Portugal
Sara Silva, Peek Health S.A., Portugal
Victor Alves, University of Minho, Portugal

In the surgical field, the patient's needs and requirements increasingly follow the newest technological developments. Nowadays it is still problematic to implement different types of technologies in operating environments due to the drawbacks that these can bring to their users and their longstanding learning process. A research was carried out with the objective of clarifying concepts and gathering some existing approaches to the solution of these problems as well as the respective technologies used. This chapter addresses a new concept of mobile applications for surgical planning using augmented reality technologies. The proposed solution aims to help the surgeon from the planning stage to the surgery intervention itself. In addition to some examples and practical demonstrations of the solution, its implementation process and system architecture are described and explained. Based on the developed prototype, the advantages of its use in a surgical context are discussed, being pointed out some improvements to be made.

Chapter 8
Recommendation System: A Potential Tool for Achieving Pervasive Health Care 111
Shashi Kant Srivastava, Indian Institute of Management Indore, India
Sudipendra Nath Roy, Indian Institute of Management Indore, India

Health is the most critical but very less celebrated application area of recommendation system. The purpose of this work is to put forward the present development and potential future applications of the recommendation system for the physical health of an individual and community. These recommendations are aimed to mitigate the probable future health risks. Present chapter ensembles the existing literature to illustrate the current applications of the subject. Furthermore, this put forward future scope and knowledge boundary for health recommendation system research. Because of present innovations i.e. wearable health technologies, the application of recommendation system for health has become possible. The present chapter evaluates the existing wearable health technologies and its suitability for the deployment of a responsive health recommendation system.

Chapter 9
Real-Time Healthcare Intelligence in Organ Transplantation: Real-Time Intelligence in Organ Transplantation 128
Bruno Fernandes, University of Minho, Portugal
Cecília Coimbra, University of Minho, Portugal
António Abelha, University of Minho, Portugal

Organ transplantation is the best and often the only treatment for patients with end-stage organ failure. However, the universal shortage of deceased donors results in a worrying situation that must be addressed. Brain dead donors constitute the largest share of organ donors, but identifying a patient that may progress to brain death can be a complex task. Therefore, the urgent need of intelligent solutions to support the decision-making process is crucial in critical areas as the organ transplantation is. This work aims at acquiring knowledge on the potential organ donor criteria for further detection and implementing a platform to assist the process of identification of potential organ donors at Centro Hospitalar do Porto – Hospital de Santo António. The developed system is currently implemented and displays a steady and competent behavior providing consequently a way to have more control of the information needed for the decision-making process

Chapter 10
Advanced Issues of Health Informatics and Clinical Decision Support System in Global Health Care 153
Kijpokin Kasemsap, Suan Sunandha Rajabhat University, Thailand

This chapter indicates the advanced issues of health informatics; the advanced issues of Clinical Decision Support System (CDSS); CDSS and Computerized Physician Order Entry (CPOE); the false positive alerts in CDSS; and CDSS and biomedical engineering. Health informatics and CDSS are the advanced health care technologies with the support of many technological fields. Health informatics and CDSS apply various computerized devices to provide enhanced health-related outcomes in terms of problem solving, analytical thinking, and decision making. Health informatics and CDSS help clinicians and health care providers to make complex information useful in supporting clinical decisions, thus delivering the best standard of care for each patient. The chapter argues that utilizing health informatics and CDSS has the potential to increase health outcomes and reach strategic goals in global health care.

Chapter 11
Applied Business Intelligence in Surgery Waiting Lists Management 171
Cristiana Neto, University of Minho, Portugal
Inês Dias, University of Minho, Portugal
Maria Santos, University of Minho, Portugal
Hugo Peixoto, University of Minho, Portugal
José Machado, University of Minho, Portugal

With the advent of computer science in hospitals, Electronic Health Record comes up, with the aim of bringing the new information technologies to the hospital environment with the promise not only to replace the paper process, but also to improve and provide better patient care. The operationalization of the EHR in supporting evidence-based practice, complex and conscientious decision-making, and improving the quality of healthcare delivery has been supported by the Business Intelligence (BI) technology. Since the beginning of the 1990s, the Portuguese health system has been confronted with a chronic problem, waiting time for surgery, due to inability to respond to demand for surgical therapy. Therefore, using business intelligence and information, obtained with the construction of dashboards, can help, for example, allocating hospital resources and reducing waiting times.

Chapter 12
Pervasive Business Intelligence Platform to Support the Decision-Making Process in Waiting Lists 186
Marisa Esteves, University of Minho, Portugal
Filipe Miranda, University of Minho, Portugal
António Abelha, University of Minho, Portugal

In recent years, the increase of average waiting times in waiting lists is an issue that has been felt in health institutions. Thus, the implementation of new administrative measures to improve the management of these organizations may be required. Hereupon, the aim of this present work is to support the decision-making process in appointments and surgeries waiting lists in a hospital located in the north of Portugal, through a pervasive Business Intelligence platform that can be accessed anywhere and anytime by any device connected within the hospital's private network. By representing information that facilitate the analysis of information and knowledge extraction, the Web tool allows the identification in real-time of average waiting times outside the outlined patterns. Thereby, the developed platform permits their identification, enabling their further understanding in order to take the necessary measures. Thus, the main purpose is to enable the reduction of average waiting times through the analysis of information in order to, subsequently, ensure the satisfaction of patients.

Chapter 13
Business Intelligence for Nutrition Therapy 203
Rita Reis, University of Minho, Portugal
Ana Mendonça, University of Minho, Portugal
Diana Lisandra Azevedo Ferreira, University of Minho, Portugal
Hugo Peixoto, University of Minho, Portugal
José Machado, University of Minho, Portugal

The assessment of health status in communities throughout the world is a massive information technology challenge. Data warehousing provides a flexible environment to support the business management and serve as an integrated repository for data. With the addition of models and analytic tools that have the potential to provide actionable information resources and support effective problem identification, critical decision-making, and strategy formulation, implementation, and evaluation. Of particular interest are the factors of influence like the patient's height or weight and its impact on processes and results. A multidimensional process is a way to discover health care processes according to certain factors of influence. This study aims to implement a data warehousing environment for decision support, in the context of nutrition evaluation, to integrate data obtained from a health care facility. This paper highlights the implementation of Business Intelligence in health care settings allows searching and interpreting stored information to support decisions concerning people's life.

Chapter 14
Indian Healthcare Service Management Through Data Mining: Datamining for Healthcare Services 219
Manaswini Pradhan, Fakir Mohan University, India

The main intention of our method is to provide better Healthcare services over the rural areas in terms of prediction of the chief hospitals with required basic facilities around that particular area. Accordingly, a Questionnaire survey is made for collecting the relevant hospital data around the Odisha region. Then, the concept of data mining is utilized in order to extract the data from the Questionnaire. Further, Incremental Spanning algorithm is introduced here for the mining of data from the Questionnaire. In the Questionnaire, appropriate score values were assigned for each category based on the requirement. Moreover, the hospital satisfying all the required components within the Questionnaire have to be determined for predicting the better hospitals. The Genetic Algorithm is introduced so as to determine the maximum of the score values obtaining for the input hospital data. Finally, the ranking of first five supreme hospitals is determined around the Odisha region.

Compilation of References 234

About the Contributors 279

Index 284

Preface

Varshney (2009) defined *Pervasive HealthCare (PHC)* as a "conceptual system of providing healthcare to anyone, at any time, and anywhere by removing restraints of time and location while increasing both the coverage and the quality of healthcare." This approach is based on information that is stored and available online (Mikkonen et al., 2002). However, although the PHC has the potential to reduce costs, improve service quality and facilitate the treatment to the patient, it also faces many technical and administrative obstacles (Varshney, 2003), such as resistance to change and significant changes in technology and systems.

Mobile Health (mHealth) is the practice of medicine and public health supported by mobile devices. It is referenced by the use of mobile communication devices, such as mobile phones, tablet computers or patient monitors, for health services and information. mHealth covers the use of mobile telecommunication and multimedia technologies as they are integrated within increasingly wireless and mobile healthcare delivery systems being them the main support of pervasive healthcare.

Several topics are addressed from multiple angles having as main focus the Next-Generation Mobile and Pervasive Healthcare Solutions. This book presents significant achievements in a full range of health delivery settings, providing decision support anywhere and anytime to acute and long-term healthcare taking as based pervasive or mobile computing.

This book promotes the cross-fertilization of health informatics information and knowledge across professional and geographical boundaries, serving as the catalyst for ubiquitous worldwide health information infrastructures for patient care and health research. The fourteen chapters are divided into two big topics Technological Trends and Data Science. These two themes address the following fields: Internet of Things, Bring Your Own Device, and mHealth, Pervasive HealthCare, Augmented Reality, Business Intelligence, Data Mining and Decision Support.

TECHNOLOGICAL TRENDS

New technological trends arise every year. In this context, some technologies have more success than another. Healthcare is a critical area where nothing can fail by consequence these technologies are strongly explored and tested before their deployment in health institutions. Some of these trends are associated with pervasive and mobile solutions as is Internet of Things, Augmented Reality and Bring Your Own Device.

Internet of Things (IoT) represents a network of physical objects or things embedded with electronics, software, sensors, and network connectivity (Babu et al., 2016) IOT enables these objects to collect and exchange data in real-time and allows a universal data access from any connected device over the Internet (Fernandez & Pallis, 2014). This new paradigm, the Internet of Things (IoT), has broad applicability in several areas, including healthcare. IOT is transforming the health industry and has numerous applications from remote monitoring to smart sensors and medical device integration. IOT is redefining the process how apps, devices and people interact and connect with each other with the goal to deliver healthcare solutions (Fernandez & Pallis, 2014).

IOT have several technologies and devices able to provide a new dimension to the world of information and communication. They can use Radio Frequency Identification (RFID) sensors, actuators, cell phones, Near Field Communication (NFC), artificial intelligence, and nanotechnologies. The use of this type of technologies allows the creation of knowledge from vast amounts of data (Babu et al., 2016) and has the potential to use these data not only to keep patients safe and healthy but also to improve how physicians deliver care (Fernandez & Pallis, 2014).

Bring Your Own Device (BYOD) concept can take advantages of their combination with IOT solutions. BYOD is a very popular topic in information technology because this approach allows the employees to bring their personal devices (smartphones, tablets and laptop computers) into the organization. They also can use them to access to the organization information. The use of personal devices at work is beneficial because it can provide more productivity, flexibility, freedom and choice to the employees (Singh, 2012).

Although the benefits of BYOD and IOT are clear, these trends bring many concerns to the organizations (Mansfield-Devine, 2012). Healthcare is one of the main preoccupation areas due to the fact they can interfere with patient safety and privacy.

The use of BYOD has significantly improved health services with the appearance of mHealth and Pervasive Healthcare. Pervasive solutions allow for delivering health services with quality care anywhere and anytime for anyone. PHC also permits the access to real-time and patient-centered records instantly and securely to authorized users.

mHealth brings new challenges and opportunities to healthcare. The increased use and diffusion of mobile platforms can provide assistance closer to the health providers. A centralized mobile platform can take advantage of the vast amount of data available to help the end user to increase their healthcare understanding.

To create a virtual reality allied to the use of pervasive solutions new concept emerged recently. Augmented Reality (AR) explores the human-computer interaction technology. One of the primary goals is to make the computer interface invisible to the use. It also tries to allow interaction with the computer as natural as interacting with real world objects by removing the separation between the digital and physical (Billinghurst, Clark, & Lee, 2015).

Nowadays the researching in AR involves the use of wearable computers and augmented reality technology (Barfield, 2015). In the healthcare area, AR can be employed, for example, to solve problems associated with the implementation of different types of technologies in operating environments to test and analyze drawbacks.

DATA SCIENCE

The introduction of new technologies in healthcare lead to a new reality: the existence of an enormous amount of data. "Health informatics explores dedicated software, hardware devices, and sophisticated computer networks with the capacity to gather, evaluate, and transmit the medical information" (Kasemsap, this volume). Nowadays organizations collect a huge amount of data provided by sensors. The data can be, for example, collected in real-time from the sensors connected to the patients. After the data processing phase, the clinicians want to turn the data into knowledge and support the decision-making process. To a better decision, they explore the use of Business Intelligence.

Business intelligence represents data that facilitate the analysis of information and knowledge extraction. Business Intelligence can achieve valuable results when the institutions are using Electronic Health Record (EHR). EHR brings new information technologies to the hospital environment to improve and provide better patient care. The use of EHR is a benefit to BI because it is supported by an evidence-based practice, complex and conscientious decision-making, and improving the quality of healthcare delivery. The data used in BI systems are collected and prepared to be integrated into a Data Warehouse (DW). DW is a repository for data that provides a flexible environment to support the business management. A correct usage of the models and analytic tools has the potential to provide useful information resources to a critical decision-making and support efficient problem identification and consequently strategy formulation, implementation, and evaluation. Institutions may use Data Mining (DM) to extract knowledge provided by the sensors. DM is the process of exploring datasets to bring out knowledge and significant information (Larose, 2014). Health informatics helps the clinicians to make complex information useful in supporting decisions, thus providing the best care for each patient.

Decision support systems are used to consume and explore the results provided by the BI and DM applications as is for example pervasive BI. Clinical Decision Support Systems (CDSS) allows for analyzing data and help clinicians and healthcare providers to make clinical decisions.

ORGANIZATION OF THE BOOK

The book is organized into 14 chapters. A brief description of each of the chapters follows:

Chapter 1 presents an approach to move the routines of medical checks from a hospital to the patient's home by using the Internet of Things (IoT). This chapter aims to describe a computer platform based on IoT for the remote monitoring of patients in critical condition. The chapter also approaches the current advances and challenges of conceiving and developing a set of technology-centric, targeting issues relevant to underdeveloped countries, particularly in regards to Brazil's health infrastructure.

Chapter 2 addresses the use of IOT in healthcare. This chapter presents pervasive healthcare systems (PHC) focusing on security and data integrity of pervasive environments. In this chapter it is stated that the ubiquitous sensing enabled by wireless sensor networks (WSN) technologies, in particularly the wireless medical sensor network (WMSN), might be one important key success factor in the modern health care system.

Chapter 3 introduces some benefits of Bring Your Own Device (BYOD) to society. This chapter identified those benefits as well the advantages and disadvantages of BYOD usage in the healthcare institutions. A SWOT analysis of BYOD usage in healthcare is also addressed. As a result, a comparison between the benefits between organizations and healthcare system is provided. This chapter concluded that the organization who embraces BYOD policies found their employees happier, more productive, and more collaborative. The patients also can benefit with the introduction of BYOD in healthcare.

Chapter 4 stated that the improved user experience could vastly increase the volume and quality of knowledge gained from the available resources. The end user could potentially enhance their healthcare understanding by using a centralized mobile platform. This chapter presents a mHealth solution incorporating the features of interest to provide a single portal for the dissemination of healthcare information.

Chapter 5 reveals the overview of mobile health systems; the adoption of mobile health systems; mobile health systems and patient monitoring; the overview of mobile health technology; the advanced issues of Electronic Health Record (EHR); and the challenges of EHR in global health care. The chapter argues that applying mobile health systems and EHR has the potential to improve health care efficiency and gain sustainable competitive advantage in global health care.

Chapter 6 shows the use of pervasive computing in Neonatal care units. This chapter is focused on sections devoted to intensive care that requires an individualized medical prescription, based on body weight and gestational age making them among the hospital settings where treatment errors are most likely to occur. Sabichão the tool mentioned in this chapter have sought, over the last years, to aid clinical decision-making to reduce clinical error. The increased use and dissemination of mobile platforms allows available assistance closer to the health providers and their practice. This chapter describes a Framework that seeks to present itself as a more efficient and ubiquitous alternative to an existing clinical decision support system.

Chapter 7 deals with the process of implementing different types of technologies in operating environments. In this chapter, a research work was carried out with the objective of clarifying concepts and gathering some existing approaches to the solution of these problems as well as the respective technologies used. This chapter addresses a new concept of mobile applications for surgical planning using augmented reality technologies. The proposed solution aims to help the surgeon from the planning stage to the surgery intervention itself. As a result, some examples and practical demonstrations of the solution, its implementation process and system architecture are described and explained.

Chapter 8 put forward the present development and potential future applications of the recommendation system for the physical health of an individual and community. The chapter collects the existing literature to illustrate the current applications of the subject. Furthermore, this chapter put forward future scope and knowledge boundary for health recommendation system research. The present chapter evaluates the existing wearable health technologies and its suitability for the deployment of a responsive health recommendation system.

Chapter 9 presents a real-time intelligent system to support the decision-making process in organ transplantation and increase the number of deceased donors. This chapter presents a work that aims to acquire knowledge of the potential organ donor criteria for further detection and to implement a platform to assist the process of identification of potential organ donors at Centro Hospitalar do Porto – Hospital de Santo António. The developed system is currently implemented and displays a steady and competent behavior providing consequently a way to have more control of the information needed for the decision-making process

Chapter 10 indicates the issues of health informatics the advanced issues of Clinical Decision Support System (CDSS); CDSS and Computerized Physician Order Entry (CPOE); the false positive alerts in CDSS; and CDSS and biomedical engineering. The chapter argues that using health informatics and CDSS has the potential to increase health outcomes and reach strategic goals in global health care.

Chapter 11 provides an analysis about applying Business Intelligence in Surgery Waiting Lists Management. The central concern of this chapter is the waiting time for surgery, due to inability to respond to demand surgical therapy. This chapter presents a solution using business intelligence and information, obtained with the construction of dashboards that can help, for example, allocating hospital resources and reducing waiting times. The solution proposed intends not only to replace the paper process but also to improve and provide better patient care.

Chapter 12 addresses the issues associated with the increase of average waiting times in waiting lists in health institutions. The aim of this chapter is to develop a platform able to support the decision-making process in appointments and surgeries waiting lists in a hospital located in the north of Portugal. A pervasive Business Intelligence platform that can be accessed anywhere and anytime by any device connected to the hospital's private network was developed. The main purpose of this work is reducing of average waiting times through the analysis of information to, subsequently, ensure the satisfaction of patients.

Chapter 13 explores the Nutrition Therapy factors of influence like the patients' height or weight and its impact on processes and results. This chapter presents a data warehousing environment for decision support, in the context of nutrition evaluation, to integrate data obtained from a healthcare facility. This chapter highlights how the implementation of Business Intelligence in healthcare settings allows searching and interpreting stored information to support decisions concerning people's life.

Chapter 14 presents a method that aims to provide better healthcare services for rural areas by predicting the best chief hospitals with required infrastructure around Odisha region. Data mining tools and Incremental Spanning are utilized to extract the data from a Questionnaire produced in this region. The hospital which satisfies all the required components must be used for predicting purposes. Genetic Algorithms were applied to determine the maximum of the score values for the input hospital data. As results, the study produced the ranking of first five supreme hospitals at Odisha region.

CONCLUSION

This book addresses important topics in the pervasive healthcare area. New significant trends are introduced and discussed. This book intends to disseminate new knowledge, useful to promote healthcare quality in the patient best interest and supporting the decision making anywhere and anytime. It is expected that this book can induce a strong impact on the healthcare institutions bringing a set of new and innovative contributions to the community.

Pervasiveness as a novel approach for information systems' development is intensely explored in this book. Special attention was given to questions as i) how to make technologies omnipresent; ii) how to provide data anywhere and anytime promoting a full interaction among the physicians, nurses, patients and information systems.

The target audience of this book includes professionals and researchers working in the field of healthcare and information systems. Moreover, the book provides insights and decision support knowledge achieved with the development of mobile and pervasive healthcare solutions.

REFERENCES

Babu, B. S., Srikanth, K., Ramanjaneyulu, T., & Narayana, I. L. (2016). IoT for Healthcare. *International Journal of Science and Research, 5*(2).

Barfield, W. (Ed.). (2015). *Fundamentals of wearable computers and augmented reality*. CRC Press. doi:10.1201/b18703

Billinghurst, M., Clark, A., & Lee, G. (2015). A survey of augmented reality. *Foundations and Trends® Human–Computer Interaction, 8*(2-3), 73-272.

Fernandez, F., & Pallis, G. C. (2014, November). Opportunities and challenges of the Internet of Things for Healthcare: Systems engineering perspective. In *Wireless Mobile Communication and Healthcare (Mobihealth), 2014 EAI 4th International Conference on* (pp. 263-266). IEEE.

Larose, D. T. (2014). *Discovering knowledge in data: an introduction to data mining*. John Wiley & Sons. doi:10.1002/9781118874059

Mansfield-Devine, S. (2012). Interview: BYOD and the enterprise network. *Computer Fraud & Security, 2012*(4), 14–17. doi:10.1016/S1361-3723(12)70031-3

Mikkonen, M., Va, S., Ikonen, V., & Heikkila, M. O. (2002). User and concept studies as tools in developing mobile communication services for the elderly. *Personal and Ubiquitous Computing, 6*(2), 113–124. doi:10.1007/s007790200010

Pereira, A., Portela, F., Santos, M. F., Abelha, A., & Machado, J. (2016). Pervasive business intelligence: A new trend in critical healthcare. *Procedia Computer Science, 98*, 362–367. doi:10.1016/j.procs.2016.09.055

Singh, N. (2012). BYOD genie is out of the bottle–"Devil or angel. *Journal of Business Management & Social Sciences Research, 1*(3), 1–12.

Varshney, U. (2003). Pervasive healthcare. *Computer, 36*(12), 138–140. doi:10.1109/MC.2003.1250897

Varshney, U. (2009). *Pervasive healthcare computing: EMR/EHR, wireless and health monitoring*. Springer Science & Business Media. doi:10.1007/978-1-4419-0215-3

Chapter 1
Promoting Better Healthcare for Patients in Critical Condition:
An IoT-Based Solution to Integrate Patients, Physicians, and Ambulance Services

Itamir Barroca
UFRN, Brazil

Gibeon Aquino
UFRN, Brazil

Maria Alzete Lima
UFRN, Brazil

ABSTRACT

The high cost of healthcare services, the aging population and the increase of chronic disease is becoming a global concern. Several studies have indicated the need to minimize the process of hospitalization and the high cost of patient care. A promising trend in healthcare is to move the routines of medical checks from a hospital to the patient's home. Moreover, recent advances in microelectronics have boosted the advent of a revolutionary model involving systems and communication technology. This new paradigm, the Internet of Things (IoT), has a broad applicability in several areas, including healthcare. Based on this context, this chapter aims to describe a computer platform based on IoT for the remote monitoring of patients in critical condition. Furthermore, it is planned to approach the current advances and challenges of conceiving and developing a set of technology-centric, targeting issues relevant to underdeveloped countries, particularly in regards to Brazil's health infrastructure.

DOI: 10.4018/978-1-5225-2851-7.ch001

INTRODUCTION

The high cost of healthcare services, the aging population and the increase of chronic disease are becoming a global concern. Several studies have indicated the need for strategies to minimize the institutionalization process and the effects of the high cost of patient care (Hochron, & Goldberg, 2015). A promising trend in health treatments is to move the routines of hospital medical checks to the patient's home. However, the public health system in Brazil still lacks accessible technologies that facilitate the patient monitoring process in this situation (Mendes, 2010).

On the other hand, recent advances in microelectronics, wireless, sensing and information have fueled the advent of a revolutionary model involving systems and communication technology, enabling smarter ways to "make things happen". This new paradigm, known as the Internet of Things (IoT), has a broad applicability in several areas, including health. In this trend, it is estimated that by 2020 there will be around 20 billion "things" connected (Gartner, 2015) and uniquely identifiable (Gubbi et al.., 2013). These "things" promote the basic idea of IoT that is pervasive computing around this range of devices, such as RFID tags, sensors, actuators, mobile phones, etc. (Atzori et al.., 2010). It can act as the backbone of the health system for information sharing (Abinaya & Swathika, 2015). The field of health in particular is expected to see the development and application of this trend as part of its future because it has the ability to allow hospitals to operate more efficiently and patients to receive better treatment. A type of healthcare application which will be focused on in conjunction with this new paradigm is the application of mobile health. The main objective of mobile health is to allow for the remote monitoring of the health status and the treatment of patients from anywhere (López, Fernández, Jara & Skarmeta, 2013).

In this context, the potential for change in the quality of life that can be promoted by IoT is unquestionable. Creating integrated utilities will lead to a qualitative change in the services to integrate information systems, computing and communication with extensive control (Yinong, 2016). Therefore, there is an urgent need for the development of technologies and applications related to IoT infrastructure for health care. Currently, the process of early hospital discharge of critically ill patients has enjoyed the support of this new technology to ensure the case management through remote monitoring of patients who remain under home confinement and are still considered critical. Therefore, the rapid recognition of changes in conditions that are associated with complications is crucial to improving the survival of patients by the possibility of hemodynamic instability (Jiang et al., 2016)

Although they remain under health team care or are receiving regular follow-up visits, patients in home hospitalization are encouraged to perform a daily evaluation with self-monitoring of their vital signs and patterns related to their health condition (Kotsimbos, Williams, & Anderson, 2012). Moreover, although everyone receives instructions for detecting and reporting changes in the critical state for home self-monitoring, many patients find it challenging to identify the critical threshold values, i.e. the lower or upper limits of blood pressure, and recognize changes in their own personal baselines (Dabbs et al., 2009). Considering the amount of monitored data, it is hard to engage the patient in self-management; it is essential, therefore, to send this information to the care providers (Hendriks & Rademakers, 2014; Coulter, 2012).

Thus, Brazilian researcher groups seek to develop a computational solution in order to improve the remote care of the patient in a critical situation, which is expected to extend the health care of patients in hospital critical situation for their homes. The hypothesis put forward is that the technology will help maintain the supported self-care and remote management case. It therefore foresees overcoming the constraints identified in the process of institutionalization of people in a critical health situation. Finally, this chapter describes a computer platform based on IoT for the remote monitoring of patients in critical condition. It involves embedding sensors in patients, physicians, clinical staff, medical equipment and physical spaces in order to monitor, track and alert. Moreover, it is planned to approach the current advances and challenges of conceiving and developing a set of technology-centric strategies with the aim of making possible the effective application of affordable technologies in this kind of monitoring, targeting issues relevant to underdeveloped countries, particularly in regards to Brazil's current health infrastructure. The following sections describe the background of this research, the challenges and opportunities related to this topic, the proposed technology-based healthcare platform, future research directions and the conclusion.

BACKGROUND

Global projections indicate the need for strategies to minimize the effects of chronic health problems that can lead the individual to lose the ability to perform daily routine activities. There is a need for health promotion behaviors that offer new remote management options for patient cases with chronic diseases in critical condition. In Brazil, more than 70% of spending on health care is for the treatment of chronic diseases, which is seen as most alarming since they have the greatest potential for an increase in government spending (Brazil, 2013).

The services which serve patients in critical health situation are often overcrowded. Another problem is the growth of patients who require specialized care, such as intensive care, resulting in an insufficient number of vacancies (Brazil, 2013). These people need continuous monitoring to assess multiparameters from pulse pressure to oxygen saturation and electrocardiographic trace. However, insufficient material resources are considered the main difficulty in these sectors (Zandomenighi, Moorish, Oliveira & Martins, 2014). The strategies identified by developing countries is to build more hospitals, train an adequate number of doctors and equip health facilities with high-quality diagnostic instruments. However, this approach is a process that takes time and requires many resources (Hindia, Rahman, Ojukwu, Hanafi, & Fattouh, 2016). The best approach would be to propose a remote monitoring system with the ability to automatically communicate with the service providers, produce alerts to assist whenever necessary (Benlamri, & Docksteader, 2010; Constantinescu, Kim, & Feng, 2012; Pitsillides et al.., 2006;. Gorp, & Comuzzi, 2014), and integrate with emergency medical services.

The search for solutions has indicated that new devices designed for use in health service as mobile apps showed a reduced response time of nurses and doctors from thirty to five minutes, and a 20% reduction in waiting time in the emergency and medical observation units that saved $720,000, among other benefits (Hochron, & Goldberg, 2015). Thus, if a device with a sensor detecting conditions which reflect the individual's health status is configured to communicate with a portable computing device, an all care schedule can be operated efficiently. Currently, most people have access to these mobile devices, and these devices have become quite affordable (Hochron, & Goldberg, 2015). It is possible to think of a "surveillance system in mobile health," so you can easily reach large numbers of people with better planning of medical care. The problem goes beyond questions related to healthcare spending and is becoming a common concern, since with the global aging population and the increase of chronic diseases, people will demand more robust equipment to survive (Pang, 2013). The solution found by developed countries is to reduce the number of rooms in hospitals and increase the proportion of home health treatments (Prescher et al., 2014).

In Brazil, the Home Care is inserted in the proposed National Health System as a consolidated strategy in primary care and currently takes dimensions complementary to hospital care. It is characterized by a set of health promotion, prevention, and treatment of home provided diseases, ensuring continuity of care and integrated into health care networks (Brazil, 2013). In accordance with the logic of a health service organization, it seeks to insert, in the home environment, the remote monitoring system consisting of the patient's health parameters, daily measurements and its transmission to mobile phones belonging to the responsible healthcare professionals (Prescher et al., 2014; Brennan et al., 2010). Adherence to this complementary monitoring modality by the patient can be considered as a strategy for the adoption of continued care. Still, with regards to the Brazilian context, groups of researchers have made efforts to integrate a data mobile platform related to critical patients with minimally invasive monitoring. They seek strategies to help to promote health in order to suit the modern quotidian permeation of technology, trying to offer easy access to remote monitoring technology, promoting better integration between healthcare networks, care in the home environment and operationalizing the remote monitoring of patients in critical condition. Thus, it is intended to reduce public spending by reducing admissions numbers.

Despite concerns about security and privacy risks, remote monitoring is considered a tool to promote patient-centered care (Filkins, et al., 2016;. Sieverink, Siemons, Braakman-Jansen & Van Gemert-Pijnen, 2016). The use of mobile technology in healthcare can lead to a great revolution in digital health. Currently, the concept of mobile health (or mHealth) broadly describes the use of telecommunication technologies that deliver health actions to promote the welfare of patients (Dwivedi, 2016).

CHALLENGES AND OPPORTUNITIES

The health care environment is facing a challenge of raising the quality of services alongside new requirements for minimal resource utilization. At the same time, society is requiring more services due to demographic changes and the prevalence of chronic disease which puts the individual into critical health conditions. In the United States, it is expected that the growth in direct costs related to cardiac insufficiency will grow from $21 billion in 2012 to $53 billion in 2030 (Heidenreich et al., 2015). Most of these costs are related to hospitalization, which accounts for 4,800,000 hospital admissions annually (Piccini et al., 2016).

The technology information and communication systems were considered to be important tools to help solve these challenges (Chen, Kennedy, Sales, & Hofer, 2013; Jogh et al., 2012). However, traditional remote management by telephone failed to improve results and reduce readmission (Chaudhry et al., 2014). In contrast, the results of automatic remote monitoring (MR) have been more favorable, showing better outcomes (Hindricks et al., 2014; Saxon et al., 2015; Varma et al., 2015; Portugal et al., 2016). In previous analyses regarding the ambulatory treatment efficiency, the use of remote monitoring has reduced medical and nurse actions and the costs associated with displacement of patients, as compared to the traditional method (Heidbuchel et al., 2015; Varma et al., 2015).

However, the benefits of remote monitoring can go beyond efficiency in patient care, since this modern technology enables early intervention to prevent the morbidity of the patient and prevent or potentially reduce hospitalization, with profound implications for health costs, time in the trial, clinical decisions and a shorter length of stay. In a recent cohort study of 490,000 patients, where 37% (34,259) used remote monitoring compared with the traditional method, there was a 31% reduction in the cost of hospitalization and 23% fewer readmissions within 30 days (Piccini et al., 2016).

Despite evidence that remote monitoring offers several potential advantages to patients, including early detection of arrhythmia, a malfunction or organ system failure (Crossley et al., 2011; Varma et al., 2010), initiatives using remote monitoring are still scarce. In particular, patients with atrial fibrillation history, stroke and early diagnosis of myocardial infarction are the biggest beneficiaries of this method. Oral anticoagulation, for example, is often underutilized in patients with atrial fibrillation history; the possibility of early detection of more episodes of this fibrillation increases with the appropriate use of oral anticoagulation and the patients' chance of survival increases as a consequence (Piccini et al., 2016).

In order to face the challenges in the management of seriously ill patients' cases and deal with the issue of cost reduction in the hospitalization process with the support of continuous monitoring services, the paradigm of the architecture used to build smart applications that perform data processing through mobile devices is used. These devices are incorporated into the components used to support the decision-making process based on the professionals' knowledge. Mobile devices may allow an accurate and continuous analysis of the patient's health status to be performed locally, minimizing the transmission network, avoiding communication delays or interruptions and maintaining appropriate levels of security and privacy (Minutolo, Esposito, & Pietro, 2016). Therefore, it can act as a decision support system, capable of automatically processing and correlating large volumes of monitored physiological parameters, detecting suspicious changes and providing alarms in response to the worsening of the patient's condition, as well as suggestions on possible actions. It can facilitate diagnosis and personalized treatments, predict the patient's condition based on the observation of several monitored levels and empower patients to actively participate in their health (Minutolo, Esposito, & Peter, 2016).

It is important to note that there are many barriers to the implementation of patient management for the remote system, including the refusal of the patient, the lack of access to technology for remote monitoring and access to telecommunications, lack of infrastructure in health services, lack of resources and institutional support. Eliminating these hurdles with an awareness of the professional on the importance of continuous remote monitoring is essential to improving care in health and meeting the new challenges imposed by the advances of technology and health.

A TECHNOLOGY-BASED HEALTHCARE PLATFORM

This section presents the technology-based healthcare platform describing the aspects of design and requirements, the actors and use cases that guided its development. It also explains the platform's architecture considering its modules, their relationship, components and protocols.

Design Issues and Requirements

The main goal of the proposed technology-based healthcare platform is to provide remote monitoring for patients in a critical situation, and it was developed considering the necessity to transfer the healthcare from the hospital (hospital-centric) to home (home-centric). This platform is IoT-based and integrates patients, physicians and ambulance services in order to promote better care and rapid preventive and reactive urgent actions. Regarding requirements, this platform has *Remote Patient and Ambient Monitoring, Patient Healthcare Data Management, Patient Health Condition Management and Emergency and Crisis Management.* Figure 1 presents the relationship between these requirements:

Figure 1. The relationship between requirements

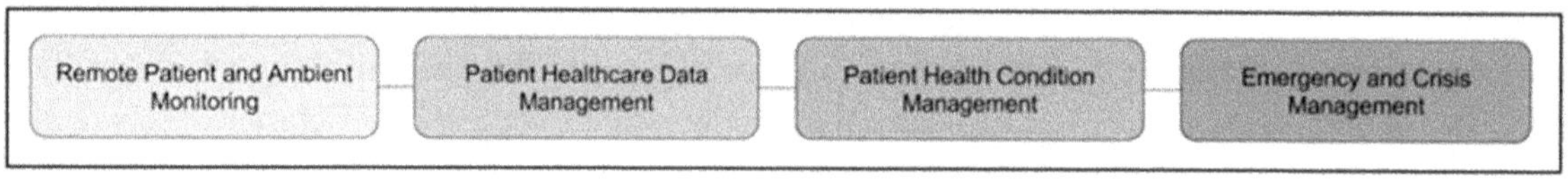

The *Remote Patient and Ambient Monitoring* involves the acquirement of data from sensors attached to the patient's body and in the ambient (patient's home). The acquired data from the sensors are used by clinical staff (physician and nurses) for healthcare treatment and emergency alert purposes. Thus, the sensors attached to the patient body provide information about:

1. **Electrocardiogram (ECG)** (Maglogiann, 2012; Jara et al., 2013; Yang et al., 2014; Maksimović et al., 2015): Recording of the electrical activity of the heart in the form of specific waves. The ECG monitoring can be used to monitor the heart rate of a patient, assess the effects of an illness or injury on the function of the pacemaker, and evaluate the response after a physician's procedure. The ECG can give information about the orientation of the heart, conduction disturbances, electrical effects of medications and electrolytes, the mass of the heart muscle and the presence of ischemic damage. However, to evaluate the effectiveness of the mechanical activity of the heart the pulse and blood pressure of the patient is evaluated (Aehlert, 2011).
2. **Blood Pressure** (Jara et al., 2013; Raad et al., 2015; Maksimović et al., 2015): Recorded as a ratio between two numbers, systolic - the top number, which is also the higher of the two numbers, measures the pressure in the arteries when the heart beats (when the heart muscle contracts); diastolic - the bottom number, which is also the lower of the two numbers, measures the pressure in the arteries between heartbeats (when the heart muscle is resting between beats and refilling with blood) (American Heart Association, 2016). For example: Read as 140X90 mmHg (millimeters of mercury). Can be decisive in the early identification of cardiac and vascular problems (Vidal-Petiot et al., 2016). In cases of high pressure, their control reduces the risk of cardiovascular events and death (Zanchetti, Thomopoulos, & Parati, 2015; Ettehad et al., 2016). Similarly, a reduction in blood pressure may not be compatible with survival and vasoactive drugs need to be administered urgently (Vidal-Petiot et al., 2016).
3. **Blood Glucose** (Poenaru, et al., 2013): Monitoring is the main tool you have to check patient diabetes control (American Diabetes Association, 2016). Population data indicate that 30-40% of people with type 1 diabetes experience an average of 1 to 3 episodes of severe hypoglycemia each year. With self-monitoring and patient education and care, the patient may benefit from a controlled glycemic rate with individual goals set by the team of health professionals. During the last decade, the introduction of continuous glucose monitoring to facilitate the self-administration has shown an improvement in glucose control and reduced exposure to hypoglycemia (Bolinder et al. 2016). Experience shows the beneficial effect of continuous monitoring of blood glucose (Thabit, Bally, & Hovorka, 2016).
4. **Heart Rate** (van der Valk et al., 2015; Raad et al., 2015; Gia et al., 2014; Khattak et al., 2014): The number of heartbeats per unit of time, usually per minute. The heart rate is based on the number of contractions of the ventricles (the lower chambers of the heart) (Medicinet, 2016). It refers to the number of heartbeats per unit time, usually expressed as beats per minute (bpm) (American Heart

Association 2016). The heart rate variability has been used as a noninvasive means of assessing the neural control of the heart and is used to identify hemodynamic problems. In other words, the pulse rate translates cardiac function; its monitoring is important because even in sinus rhythm it can face a paroxysmal fibrillation which can lead to widespread uncontrolled cardiac electrical activity and impair heart function (Port et al., 2015). Importantly, there are variations as to its value, for what may be appropriate for one patient may not be suitable for others, for example, heart failure patients with left ventricular ejection usually preserved need a low heart rate (Gelder et al., 2016). This allows the care team to plan individualized intervention, including programming the alarm system.

5. **Oxygen Saturation** (Maglogiann, 2012; Sebestyen et al., 2014; Chiuchisan et al., 2014; Raad et al., 2015): It is especially useful to detect hypoxemia associated with critical problems such as cardiovascular ones (Ewer, 2014). The oxygen uptake occurs primarily in the lungs, constituting the first step in the process of oxygen to the tissues. The oxygen taken up in the lungs is transported in the blood in two ways: by dissolving in plasma and also combined with hemoglobin. Hemoglobin is capable of carrying 98-99% of all oxygen in the blood and can be viewed through the oxygen saturation measured by pulse oximetry. The arterial oxygen saturation is determined as a percentage, on average it is in the range of 95% to 100%. There may be some changes and false readings of oxygen saturation, which are usually caused by chills, hypotension, low perfusion and edema (Bezerbashi et al., 2016).
6. **Temperature** (Ray et al., 2015; Tabish et al., 2014): The human being is homeothermic, i.e. has the ability to maintain body temperature within a certain predetermined range despite variations in the thermal environment - thermal homeostasis (Gasparrini et al., 2015). Increased body temperature may indicate increased cell metabolism, consumption of O2 and CO2 production, demands on the heart and lungs and additional stress to the cardiopulmonary system and infectious processes, and therefore may justify a continued investigation in critically ill patients (Cahill, & Prendergast, 2016). Measured in degrees Celcius (° C), it is taken by means of a catheter close to the skin in the axillary region (Hall, 2006) continuously.
7. **Breathing Rate** (Castillejo et al., 2013; Chiuchisan, et al., 2014): It is measured by the respiratory motion for one minute, measured in rpm. It demonstrates not only lung function but can denote problems in other systems, such as neurological and cardiac (Cahill, & Prendergast, 2016; Goligher, Ferguson, & Brochard, 2016; Ferguson et al., 2013).
8. **Capnography**: Capnography is a graphical display of the carbon dioxide concentration in exhaled and inhaled function of time, and is used to monitor ventilatory support. There is a growing recognition that capnography is rich in information regarding lung and circulatory physiology and provides insights into many diseases and treatments (Sweeney & McAuley 2016). These include inadequate matching conditions of ventilation and perfusion, such as pulmonary embolism and obstructive pulmonary diseases and adequacy of chest compressions during cardiac arrest or responsiveness in patients in shock (Nassar & Schmidt 2016; Langhan et al., 2014).

The sensors from the ambient provide information about environment temperature (Maglogiann, 2012; Yang et al., 2013; van der Valk et al., 2015), location (Maglogiann, 2012) with latitude and longitude, and humidity (Yang et al., 2013). This is important because the control of the ambient temperature and humidity can directly affect the patient's treatment. Regarding the location, it assists in the rapid response of the ambulance service. Therefore, as the patient in critical condition is at home and not in a hospital, which is a more controlled environment, this ambient information is of greater importance for effective healthcare and enriches the remote monitoring provided by this platform.

The *Patient Healthcare Data Management* records the data about the patient: name, gender, birth, contacts, address, family information, physician information (name and contacts), health insurance information, health situation and the history of monitoring sensors and emergency alerts. These data are important to physicians and nurses to understand the current situation and history of patients, and also to facilitate the accurate monitoring of health treatment.

The *Patient Health Condition Management* considers the patient healthcare data, especially the health situation and history of sensors monitoring data, to allow the definition of critical levels to the values of the sensors that are important to the rapid response in case of emergency. It also defines rules to actions considering the settled critical levels for a patient and the related alerts.

Finally, the *Emergency and Crisis Management* address the information about the patient's health condition and the services that should be alerted in case of emergency with a monitored patient in a critical situation. As this patient is at home and not in a hospital, the efficiency of a rapid response in an emergency case can be the deciding factor between life and death.

To achieve the presented requirements, this platform is composed of ten use cases, presented by the use case diagram in Figure 2 and it indicates four actors: *the hospital operator, physician and nurses, ambulance service operator and the patient and family*.

Considering the hospital operator actor, it interacts with the use cases related to patient, health insurance and clinical staff data, that are:

1. **Patients Data Management**: It allows the register of data related to *Patient Healthcare Data Management* cited before;
2. **Clinical Staff Data Management**: It allows the register of data related to the clinical staff (physician and nurse). These data include: name, contacts and specialty from physician and nurses;

Figure 2. Healthcare platform use case diagram

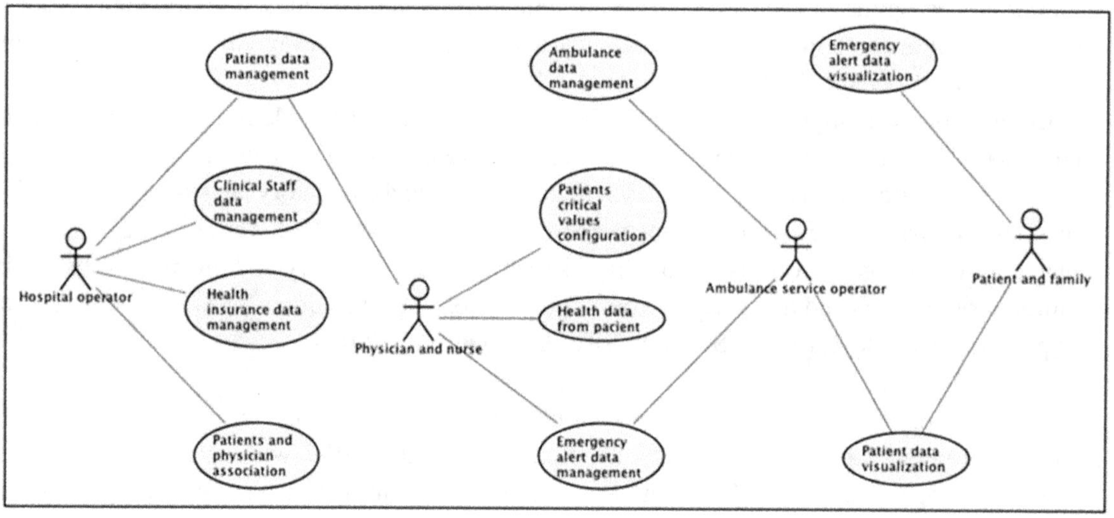

3. **Health Insurance Data Management**: It allows the register of data from the health insurance;
4. **Patient and Physician Association**: It allows the register of the responsibility of a physician with a patient.

Regarding the physician and nurse actors, they can use the patients data management, and interact with others use cases related to *Remote Patient and Ambient Monitoring*, *Patient Healthcare Data, Patient Health Condition Management* and *Emergency and Crisis Management,* that are:

1. **Patients Critical Values Configuration**: it allows the definition of critical levels for the values of the sensors attached to the patient body that are considered in the alerts and notifications;
2. **Health Data From Patient**: It allows the visualization of real-time health data from the sensors deployed in any patient body and ambient;
3. **Emergency Alert Data Management**: It allows the notification and alerts to be presented and managed by physicians and nurses.

The ambulance service operator actor uses the emergency alert data management use case and interacts with others use cases related to *Emergency and Crisis Management*, that are:

1. **Ambulance Data Management**: It allows the management of data from the ambulances, such as real-time location and activation of an ambulance to an emergency.
2. **Patient Data Visualization**: It allows the visualization of real-time health data from the sensors deployed in a single patient body and ambient, besides his home location.

Finally, the patient and family actor uses the patient data visualization use case and interacts with the emergency alert data visualization, related to *Emergency and Crisis Management.* The emergency alerts and patient data regards only to itself, in a case of a patient, or his familiar, in a case of a family.

Thus, the proposed platform was developed considering the presented requirements, actors, and use cases. It provides integration between patients, physician and ambulance services, for efficient patients' healthcare in critical condition. In the following subsection, the architecture overview is presented with details of these platform modules.

Architecture Overview

The healthcare platform architecture, presented in Figure 3, is composed of five modules: *Patient's Home, Cloud Health Infrastructure, Hospital, Family's Home and Ambulance Service*. These modules address the solution's functional requirements and work together to achieve the goal of remote monitoring and efficient healthcare for patients in critical condition.

Considering the *Patient's Home module*, it is mainly composed of sensors that provide body and ambient remote monitoring. The sensors attached to the patient body, described in the previous section, are part of a multi-parameter portable patient monitoring, which continuously measures his vital signs. This monitoring is configured by the clinical staff at the patient's home and does not require his intervention. Regarding security and essential performance issues, the monitor is in agreement with the standard IEC 60601-1-11:2015 (IEC 60601, 2015) that defines the basic safety and essential performance of medical

Figure 3. IoT-based platform to integrate patients, physicians, and ambulance services

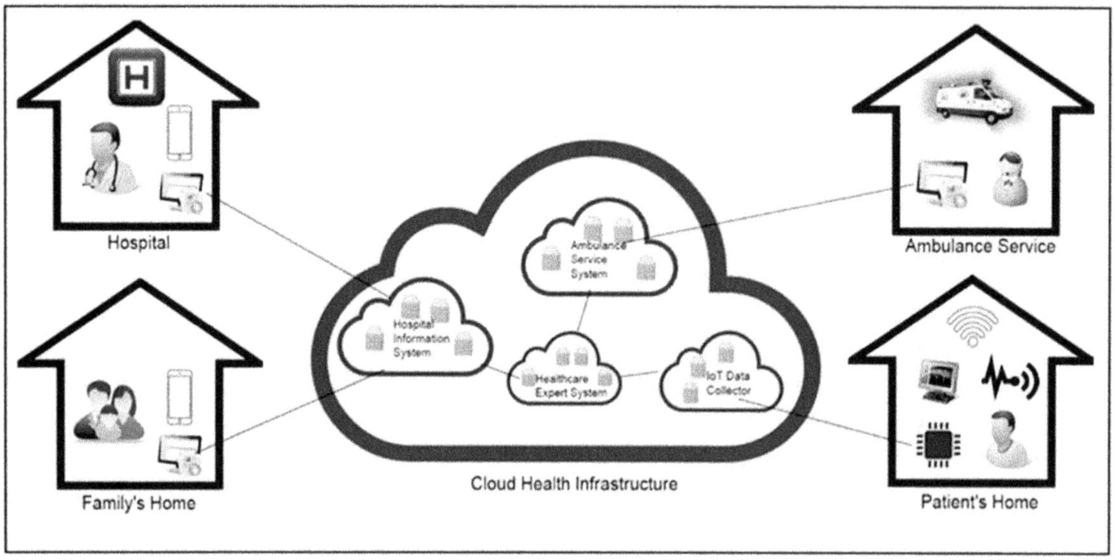

electrical equipment and medical electrical systems for use in the home healthcare environment. The sensors of the ambient monitoring, described in the previous section, are also deployed at the patient home.

Thus, this multi-parameter monitor is connected through the Internet to the *Cloud Health Infrastructure* module, as presented in Figure 4. The ambient sensors are connected to a gateway through 6LoWPAN protocol. Regarding 6LoWPAN, it is a protocol for Wireless Sensor Networks (WSNs) defined to enable IPv6 packets to be carried on top of low power wireless networks, specifically exploiting IEEE 802.15.4 protocol (Khattak et al., 2014). This gateway is also connected by the Internet to the IoT Platform of the *Cloud Health Infrastructure* module. The reason for a gateway to the sensors is because they do not have interfaces for direct connection to the Internet.

Regarding the *Cloud Health Infrastructure module*, it is composed by the IoT Data Collector, the Healthcare Expert System, the Hospital Information System and the Ambulance Service System. These systems implement the use cases described previously. The features of each system are:

1. **IoT Data Collector**: Responsible for receiving sensors' data. This is a challenge for realizing IoT due to the huge number of devices integrated into this component and their diversity in terms of data formats, protocols, nature of components, etc. (Delicato et al., 2013).
2. **Healthcare Expert System**: Configuration of the patients' critical values for alerts that are displayed in the Hospital Information and Ambulance System. These critical values are used in the rules defined by the physicians and nurses. This system provides standard mapped rules, presented in Table 1, and realizes machine learning and analytics to assist the physician in defining the appropriate critical values for each patient. Regarding the rule, it is composed of a type of sensor, a value, a critical level and its action. This action is associated with a color, according to the Manchester Triage System, that are displayed on the related information systems.

3. **Hospital Information System**: Data management of patients, clinical staff and health insurance, and the association between patients and physicians. It also provides mobile views for patient data and alerts visualization.
4. **Ambulance Service System**: Data management of emergency alert and ambulances. It also provides visualization of the patient's data.

The data received by the IoT Data Collector are used by the Healthcare Expert System, which contains rules and creates derived information to be used by the Hospital Information System and the Ambulance Service System. The Healthcare Expert System uses techniques of Machine Learning and Analytics based on the huge amount of received data to produce knowledge about the patient's health behavior. This knowledge is then stored in the computer and users call upon the computer for specific advice as needed. The computer can make inferences and arrive at a specific conclusion (Liao et al., 2005). For example, the critically ill patients, particularly those with hemodynamic instability signals, need a diagnosis and immediate treatment. This condition presents itself with signs of tissue perfusion and impaired tissue oxygenation, which is usually detected by macrocirculatory parameters or global hemodynamic measurements such as blood pressure and oxygen saturation in arterial blood (Bazerbashi et al., 2014). When a critical value is captured by this healthcare expert system, it automatically generates an alert message to the Hospital Information System, the physician, the patient's family and ambulance service system providing support for a specific decision on when and how to intervene. Thus, the patient's state of the classification system is issued together with the monitoring values. Another example is that if the data from the sensors show that the patient's heart rate is zero, it can translate this as a heart attack. Therefore, this Healthcare Expert System also notifies the Hospital Information System, the physician, the patient's family and Ambulance Service System.

Figure 4. The connections between the multi-parameter monitor and ambient sensors

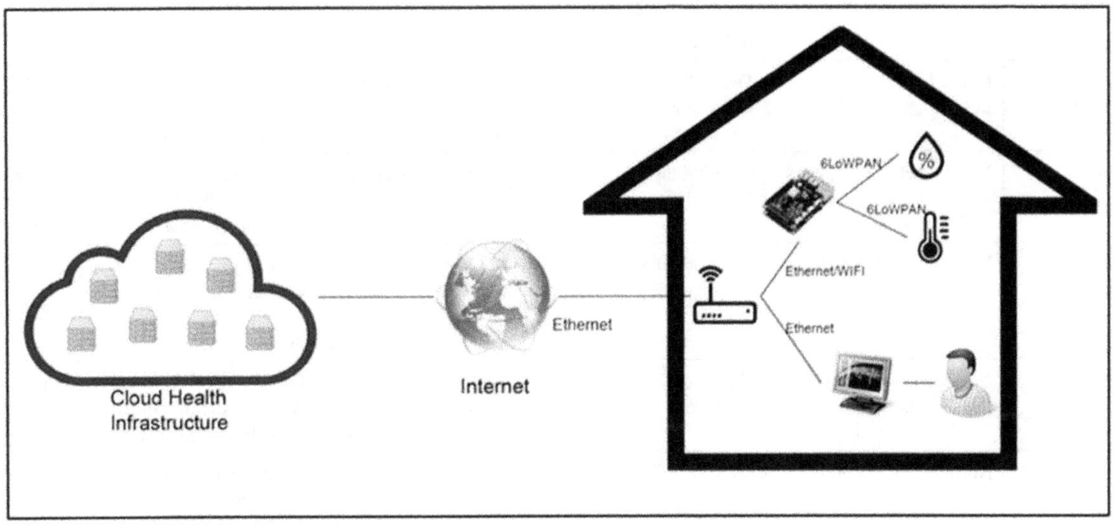

Moreover, the Healthcare Expert System also provides an API to make the patient's information available to authorized third party systems, taking into account privacy and ethics. This API is composed of RESTFul Web Services (Oracle, 2016) and the uses JSON (JSON, 2016). The purpose of this API is to facilitate the development of new solutions with the use of this data to promote innovation in the healthcare area. As a result, companies and researchers can benefit from this use.

The *Hospital module* is used by physicians, nurses and clinical staff, and it uses the hospital information system. This system contains the records of patients including information about age, gender, name, contacts, family contact. It also provides the real-time remote monitoring of the patients in critical condition. Integrated with this Hospital Information System, there is a mobile app, where in a case of any problem with a patient, it notifies the physician responsible for him. With this notification, this mobile app also presents the real-time situation and data from the sensors, such as ECG, blood pressure, blood glucose, heart rate, oxygen saturation, temperature, and breathing rate.

The *Family's Home module* is used by the patient's family and is connected with the Hospital Information System, however the information presented is unique to their related patient. It provides a mobile app that displays real-time monitoring from the sensors connected to the patient. Finally, this mobile app displays less information than the version used by the physicians and clinical staff because some of the data from sensors require medical expertise to be understood.

Regarding the ambient monitoring provided by this platform, all data from the sensors - temperature, location, and humidity - are presented at the hospital information system and its mobile apps, and at the ambulance service system. This monitoring is important because the control of the ambient temperature and humidity can directly affect the patient health treatment.

Table 1. Rules of the expert system

Sensor	Value	Critical Level	Action
ECG	Alteration of the electrocardiographic trace.	Irregular electrical activity, ventricular fibrillation supra or infra of ST asystole.	Red alarm issued to the medical staff on the Hospital Information System and Physician mobile app. If asystole, it alerts the ambulance service system and the ambulance mobile app.
Blood Pressure	Normal is 120 X 80 mmHG	Over 140X90mmHg or under 90X60mmHg.	Green alert issued to the family mobile app. Considering the patient history, a red alert can be issued to the medical staff in the Hospital Information System and Physician mobile app.
Blood Glucose	Normal between 100 and 126mgdL	Over 200mg/dL or under 60 mg/dL.	Green alert issued to the family mobile app. Considering the patient history, a red alert can be issued to the medical staff in the Hospital Information System and Physician mobile app.
Heart rate	Normal between 60 and 100bpm	Under to 60bpm or over a 100 bpm	Red alarm issued to the medical staff on the Hospital Information System and Physician mobile app. Considering the patient history, it can alert the ambulance service system and the ambulance mobile app.
Breathing rate	Normal between 16rpm and 20rpm	Under to 12rpm or over to 35rpm	Green alert issued to the family mobile app. Considering the patient history and clinical staff programming, it can alert the ambulance service system and the ambulance mobile app.
Temperature	Normal between 36°C and 37.5°C	Over 37.5°C	Green alert issued to the family mobile app. Considering the patient history and in cases of desirable hypothermia, clinical staff can program the threshold.
Capnography	Normal between 35mmHg and 45mmHg	Under to 35mmHg or over to 55mmHg	Red alarm issued to the medical staff on the Hospital Information System, Physician mobile app, the ambulance service system and the ambulance mobile app.

The *Ambulance Service module* is connected to the Ambulance Service System and is used by operators. The ambulances have a mobile app that is connected to the Ambulance Service System, using 3G/4G, to receive real-time information about the body and ambient monitoring sensors, emergency alarms and patient's situation. It is important to emphasize that the monitored location data from the patient is a key point for an effective response to the ambulance service.

Considering the presented modules of this platform and it purpose, there are important requirements that need to be addressed: privacy (Maglogiann, 2012; Sebestyen et al., 2014; Ray, 2015), security (Świątek & Rucinski, 2013; Fan et al., 2014; Hassan, 2014; Gao et al., 2015), interoperability (Jara et al., 2013; Castillejo et al., 2013; Gia et al., 2015), scalability (Maglogiann, 2012; Jara et al., 2013; Mohammed et al., 2014), reliability (Świątek & Rucinski, 2013; Hassan et al., 2014; Gao et al., 2015), robustness (Jara et al., 2013), ubiquity (López et al., 2013), portability (Mohammed et al., 2014), performance (Mohammed et al., 2014), availability (Maglogiann et al., 2012; Jara et al., 2013; Świątek & Rucinski, 2013) and integrity (Maksimović, et al., 2015). Once all the information transmitted from the sensors to the systems and mobile apps are sensible, there is a need for privacy in this communication. To assure privacy, this platform uses encryption. There is also the special need for security, which is guaranteed mainly by authentication (Maksimović et al., 2015). The IoT platform from the Cloud Health Infrastructure module assures scalability, integrity, portability and interoperability between the different types of the connected monitoring devices. The expert system of this module addresses the need for ubiquity, considering the defined rules and the customization feature. Finally, the proposed platform and its modules organization aim to achieve good performance, robustness, reliability, and availability regarding the information about patient monitoring.

FUTURE RESEARCH DIRECTIONS

With the use of a technology-based healthcare approach, there is an unprecedented opportunity for improving the quality and efficiency of healthcare. Consequently, this will improve the wellness of all citizens and lead to a better application of governments' financial resources. However, to effectively implement this strategy there are still big challenges that need to be addressed by research and innovation.

To effectively implement and adopt a technological approach based on IoT for remote healthcare, several non-functional issues need to be addressed. One of the most important aspects of healthcare is the safety of the solution. The safety in this context involves several factors, particularly: reliability, availability, security, integrity within a long-time-period. In software engineering, the ability to deal with these requirements is known as dependability. The exploration of dependability issues in the context of IoT is a very young and fertile research topic, creating an excellent opportunity to develop science and innovation involving both industry and academics. The engineering challenges - of conceiving and developing a set of technology-centric strategies to address the dependability requirement in healthcare applications based on the IoT infrastructure - is an open field for academics. Moreover, how to address dependability in healthcare applications based on the IoT infrastructure and targeted at underdeveloped countries, for example Brazil, is a big challenge due to the absence of basic health infrastructure that is generally found in developed countries.

Another key issue related to the proposed approach is the challenge of handling a huge volume of data produced by the different elements of the platform. In particular, the patient's home component has the capacity of collecting data from several sensors repeatedly during the day in a short period of time.

It might produce a huge volume of data if we consider several patients being monitored at the same time. That produced data must be evaluated in real-time in order to detect a patient's health anomalies. Moreover, a historical data analysis of patient's health measures must be performed in order to detect patterns and anomalies, build a health profile of critical patients and make predictive analyses to prevent critical situations and more. Due to the abovementioned characteristics involving the proposed platform, it represents a rich field to apply, evaluate and evolve the techniques of the recent area known as Big Data.

Interoperability is also an open research problem, mainly when faced information technology systems in medical context. This ability allows different information systems, healthcare devices, and software applications to communicate, exchange data, and use the shared information across physicians, hospital, pharmacy, ambulance, and patient regardless of the application or application vendor. Despite the clear benefits of this capacity, i.e. improving the quality, safety, efficiency, and efficacy of healthcare delivery, the reality shows that currently, it is far from being achieved. Several issues must be addressed involving communication protocols, connectivity interfaces, open standards for healthcare data to reach an effectivity level of interoperability to allow the electronic exchange of patient's measures among all IT parties involved.

Finally, the use of remote monitoring is emerging as an opportunity to address resource shortages, health workers' overload, and an increased prevalence of chronic disease. However, assuring the long term effectiveness of remote monitoring and its impact on health indicators is a challenge to be overcome by experimental research on usability and clinical effects, to support medical decisions that can be subsidized based on remote monitoring.

CONCLUSION

To effectively implement this proposed platform in Brazil there are still big challenges not generally observed in developed countries that need to be addressed by research and innovation. Although the Brazilian constitution declares that healthcare is an official government responsibility and that it is the right of every citizen to have free public access to it, nevertheless government hospitals are often crowded, waiting times for appointment and treatment are lengthy, and the facilities are often inadequate. Indeed, healthcare is one of the worst problems in Brazil, ranking above violence and education.

On the other hand, the recent advances in IoT applied to healthcare is promoting a powerful environment for a disruptive innovation in the health research field as well as in the computer science area. This current scenario creates several opportunities to improve the effectiveness and efficiency of the use of national health infrastructure. Improving the quality and efficiency of the care for patients in a critical situation through the exploitation of technological "smart" solutions would promote substantial results in terms of welfare for the patients. The deployment of remote monitoring solutions for healthcare is not science fiction. The current advances in technology demonstrate that its development and deployment are viable and, in specific scenarios, it is already a reality. Some companies are already focused on the development of solutions for remote patient monitoring (RPM) and, at the same time, several types of research are being conducted to develop this field.

The proposed platform was described focusing on the patient's home care, but it can be easily evolved to also consider the patients inside the hospital in addition to other use cases involving health professionals, medical devices, information systems and other actors. With the use of a technology-based healthcare approach, there is an unprecedented opportunity for improving the quality and efficiency of the public health system in Brazil. Consequently, this will improve the wellness of all citizens and a better application of government financial resources. Moreover, the study, development, and deployment of appropriate technology-focused solutions addressing the specific issues and peculiarities of public Brazilian healthcare is an excellent opportunity to develop science and innovation as well as inducing economic and social development.

Although patient monitoring technology is introduced as one solution to increase the quality and efficiency of the public health system, there is a real barrier in Brazil due to the absence (or inadequate availability) of basic technological infrastructure, which is the premise for this proposal. For this reason, the biggest challenge in an underdeveloped country is related to the influencing of public policy to make available the basic elements needed to make feasible remote healthcare for patients in a critical condition.

REFERENCES

Abinaya, V. K., Kumar, V., & Swathika, . (2015). Ontology Based Public Healthcare System in Internet of Things (IoT). *Procedia Computer Science, 50*, 99–102. doi:10.1016/j.procs.2015.04.067

Aehlert, B. (2011). *ACLS Advanced Cardiac Life Support, Study Guide* (4th ed.). Mosby.

American Diabetes Association. (2016). *Checking Your Blood Glucose*. Retrieved September 14, 2016, from http://www.diabetes.org/living-with-diabetes/treatment-and-care/blood-glucose-control/checking-your-blood-glucose.html

American Heart Association. (2016). *Understanding Blood Pressure Readings*. Retrieved September 14, 2016, from http://www.heart.org/HEARTORG/Conditions/HighBloodPressure/AboutHighBloodPressure/Understanding-Blood-Pressure-Readings_UCM_301764_Article.jsp

Atzori, L., Iera, A., & Morabito, G. (2010). The internet of things: A survey. *Computer Networks, 54*(15), 2787–2805. doi:10.1016/j.comnet.2010.05.010

Bazerbashi, H., Merriman, K. W., Toale, K. M., Chaftari, P., Carreras, M. T. C., Henderson, J. D., & Rice, T. W. et al. (2014). Low tissue oxygen saturation at emergency center triage is predictive of intensive care unit admission. *Journal of Critical Care, 29*(5), 775–779. doi:10.1016/j.jcrc.2014.05.006 PMID:24973103

Benlamri, R., & Docksteader, L. (2010). MORF: A mobile health-monitoring platform. *IT Professional, 3*(3), 18–25. doi:10.1109/MITP.2010.3

Bolinder, J., et al. (in press). Novel glucose-sensing technology and hypoglycaemia in type 1 diabetes: a multicentre, non-masked, randomised controlled trial. *Lancet.*

Brasil. (2013). *Ministério da Saúde. Secretaria de Atenção à Saúde. Departamento de Atenção Especializada. Manual instrutivo da Rede de Atenção às Urgências e Emergências no Sistema Único de Saúde (SUS)*. Brasília, DF: Editora do Ministério da Saúde.

Brennan, T. (2010). Gestão da doença para promover o controle da pressão arterial entre os afro-americanos. *Popul Manag Saúde, 13*(2), 65–72.

Cahill, T. J., & Prendergast, B. D. (2016). Infective endocarditis. *Lancet*, *387*(10021), 882–893. doi:10.1016/S0140-6736(15)00067-7 PMID:26341945

Castillejo, P., Martinez, J. F., Rodriguez-Molina, J., & Cuerva, A. (2013). Integration of wearable devices in a wireless sensor network for an E-health application. *IEEE Wireless Communications*, *20*(4), 38–49. doi:10.1109/MWC.2013.6590049

Chaudhry, S. I., Mattera, J. A., Curtis, J. P., Spertus, J. A., Herrin, J., Lin, Z., & Krumholz, H. M. et al. (2010). Telemonitoring in patients with heart failure. *The New England Journal of Medicine*, *363*(24), 2301–2309. doi:10.1056/NEJMoa1010029 PMID:21080835

Chen, L. M., Kennedy, E. H., Sales, A., & Hofer, T. P. (2013). Use of health IT for higher-value critical care. *The New England Journal of Medicine*, *368*(7), 594–597. doi:10.1056/NEJMp1213273 PMID:23363474

Chiuchisan, I., Costin, H. N., & Geman, O. (2014, October). Adopting the internet of things technologies in health care systems. In *Electrical and Power Engineering (EPE), 2014 International Conference and Exposition on* (pp. 532-535). IEEE. doi:10.1109/ICEPE.2014.6969965

Constantinescu, L., Kim, J., & Feng, D. D. (2012). SparkMed: A framework for dynamic integration of multimedia medical data into distributed m-health systems. *IEEE Transactions on Information Technology in Biomedicine*, *16*(1), 40–52. doi:10.1109/TITB.2011.2174064 PMID:22049371

Coulter, A. (2012). Patient engagement—what works? *The Journal of Ambulatory Care Management*, *35*(2), 80–89. doi:10.1097/JAC.0b013e318249e0fd PMID:22415281

Crossley, G. H., Boyle, A., Vitense, H., Chang, Y., & Mead, R. H. (2011). CONNECT Investigators. The CONNECT (Clinical Evaluation of Remote Notification to Reduce Time to Clinical Decision) trial: The value of wireless remote monitoring with automatic clinician alerts. *Journal of the American College of Cardiology*, *57*(10), 1181–1189. doi:10.1016/j.jacc.2010.12.012 PMID:21255955

Dabbs, A. D., Myers, B. A., Mc Curry, K. R., Dunbar-Jacob, J., Hawkins, R. P., Begey, A., & Dew, M. A. (2009). User-centered design and interactive health technologies for patients. *Computers, Informatics, Nursing*, *27*(3), 175–183. doi:10.1097/NCN.0b013e31819f7c7c PMID:19411947

Delicato, F. C., Pires, P. F., & Batista, T. (2013). *Middleware solutions for the Internet of Things*. Springer London. doi:10.1007/978-1-4471-5481-5

Dwivedi, S. (2016). Reshaping Medical Practice and Care with Health Information Systems. In R. Misra (Ed.), *The Benefits and Challenges of Using Mobile-Based Tools in Self-Management and Care* (pp. 1–13). University of Hull. doi:10.4018/978-1-4666-9870-3

Ettehad, D., Emdin, C. A., Kiran, A., Anderson, S. G., Callender, T., Emberson, J., & Rahimi, K. et al. (2016). Blood pressure lowering for prevention of cardiovascular disease and death: A systematic review and meta-analysis. *Lancet*, *387*(10022), 957–967. doi:10.1016/S0140-6736(15)01225-8 PMID:26724178

Ewer, A. K. (2014, August). Pulse oximetry screening: Do we have enough evidence now? *Lancet*, *384*(9945), 725–726. doi:10.1016/S0140-6736(14)60575-4 PMID:24768154

Fan, Y. J., Yin, Y. H., Da Xu, L., Zeng, Y., & Wu, F. (2014). IoT-based smart rehabilitation system. *IEEE Transactions on Industrial Informatics, 10*(2), 1568-1577.

Ferguson, N. D., Cook, D. J., Guyatt, G. H., Mehta, S., Hand, L., Austin, P., & Meade, M. O. et al. (2013). High-Frequency Oscillation in Early Acute Respiratory Distress Syndrome. *The New England Journal of Medicine*, *368*(9), 795–805. doi:10.1056/NEJMoa1215554 PMID:23339639

Filkins, B. L. (2016). Privacy and security in the era of digital health: What should translational researchers know and do about it?. *Am J Transl Res.*, *8*(3), 1560–1580. PMID:27186282

Gao, R., Zhao, M., Qiu, Z., Yu, Y., & Chang, C. H. (2015, June). Web-based motion detection system for health care. In *Computer and Information Science (ICIS), 2015 IEEE/ACIS 14th International Conference on* (pp. 65-70). IEEE.

Gartner. (2015). *Gartner says 6.4 billion connected ''things''will be in use in 2016, up 30 percent from 2015*. Retrieved June 10, 2016, from Http://www.gartner.com/newsroom/id/3165317

Gasparrini, A., Guo, Y., Hashizume, M., Lavigne, E., Zanobetti, A., Schwartz, J., & Armstrong, B. et al. (2015). Mortality risk attributable to high and low ambient temperature: A multicountry observational study. *Lancet*, *386*(9991), 369–375. doi:10.1016/S0140-6736(14)62114-0 PMID:26003380

Gelder, I. C. V. (2016). Rate control in atrial fibrillation. *Lancet*, *388*(10046), 818–828. doi:10.1016/S0140-6736(16)31258-2 PMID:27560277

Gia, T. N., Thanigaivelan, N. K., Rahmani, A. M., Westerlund, T., Liljeberg, P., & Tenhunen, H. (2014, October). Customizing 6LoWPAN networks towards Internet-of-Things based ubiquitous healthcare systems. In NORCHIP, 2014 (pp. 1-6). IEEE.

Goligher, E. C., Ferguson, N. D., & Brochard, L. J. (2016). Clinical challenges in mechanical ventilation. *Lancet*, *387*(10030), 1856–1866. doi:10.1016/S0140-6736(16)30176-3 PMID:27203509

Gorp, V. P., & Comuzzi, M. (2014). Lifelong personal health data and application software via virtual machines in the cloud. *IEEE Journal of Biomedical and Health Informatics*, *18*(1), 36–45. doi:10.1109/JBHI.2013.2257821 PMID:24403402

Gubbi, J., Buyya, R., Marusic, S., & Palaniswami, M. (2013). Internet of things (iot): A vision, architectural elements, and future directions. *Future Generation Computer Systems*, *29*(7), 1645–1660. doi:10.1016/j.future.2013.01.010

Hall, J. E. (2006). *Guyton and Hall Textbook of Medical Physiology (12th ed.)*. Elsevier.

Hassan, M. M., Albakr, H. S., & Al-Dossari, H. (2014, November). A Cloud-Assisted Internet of Things Framework for Pervasive Healthcare in Smart City Environment. In *Proceedings of the 1st International Workshop on Emerging Multimedia Applications and Services for Smart Cities* (pp. 9-13). ACM. doi:10.1145/2661704.2661707

Heidbuchel, H., Hindricks, G., Broadhurst, P., Van Erven, L., Fernandez-Lozano, I., Rivero-Ayerza, M., & Annemans, L. et al. (2015). EuroEco (European Health Economic Trial on Home Monitoring in ICD Patients): A provider perspective in five European countries on costs and net financial impact of follow-up with or without remote monitoring. *European Heart Journal*, *36*(3), 158–169. doi:10.1093/eurheartj/ehu339 PMID:25179766

Hendriks, M., & Rademakers, J. (2014). Relationships between patient activation, disease-specific knowledge and health outcomes among people with diabetes; a survey study. *BMC Health Services Research, 14*(1), 393. doi:10.1186/1472-6963-14-393 PMID:25227734

Hindia, M.N., Rahman, T.A., Ojukwu, H., Hanafi, E.B., & Fattouh, A. (2016). Enabling Remote Health-Caring Utilizing IoT Concept ov er LTE-Femtocell Networks. *Lista Jornal PLoS One, 11*(5).

Hindricks, G., Taborsky, M., Glikson, M., Heinrich, U., Schumacher, B., Katz, A., & Søgaard, P. et al. (2014). Implant-based multiparameter telemonitoring of patients with heart failure (IN-TIME): A randomised controlled trial. *Lancet, 384*(9943), 583–590. doi:10.1016/S0140-6736(14)61176-4 PMID:25131977

Hochron, S., & Goldberg, P. (2015). Driving physician adoption of mHeath solutions. *Healthcare Financial Management, 69*(2), 36–39. PMID:26665538

IEC 60601. (2015). *IEC 60601-1-11:2015 RLV Redline version.* Retrieved October 11, 2016, from https://webstore.iec.ch/publication/22261

Jara, A. J., Zamora-Izquierdo, M. A., & Skarmeta, A. F. (2013). Interconnection framework for mHealth and remote monitoring based on the Internet of Things. *IEEE Journal on Selected Areas in Communications, 31*(9), 47–65. doi:10.1109/JSAC.2013.SUP.0513005

Jiang, Y., Sereika, S. M., Dabbs, A. D., Handler, S. M., & Schlenk, E. A. (2016). Using mobile health technology to deliver decision support for self-monitoring after lung transplantation. *International Journal of Medical Informatics, 94*, 164–171. doi:10.1016/j.ijmedinf.2016.07.012 PMID:27573324

JSON. (2016). *Introducing JSON.* Retrieved September 14, 2016, from http://www.json.org/

Khattak, H. A., Ruta, M., Di Sciascio, E., & Sciascio, D. (2014, January). CoAP-based healthcare sensor networks: A survey. In *Proceedings of 2014 11th International Bhurban Conference on Applied Sciences & Technology (IBCAST)* (pp. 499-503). IEEE. doi:10.1109/IBCAST.2014.6778196

Kotsimbos, T., Williams, T. J., & Anderson, J. P. (2012). Update on lung transplantation: Programmes, patients and prospects. *European Respiratory Review, 21*(126), 271–305. doi:10.1183/09059180.00006312 PMID:23204117

Langhan, M. L., Kurtz, J. C., Schaeffer, P., Asnes, A. G., & Riera, A. (2014). Experiences with capnography in acute care settings: A mixed-methods analysis of clinical staff. *Journal of Critical Care, 29*(6), 1035–1040. doi:10.1016/j.jcrc.2014.06.021 PMID:25129575

Liao, S. H. (2005). Expert system methodologies and applications—a decade review from 1995 to 2004. *Expert Systems with Applications, 28*(1), 93–103. doi:10.1016/j.eswa.2004.08.003

López, P., Fernández, D., Jara, A. J., & Skarmeta, A. F. (2013, March). Survey of internet of things technologies for clinical environments. In *Advanced Information Networking and Applications Workshops (WAINA), 2013 27th International Conference on* (pp. 1349-1354). IEEE. doi:10.1109/WAINA.2013.255

Maglogiann, D. I. (2012). Bringing IoT and Cloud Computing towards Pervasive Healthcare Charalampos. *Sixth International Conference on Innovative Mobile and InternetServices in Ubiquitous Computing.*

Maksimović, M., Vujović, V., & Perišić, B. (2015, June). A custom internet of things healthcare system. In *2015 10th Iberian Conference on Information Systems and Technologies (CISTI)* (pp. 1-6). IEEE. doi:10.1109/CISTI.2015.7170415

Mattern, F., & Floerkemeier, C. (2010). From the Internet of Computers to the Internet of Things. In *From active data management to event-based systems and more* (pp. 242–259). Springer Berlin Heidelberg. doi:10.1007/978-3-642-17226-7_15

Medicinet. (2016). *Definition of Heart Rate*. Retrieved September 17, 2016, from http://www.medicinenet.com/script/main/art.asp?articlekey=3674

Mendes, E.V. (2010). As redes de atenção à saúde. Ciênc. *saúde coletiva, 15*(5), 2297-2305.

Minutolo, A., Esposito, M., & Pietro, G. D. (2016). Design and validation of a light-weight reasoning system to support remote health monitoring applications. *Engineering Applications of Artificial Intelligence, 41*, 232–248. doi:10.1016/j.engappai.2015.01.019

Mohammed, J., Lung, C. H., Ocneanu, A., Thakral, A., Jones, C., & Adler, A. (2014, September). Internet of Things: Remote patient monitoring using web services and cloud computing. *Chest, 149*(2), 576–585.

Oracle. (2016). *What Are RESTful Web Services?*. Retrieved September 14, 2016, from http://docs.oracle.com/javaee/6/tutorial/doc/gijqy.html

Pang, Z. (2013). *Technologies and architectures of the internet-of-things (iot) for health and well-being.* Retrieved June 13, 2016, from http://kth.diva-portal.org/smash/get/diva2:621384/FULLTEXT01.pdf

Piccini J.P., et al. (in press). Impact of remote monitoring on clinical events and associated health care utilization: A nationwide assessment. *Heart Rhythm.*

Pitsillides, A. (2006). DITIS: A collaborative virtual medical team for home healthcare of cancer patients M-Health. Springer.

Poenaru, E., & Poenaru, C. (2013, November). A structured approach of the Internet-of-Things eHealth use cases. In E-Health and Bioengineering Conference (EHB), 2013 (pp. 1-4). IEEE. doi:10.1109/EHB.2013.6707299

Portugal, G., Cunha, P., Valente, B., Feliciano, J., Lousinha, A., Alves, S., & Ferreira, R. C. et al. (2016). Influence of remote monitoring on long-term cardiovascular outcomes after cardioverter-defibrillator implantation. *International Journal of Cardiology, 222*, 764–768. doi:10.1016/j.ijcard.2016.07.157 PMID:27521554

Prescher, S. (2014). Wird Telemonitoring von Patienten mit chronischer Herzinsuffizienz angenommen?. *Dtsch Patienten, 139*(16), 829–834.

Raad, M. W., Sheltami, T., & Shakshuki, E. (2015). Ubiquitous Tele-health System for Elderly Patients with Alzheimers. *Procedia Computer Science, 52*, 685–689. doi:10.1016/j.procs.2015.05.075

Ray, P. P. (2015, January). Internet of Things for Sports (IoTSport): An architectural framework for sports and recreational activity. In *Electrical, Electronics, Signals, Communication and Optimization (EESCO), 2015 International Conference on* (pp. 1-4). IEEE.

Saxon, L. A., Hayes, D. L., Gilliam, F. R., Heidenreich, P. A., Day, J., Seth, M., & Boehmer, J. P. et al. (2010). Long-term outcome after ICD and CRT implantation and influence of remote device follow-up: The ALTITUDE survival study. *Circulation*, *122*(23), 2359–2367. doi:10.1161/CIRCULATIONAHA.110.960633 PMID:21098452

Sebestyen, G., Hangan, A., Oniga, S., & Gál, Z. (2014, May). eHealth solutions in the context of Internet of Things. *Proc. IEEE Int. Conf. Automation, Quality and Testing, Robotics (AQTR 2014)*, 261-267. doi:10.1109/AQTR.2014.6857876

Sieverink, F., Siemons, L., Braakman-Jansen, A., & Van Gemert-Pijnen, L. (2016). Internet of Things & Personalized Healthcare. *Studies in Health Technology and Informatics*, *221*, 129. PMID:27071903

Sweeney, R.M., McAuley, D.F. (in press). Acute respiratory distress syndrome. *Lancet*.

Świątek, P., & Rucinski, A. (2013, October). IoT as a service system for eHealth. In *e-Health Networking, Applications & Services (Healthcom), 2013 IEEE 15th International Conference on* (pp. 81-84). IEEE. doi:10.1109/HealthCom.2013.6720643

Tabish, R., Ghaleb, A. M., Hussein, R., Touati, F., Mnaouer, A. B., Khriji, L., & Rasid, M. F. A. (2014, February). A 3G/WiFi-enabled 6LoWPAN-based U-healthcare system for ubiquitous real-time monitoring and data logging. In *2nd Middle East Conference on Biomedical Engineering* (pp. 277-280). IEEE doi:10.1109/MECBME.2014.6783258

Thabit, H., Bally, L., & Hovorka, R. (in press). Available at a flash: a new way to check glucose. *Lancet*.

van der Valk, S., Myers, T., Atkinson, I., & Mohring, K. (2015, April). Sensor networks in workplaces: Correlating comfort and productivity. In *Intelligent Sensors, Sensor Networks and Information Processing (ISSNIP), 2015 IEEE Tenth International Conference on* (pp. 1-6). IEEE.

Varma, N., Piccini, J. P., Snell, J., Fischer, A., Dalal, N., & Mittal, S. (2015). Relationship between level of adherence to automatic wireless remote monitoring and survival in pacemaker and defibrillator patients. *Journal of the American College of Cardiology*, *65*(24), 2601–2610. doi:10.1016/j.jacc.2015.04.033 PMID:25983008

Vidal-Petiot, E., et al. (in press). Cardiovascular event rates and mortality according to achieved systolic and diastolic blood pressure in patients with stable coronary artery disease: an international cohort study. *Lancet*.

Yang, C. T., Liu, J. C., Liao, C. J., Wu, C. C., & Le, F. Y. (2013, December). On Construction of an Intelligent Environmental Monitoring System for Healthcare. In *2013 International Conference on Parallel and Distributed Computing, Applications and Technologies* (pp. 246-253). IEEE. doi:10.1109/PDCAT.2013.45

Yang, G., Xie, L., Mäntysalo, M., Zhou, X., Pang, Z., Da Xu, L., ... Zheng, L. R. (2014). A health-IoT platform based on the integration of intelligent packaging, unobtrusive bio-sensor, and intelligent medicine box. *IEEE Transactions on Industrial Informatics, 10*(4), 2180-2191.

Yinong, C. (2016). Analyzing and visual programming internet of things and autonomous decentralized systems. *Simulation Modelling Practice and Theory*, *65*, 1–10. doi:10.1016/j.simpat.2016.05.002

Zanchetti, A., Thomopoulos, C., & Parati, G. (2015). Randomized controlled trials of blood pressure lowering in hypertension: A critical reappraisal. *Circulation Research*, *116*(6), 1058–1073. doi:10.1161/CIRCRESAHA.116.303641 PMID:25767290

Zandomenighi, R. C., Mouro, D. L., Oliveira, C. A., & Martins, E. A. P. (2014). Cuidados intensivos em um serviço hospitalar de emergência: Desafios para os enfermeiros. REME rev. min. *Enferm*, *18*(2), 404–414.

Chapter 2
Internet of Things in Pervasive Healthcare Systems

Teresa Guarda
Universidad Peninsula de Santa Elena (UPSE), Ecuador

Maria Fernanda Augusto
Universidad Peninsula de Santa Elena (UPSE), Ecuador

Oscar Barrionuevo
Universidad de las Fuerzas Armadas (ESPE), Ecuador

Filipe Mota Pinto
Polytechnic Institute of Leiria, Portugal

ABSTRACT

Throughout the stunning development of wireless communication technologies, sensors and wireless sensor networks (WSN) are being used in almost every area, such as in healthcare field. The ubiquitous sensing enabled by WSN technologies, in particularly the wireless medical sensor network (WMSN), might be one important key success factor in the modern medical system. The recent advances, and wireless devices proliferation, had proved the technical feasibility of the pervasive health care systems. The data collected by sensors are very sensitive and important, and the leakage of them could compromise security and privacy. This work presents the pervasive health care systems (PHCS) focusing on security and privacy of pervasive environments.

INTRODUCTION

Nowadays, Internet of things and the ageing of world population are reshaping the world. It's expected that world population with 60 years or more reach 22% in 2050 (11% in 2009) (Department of Economic and Social Affairs of the United Nations, 2009). In the case of European Union (EU) it's projected to increase 30% in 2050 (22.5% in 2005) (Eurostat, 2008), and in United States 20.2% (13% in 2010) (Vincent & Velkof, 2010). In this context, resources and efficiency of health care services must to be improved to fulfill such group of people.

DOI: 10.4018/978-1-5225-2851-7.ch002

In 1990, the 27 EU Member States was public health expenditure averaged 5.9% of GDP, increased to 7.2% in 2010 and being expected to reach 8.5% in 2060, as result of population aging and others factors (cultural and socio-economics). This trend will be accompanied by an expected decline of working-age population from 61% to 51% of the total population. Deep structural reforms are needed to ensure the sustainability of health systems, while ensuring that all citizens have access to services (UE, 2012). The impact of these changes is visible, being conditioned by the decrease in the number of health professionals, by the increasing increase in the incidence of chronic diseases, by the requirement of the citizens of a better quality in the services and the assistance.

On the other hand, the dissemination of wireless characteristic on almost fields of technology is promising new approaches to address challenges faced by the health care sector.

Healthcare technologies had provided suitable solutions powered by the ubiquitous identification, sensing and communication capacities, whereas all system's objects may be continuously tracked and monitored (Alemdar, 2010; Portela, Santos, Silva, Machado, Abelha, & Rua, 2014).

Nowadays' scenario delivered by global connectivity of the Internet of Things (IoT), enable efficiency on collecting, management and use of all healthcare devices' information (Domingo, 2012), leveraged through intelligent and ubiquitous systems (Portela, Santos, Silva, Machado, Abelha, & Rua, 2014).

The IoT systems integrates many different types of devices, like sensing, communication, identification, networking, information management, and systems that links people and things at anytime and anywhere, through any device and media, accessing any information from any object to obtain any service in a more efficiently mode (European Commission Information Society, 2009).

The healthcare delivery model has been evolved from different perspectives from the hospital centric view, passing to hospital home balanced projected by 2020, until the home centric view to 2030 (Koop et al., 2008).

IoT is presented as a new paradigm of information and communication technology being exploited by industry, offering a huge potential to every areas (Atzori, Iera, & Morabito, 2010) in particular the healthcare system (Miorandi, Sicari, De Pellegrini, & Chlamtac, 2012). Such advances had enabled the transformation of the healthcare system view, from a career-centric view to patient-centric view (Pang, Zheng, Tian, Kao-Walter, Dubrova, & Chen, 2015).

This work, following the introduction, goes by the background concepts exposition through Internet of Things, Wireless Sensor Network, Pervasive Health Care Systems and contextualizing of the work. The focus of section three is the security and privacy in pervasive health care systems (PHCS) in of pervasive environments. The article ends by the conclusions section whereas final remarks and future work is addressed.

BACKGROUND

Internet of Things

The IoT (Guillemin & Friess, 2009) paradigm relates a world set of physical objects provided with sensors and actuator triggers connected through wireless networks over internet, setting and enabling an intelligent objects network capable to collect data, processing information and execute actions accordingly. Those objects communicate each other and with others resources (physical or virtual) expanding initial system throughout its boundaries. IoT will allow people and things to be connected Anytime, Anyplace, with Anything and Anyone, ideally using Any path/network and Any service. Also de concept of IoT can be regarded as an extension of the existing interaction between humans and applications through the new dimension of "Things" communication and integration (Vermesan, et al., 2011). The emerging of such new kind heterogeneous systems addresses and enables a myriad of applications almost in all knowledge areas (Atzori, Iera, & Morabito, 2010).

One of IoT's main technologies is Radio Frequency Identification (RFID) used to electronically address objects. Other technologies such as sensors, actuators, cell phones, Near Field Communication (NFC), artificial intelligence, nanotechnologies, can also be used in IoT, providing a new dimension to the world of information and communication. Objects equipped with these technologies exchange information among themselves, generating a huge traffic if billions of objects are interconnected. Objects capture the activities of interconnected individuals through the Internet, raising questions about security and privacy.

IoT consists in the interconnecting of the everyday objects in the real environment with the Internet, the virtual environment, making them intelligent objects. This is possible due to the use of sensors and addressable RFID tags embedded in objects, which communicate through a network, and these with the Internet (Wu, Lu, Ling, Sun, & Du, 2010).

Currently, IoT despite being very present in the daily lives of persons, some issues remain open, with concerns the standardization and architectures; acceptance by the persons; and security and privacy.

In a network of objects capturing and transmitting data about the users, privacy is one of the great challenges of IoT. In a reality where RFID tags are embedded in clothes, food and personal devices; they can be triggered to respond with their ID and other information without the user noticing that it is being monitored.

In addition to the use of RFID, IoT should include technologies such as Artificial Intelligence (AI), embedded systems and nanotechnology, which will allow machine-to-machine interconnection, leading to a new form of ubiquitous communication, in which objects can communicate with people and other objects in an independent way. A new dimension was added to the world of communication that already possessed the concepts of connectivity at any time, from anywhere, to any person, to have connectivity to anything (Xue, Li, Liu, & Liu, 2012).

Therefore, IoT might be considered as a network of networks, in which a massive number of things, objects, sensors and devices are connected through the information and communications infrastructure (ICI) providing value-added services (Stankovic, 2014). It is also possible to introduce IoT as a global network paradigm that allows communications between humans, between humans and things, and also between things, providing a unique identity to every object (Aggarwal & Das, 2012; Chiti, Fantacci, Loreti, & Pugliese, 2016). By the end the basic concept of IoT is the pervasive presence of a variety of things, as representing an instance of anything, with ability to compute and communicate each other.

Actually IoT may represent a technology based society revolution and evolution, that will include computing and communication in wireless devices and sensors at nanotechnology scale (Madakam, Ramaswamy, & Tripathi, 2015). Currently there are many areas of IoT applications: Aerospace and aviation (systems status monitoring, green operations); Automotive; Telecommunications; Intelligent Buildings (automatic energy metering / home automation / wireless monitoring); Pharmaceutical; Independent Living (wellness, mobility, monitoring of an aging population); Agriculture; Retail, Logistics, Supply Chain Management; Manufacturing, Product Lifecycle Management; Processing industries (Oil and Gas); Recycling; Insurance; Safety, Security and Privacy; Environment Monitoring; Education; Media and entertainment among many others (Campbell, et al., 2008; Parwekar & Reddy, 2013).

Thus, the scope of IoT is extensive and fairly heterogeneous. Globally the scope of IoT is structured in four general areas, since a single person, passing by groups and communities, until the industry. At level of personal IoT, the scope is a single person, and this is the area with a more aggressive growth. The group area scope is a small group of individuals, and is one of the most challenging areas. In the case of the community area the scope is a big group of individuals in a public infrastructure context, and this is an area with great potential. The scope of industrial area refers to organizations within or between, and this is the most mature part of IoT.

The goal of IoT is to improve the quality of life of people, thus contributing also to the health area, to improve patients' daily lives.

Currently there are many proposals for IoT applications in the health area, from applications that include identification and localization of patients with RFID, identification and control of medication administration, control of childhood obesity with monitoring of food, among many others.

Wireless Sensor Network

In the last decades there has been an explosive growth of computer networks and, in particular, of wireless communications, propitiated by the continuous technological advances. Thus, it has been possible to develop electronic devices of smaller size, low cost and reduced consumption, able to process information locally and communicate wirelessly (Akyildiz, Su, Sankarasubramaniam, & Cayirci, 2002).

All these factors have allowed the launching of the field of Wireless Sensor Networks (WSN). At present different types of sensors can be found, in a large number of systems and electronic devices. In most applications, these sensors act only as transducers, making the measurement of one or more variables of the environment and sending this information to a central node that is in charge of its processing (Goldsmith, 2005).

At present it is possible to acquire large quantities of sensors at reduced costs. The WSN often are implemented in places without supervision, being vulnerable to potential attacks. In addition, the sensors present some limitations in terms of autonomy, memory and processing capacity, so it is not possible to implement the measures that guarantee the reliability and confidentiality usually used in wireless networks.

A WSN consists of a set of these sensors, distributed spatially, with the aim of collecting and transmitting data, where it is not possible to do it with traditional networks, either for strategic reasons or for limitations of the environment where they are inserted, so WSN is a heterogeneous system with the purpose to computing elements, which combines tiny sensors and actuators. The sensors are small autonomously geographically distributed devices, called sensor nodes. Sensors nodes have capacity for computing, storage and communication in a network connected without cables, and installed around an object phenomenon to monitor it (Karlof & Wagner, 2003).

The communication in WSN is taken place between source and destination. The destination is called as base station or Sink. When events occur, it is the taking of measurements or any programmed activity with the phenomenon in question, the information is transformed into digital at the node itself, and transmitted outside the network, via a gateway element, to a base station that is used to collect and process data, to finally end up in a server with greater capacity that allows to compose a historical sequence or to make an analysis of the data (see Figure 1).

The areas of application of the WSN are quite distinct, as is the case of industry, smart houses, intelligent parking systems, facility monitoring, robotics, security, health, among others.

Figure 1. Wireless sensor network

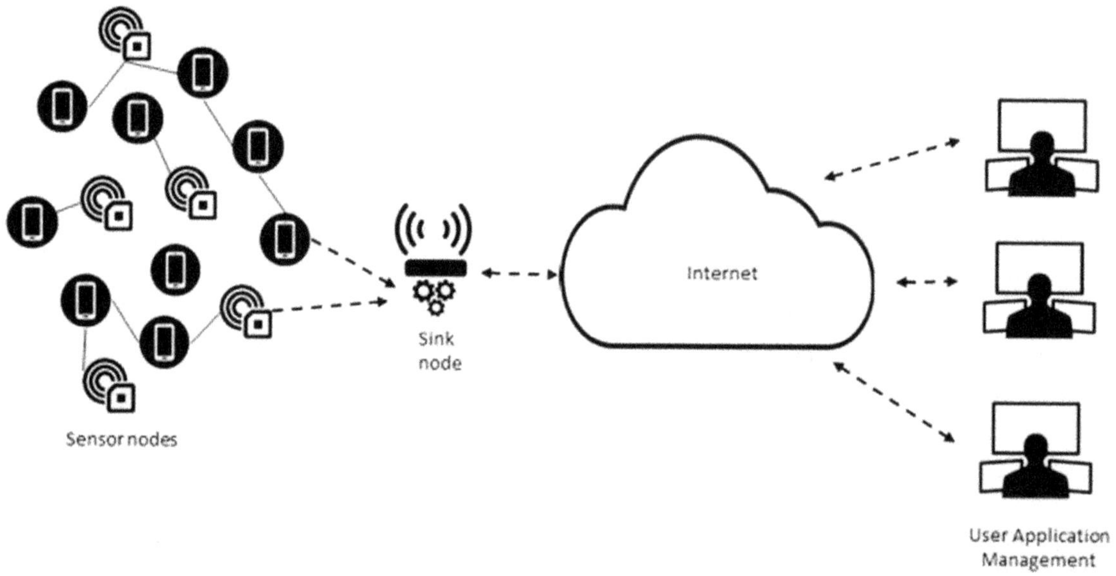

IoT for Health is a fabulous creator of opportunities, in improving the welfare of populations, allowing soften the grip of current health systems.

The connected smart devices provide information that can be used to make actionable decisions based on evidence-based models and algorithms and can have a significant impact on the delivery and operation of health services. It is an added value in preventive health, in terms of the monitoring of chronic diseases, allowing a proactive monitoring.

Pervasive Health Care Systems

Pervasive environments are heterogeneous and complex environments, consisting of several devices, such as sensors and actuators, and by applications that are incorporated in these physical environments, allowing a natural and transparent interaction with the user. These devices interconnect each other, providing a variety of user-friendly features (Satyanarayanan, 2001). The natural and transparent interaction in pervasive environments refers to the human computer interaction process (Dix, 2009; Baecker, 2014). Pervasive environments in the health area are concerned with the provision of health services to anyone, anytime, anywhere, in order to increase service coverage and quality (Varshney, 2003).

PCHS may be considered a solution and a possible future of the current healthcare services (Varshney, 2005).

PHCS are designed to provide different types of medical services and to support individual users in a personalized way (Röcker, Ziefle, & Holzinger, 2014), providing information and alerting mechanisms.

Despite the human health to be constantly evolving, there is still a long way to go. The use of IoT technologies for tracking people and objects can improve control and workflow in hospitals and clinics. With IoT applications the location of doctors, nurses, materials and patients can be optimized; as well as restricted access areas can be monitored to prevent the flow of unauthorized persons (Atzori, Iera, & Morabito, 2010), preserving security and privacy.

The World Health Organization defines eHealth as "the transfer of health resources and health care by electronic means. It encompasses three main areas: the delivery of health information, for health professionals and health consumers, through the Internet and telecommunications; using the power of IT and e-commerce to improve public health services, e.g., through the education and training of health workers; the use of e-commerce and e-business practices in health systems management" (WHO, 2017).

The fast explosion of personal eHealth, premising self-management and data collection of health conditions, are changing the way to deliver and collect health care information.

Organizations have already identified and started working on projects to address issues related to security, scalability, data collection, and interoperability (UE, 2012).

The use of PHCS for delivery of healthcare to citizens raises new challenges at security and privacy levels.

PHCS SECURITY AND PRIVACY

For assuring systems essential security requirements (confidentiality, data integrity, accountability, availability, and access control), encryption methods can be used (Pereira, et al., 2007). In the case of privacy, user's authorization in the system shouldn't be ignored and they should have control over their personal data (Ikonen & Kaasinen, 2008).

Currently, we live in a context of people-centric and urban WSN. There are a wide and diversified range of applications in the WSN, focused on monitoring the health status of individuals or patients (Al Ameen, Liu, & Kwak, 2012).

The use of WSN in health applications is growing at a rapid pace. There is a wide range of applications in use (heart rate monitor, blood pressure monitor, endoscopic capsule). In this context of increasing use of sensor technology in the health area, a new field emerged, the wireless medical sensor networks (WMSN).

Although all networks are subject to threats, wireless networks are the most susceptible to attacks, since there is no physical restriction of cabling, so the information is physically more accessible to attackers. The fact that most devices and their applications are wireless, makes security and privacy the main areas of concern, and the direct involvement of humans, increases sensitivity to security and privacy issues.

The most frequent routing protocols in the WSN are mostly oriented to energy efficiency; they are not oriented to the security problem, being subject to different types of threats and problems. Then, in absence of adequate security measures, a WSN remains vulnerable to a variety of attacks.

WSNs require a different approach to security. The hardware and energy limitations of the sensors create difficulties with respect to guaranteeing the basic characteristics of the information (Intanagonwiwat, Govindan, Estrin, Heidemann, & Silva, 2003):

1. **Availability:** Determines whether a sensor has the ability to access the network and whether messages are conveniently communicated by it;
2. **Confidentiality:** Results from the ability of a network to hide an attacker's data, so that all transmitted messages remain confidential;

3. **Integrity:** Data integrity in wireless sensor networks is necessary to ensure the reliability of transmitted data and refers to the ability to confirm that the message has not been altered during their journey through the network;
4. **Authentication:** Ensures the reliability of the message by identifying its origin.

Security and privacy issues in PHCS in the IoT context is a growing concern for organizations, new devices open doors to new forms of cyber-attack. Organizations are poised to guard against common attacks, but IoT has created a whole new world of connected devices that are a potential vulnerability to organizations, putting networks and systems at risk.

Secure routing algorithms are vital for the acceptance and use of WSN in many applications and areas. Authentication is a key factor for the reliability of the data collected, since an attacker can send information that is intentionally incorrect if it is recognized as a constituent of the network, distorting the practical results of its use. In addition, the possibility of circulating sensitive information on the network is sometimes essential, so a good encryption scheme is necessary.

Much work has been done to protect WMSN in protecting patient data during transmission, despite of advancement of WMSNs in healthcare applications have made patient monitoring more feasible.

CONCLUSION

IoT can facilitate many improvements in the health care scene. IoT can also contribute to safety in medical procedures and real time information of patients, revolutionizing procedures and unlocking new features for medical care.

WMSNs improve the quality of patient care without disturbing your comfort. A medical sensor detects the patient's sensitive body data and transmits them through wireless communication channels. The success of WMSNs depends on security. Since the wireless communication ranges are not confined, malicious threats makes more significant risks to the patient, the patient's data can be accessed in an unauthorized manner and be modified.

Many security and privacy issues in healthcare applications using WMSNs still need to be explored, and then a well-planned security mechanism should be designed for the PHCS successful.

PHCS successful is intrinsically linked to the deployment of a secure infrastructure that preserves the privacy, offering opportunities and new challenges to the industry.

REFERENCES

Aggarwal, R., & Das, M. L. (2012). RFID security in the context of internet of things. In *Proceedings of the First International Conference on Security of Internet of Things* (pp. 51-56). ACM. doi:10.1145/2490428.2490435

Akyildiz, I. F., Su, W., Sankarasubramaniam, Y., & Cayirci, E. (2002). Wireless sensor networks: A survey. *Computer Networks*, *38*(4), 393–422. doi:10.1016/S1389-1286(01)00302-4

Al Ameen, M., Liu, J., & Kwak, K. (2012). Security and privacy issues in wireless sensor networks for healthcare applications. *Journal of Medical Systems*, *36*(1), 93–101. doi:10.1007/s10916-010-9449-4 PMID:20703745

Alemdar, H., & Ersoy, C. (2010). C. E. (2010). Wireless Sensor Networks for Healthcare: A Survey. *Computer Networks*, *54*(15), 2688–2710. doi:10.1016/j.comnet.2010.05.003

Atzori, L., Iera, A., & Morabito, G. (2010). The internet of things: A survey. *Computer Networks*, *54*(15), 2787–2805. doi:10.1016/j.comnet.2010.05.010

Baecker, R. M. (2014). *Readings in Human-Computer Interaction: toward the year 2000*. Morgan Kaufmann.

Campbell, A. T., Eisenman, S. B., Lane, N. D., Miluzzo, E., Peterson, R. A., Lu, H., & Ahn, G.-S. et al. (2008). The rise of people-centric sensing. *IEEE Internet Computing*, *12*(4), 12–21. doi:10.1109/MIC.2008.90

Chiti, F., Fantacci, R., Loreti, M., & Pugliese, R. (2016). Context-aware wireless mobile autonomic computing and communications: Research trends and emerging applications. *IEEE Wireless Communications*, *23*(2), 86–92. doi:10.1109/MWC.2016.7462489

Department of Economic and Social Affairs of the United Nations. (2009). *World Population Ageing*. New York: United Nations.

Dix, A. (2009). *Human-computer interaction*. Springer.

Domingo, M. C. (2012). An Overview of the Internet of Things for People with Disabilities. *Journal of Network and Computer Applications*, *35*(2), 584–59. doi:10.1016/j.jnca.2011.10.015

European Commission Information Society. (2009). *Internet of Things Strategic Research Roadmap 2009*. Obtido de European Commission Information Society: www.internet-of-things-research.eu

Eurostat. (2008). *The Life of Women and Men in Europe: A Statistical Portrait*. Luxembourg: Eurostat.

Goldsmith, A. (2005). *Wireless communications*. Cambridge University Press. doi:10.1017/CBO9780511841224

Guillemin, P., & Friess, P. (2009). *Internet of things strategic research roadmap*. The Cluster of European Research Projects. Tech. Rep.

Ikonen, V., & Kaasinen, E. (2008). *Ethical assessment in the design of ambiente assisted living*. Assisted Living Systems – Models, Architectures and Engineering Approaches.

Intanagonwiwat, C., Govindan, R., Estrin, D., Heidemann, J., & Silva, F. (2003). Directed diffusion for wireless sensor networking. *Networking, 11*(1).

Karlof, C., & Wagner, D. (2003). Secure routing in wireless sensor networks: Attacks and countermeasures. *Ad Hoc Networks*, *1*(2), 293–315. doi:10.1016/S1570-8705(03)00008-8

Koop, C. E., Mosher, R., Kun, L., Geiling, J., Grigg, E., Long, S., & Rosen, J. et al. (2008). Future Delivery of Health Care: Cybercare. *IEEE Engineering in Medicine and Biology Magazine*, *27*(6), 29–38. doi:10.1109/MEMB.2008.929888 PMID:19004693

Madakam, S., Ramaswamy, R., & Tripathi, S. (2015). Internet of Things (IoT): A literature review. *Journal of Computer and Communications, 3*(5), 164-173.

Miorandi, D., Sicari, S., De Pellegrini, F., & Chlamtac, I. (2012). Internet of things: Vision, applications and research challenges. *Ad Hoc Networks*, *10*(7), 1497–1516. doi:10.1016/j.adhoc.2012.02.016

Pang, Z., Zheng, L., Tian, J., Kao-Walter, S., Dubrova, E., & Chen, Q. (2015). Design of a terminal solution for integration of in-home health care devices and services towards the Internet-of-Things. *Enterprise Information Systems*, *9*(1), 86–116. doi:10.1080/17517575.2013.776118

Parwekar, P., & Reddy, R. (2013). An efficient fuzzy localization approach in wireless sensor networks. *2013 IEEE International Conference* (pp. 1-6). IEEE. doi:10.1109/FUZZ-IEEE.2013.6622548

Pereira, P., Grilo, A., Rocha, F., Nunes, M., Casaca, A., & Chaudet, C. (2007). End-to-end reliability in wireless sensor networks: survey and research challenges. *EuroFGI Workshop on IP QoS and Traffic Control*, 67–74.

Portela, F., Santos, M. F., Silva, Á., Machado, J., Abelha, A., & Rua, F. (2014). Pervasive and Intelligent Decision Support in Intensive Medicine – The Complete Picture. In Lecture Notes in Computer Science (LNCS): Vol. 8649. Information Technology in Bio- and Medical Informatics (pp. 87-102). Springer.

Röcker, C., Ziefle, M., & Holzinger, A. (2014). From computer innovation to human integration: current trends and challenges for pervasive Health Technologies. Pervasive Health, 1-17.

Satyanarayanan, M. (2001). Pervasive computing: Vision and challenges. *IEEE Personal Communications, 8*(4), 10-17.

Stankovic, J. (2014). Research Directions for the Internet of Things. *Internet of Things Journal, 1*, 3-9.

UE. (2012). *eHealth Action Plan 2012-2020-Innovative healthcare for the 21st century.* UE.

Varshney, U. (2003). Pervasive healthcare. *IEEE Computer*, *36*(12), 138–140. doi:10.1109/MC.2003.1250897

Varshney, U. (2005). Pervasive healthcare: Applications, challenges and wireless solutions. *Communications of the Association for Information Systems*, *16*(1).

Vermesan, O., Friess, P., Guillemin, P., Gusmeroli, S., Sundmaeker, H., Bassi, A., et al. (2011). *Internet of Things: Global Technological and Societal Trends 1.* Academic Press.

Vincent, G. K., & Velkof, V. A. (2010). *The Older Population in the United States: 2010 to 2050: Population Estimates and Projections.* New York: United States Census Bureau.

WHO. (n.d.). *Glossary*. Obtido em 01 de 2017, de World Health Organization: http://www.who.int/trade/glossary/story021/en/

Wu, M., Lu, T., Ling, F., Sun, J., & Du, H. (2010). Research on the architecture of Internet of things. *3rd International Conference Advanced Computer Theory and Engineering (ICACTE)*, 484-485.

Xue, X., Li, G., Liu, L., & Liu, M. (2012). Perspectives on Internet of Things and Its Applications. In *2nd International Conference on Computer Application and System Modeling*. Atlantis Press. doi:10.2991/iccasm.2012.6

KEY TERMS AND DEFINITIONS

Internet of Things: Relates a world set of physical objects provided with sensors and actuator triggers connected through wireless networks over internet, setting and enabling an intelligent objects network capable to collect data, processing information and execute actions accordingly. Those objects communicate each other and with others resources (physical or virtual) expanding initial system throughout its boundaries. IoT will allow people and things to be connected Anytime, Anyplace, with Anything and Anyone, ideally using Any path/network and Any service (Guillemin & Friess, 2009).

Pervasive Health Care Systems: Pervasive environments in the health area are concerned with the provision of health services to anyone, anytime, anywhere, in order to increase service coverage and quality (Varshney, 2003).

Wireless Sensor Network: A WSN consists of a set of these sensors, distributed spatially, with the aim of collecting and transmitting data, where it is not possible to do it with traditional networks, either for strategic reasons or for limitations of the environment where they are inserted, so WSN is a heterogeneous system with the purpose to computing elements, which combines tiny sensors and actuators. The sensors are small autonomously geographically distributed devices, called sensor nodes. Sensors nodes have capacity for computing, storage and communication in a network connected without cables, and installed around an object phenomenon to monitor it (Karlof & Wagner, 2003).

Chapter 3
Benefits of Bring Your Own Device in Healthcare

Filipe Portela
University of Minho, Portugal

Ailton Moreira da Veiga
University of Minho, Portugal

Manuel Filipe Santos
University of Minho, Portugal

ABSTRACT

Bring Your Own Device (BYOD) has become very popular topic in information technology because this approach allows the employees to bring their personal devices into organization and they want to use them to access the organization information. This trend has some benefits both for organization and to employees. This paper aims to identify those benefits as well the advantages and disadvantages of BYOD usage in organization. Also, it is present a SWOT analysis of BYOD usage. It is introduced an approach about BYOD in healthcare also. Utilizing personal devices at work is beneficial to organizational employees because they are in some way satisfies, and they have more freedom and choice to use their devices. This freedom and choice can easily lead the employees to be more productivity, flexibility. The organization who embraces BYOD policies found their employees happier, more productive, and more collaborative.

1. INTRODUCTION

The growing evolution in the development and adoption of the information and communication technology initiative has also internationally evolved the trends of the Bring Your Own Device (BYOD) that is rapidly changing the operating methods of the organisations to achieve greater efficiency and productivity. In a globalised and connected world, more and more organisations employees are bringing their own devices to the workplace. Although there are cases where the organisation itself offers the mobile devices to its employees, but not all employees use these devices. They already have the device

DOI: 10.4018/978-1-5225-2851-7.ch003

itself and can use them in the workplace, i.e. this evolution brought new opportunities to employees as it allowed them to bring their own devices to the workplace and integrate them into the organisation's network instead of using the organisation's devices.

The use of personal mobile devices by employees of organisations in the workplace has become a new paradigm. Organisations with this paradigm encourage and enable their employees to bring their mobile devices into the organisational network and encourage them to use them during their activities.

The reason that motivated the development of this article is the identification and explanation of the factors or benefits that BYOD has for organisations. Therefore, the main objective of this article is to identify and explain the benefits, advantages, and disadvantages that organisations might have with the implementation of BYOD policies. This new approach has provided significant evidence of the benefits to organisations both from the organisation's employees, but also from the organisation itself.

This article will present and discuss the main benefits, advantages, and disadvantages, and SWOT analysis that this approach has for both employees and the organisation itself. Also, BYOD in healthcare is presented. With this, it is intended to identify the firm readiness that this approach brings to the organisations.

The structure of the article is: the first chapter is the introductory chapter, the second chapter presents a background study, the third chapter is the introduction of the BYOD approach. Also, in this chapter, the benefits, advantages, and disadvantages of this approach for organisations are explained. The fourth chapter presents a SWOT analysis of BYOD for organisations. The fifth chapter presents a brief introduction of benefits of BYOD in healthcare. Finally, the sixth chapter, which is the final chapter, presenting the conclusions and the final considerations in the article.

2. BACKGROUND

By applying BYOD policies in an organisation, it is required some knowledge about its background. This background knowledge is about pervasive / ubiquitous computing, and information in real time because organisation employees need information in real time to develop their works.

Pervasive also called ubiquitous computing, is the growing trend of embedding computational capability into everyday objects to make them effectively communicate and perform useful tasks in a way that minimises the end user's need to interact with computers as computers. Pervasive computing devices are network-connected. The terms pervasive / ubiquitous signify "existing everywhere", basically devices that use pervasive/ ubiquitous computing are totally connected and consistently available (Media, n.d.).

Ubiquitous Computing is a paradigm in which the processing of information is linked with each activity involving connected devices; it can occur at any time, on any device, at any location, and in any format (Media, n.d.; Sen, n.d.).

The idea behind using BYOD in the organisation with pervasive and ubiquitous computing is to provide a real-time smart environment for accessing information and application through a new class of ubiquitous, intelligent devices that can facilitate the work when and where it is needed. This situation means that pervasive and ubiquitous computing can be the first step to having right BYOD policies implemented at the organisation.

The evolving concepts of pervasive computing, ubiquitous computing and ambient intelligence are increasingly influencing healthcare and medicine. Because of its ubiquitous and unobtrusive analytical, diagnostic, supportive, information and documentary functions, pervasive computing is predicted to improve traditional healthcare. Some of its capabilities, such as remote, automated patient monitoring and diagnosis, may make pervasive computing an advanced tool regarding the home care and may enhance patient self-care and independent living. Automatic documentation of activities, process control or the right information in specific work situations as supplied by pervasive computing are expected to increase the effectiveness as well as the efficiency of healthcare providers (Braga et al., 2016; Orwat, Graefe, & Faulwasser, 2008; Pereira, Portela, Santos, Machado, & Abelha, 2016; Portela, Santos, Machado, Abelha, & Rua, 2017).

Pervasive healthcare is able to reach the necessary quality of the service at any moment and by any anyone, regardless of its location and position, along with other restrictions. Pervasive Healthcare is characterised by having heterogeneous information, a dynamic number of interesting parts (stakeholders), and by ubiquitous computing, that connects perfectly the digital infrastructures in our daily lives (Pereira et al., 2016).

3. BRING YOUR OWN DEVICE

Bring your own Device (BYOD) is a subset of the consumerization of Information Technologies (IT). Consumerization of IT refers to private or personally owned IT resources, such as computer device or software that are used for business proposes. This consumerization of IT in the workplace is in some places referred to as BYOD. It allows employees to employ the technologies of their choice and bring them to their workplaces to perform the daily business task. BYOD refers to the use of these personal devices for business proposes and reflects a blurring of the line between personal and business use on the same device (Scarfo, 2012; Singh & Phil, 2012; Bais, 2016).

Figure 1 shows a simple architecture of BYOD in the organisation, in which is possible to see the organisation IT structure which is present one BYOD solution that deals with mobile devices that are brought to the organisation. The solution present here is Mobile Device Management (MDM) that is responsible for the management of mobile devices that interact with the organisations IT. On the BYOD side, there are mobile devices that are divided into two parts, one referring to personal space and other referring to organisational space. In the case of organisational space, there is also an MDM-Agent that works together with MDM on the infrastructure side of the organisation.

There is no formal description or definition of BYOD programme and BYOD policies as it depends upon the organisation to define its BYOD agenda and the boundaries related to it. Garba on his research papers (Bello Garba, Armarego, & Murray, 2015) proposes that a BYOD programs in any organisation should consider six building blocks stated below:

- Information security and their standards and procedures;
- Information privacy and their principles;
- Information safety and technical privacy controls;
- Liabilities;
- Awareness and training programs;
- BYOD user perception and behaviour.

Figure 1. Simple BYOD in organization
Adapted from Ocano, Ramamurthy, and Wang (2015) and Wang, Wei, and Vangury (2014)

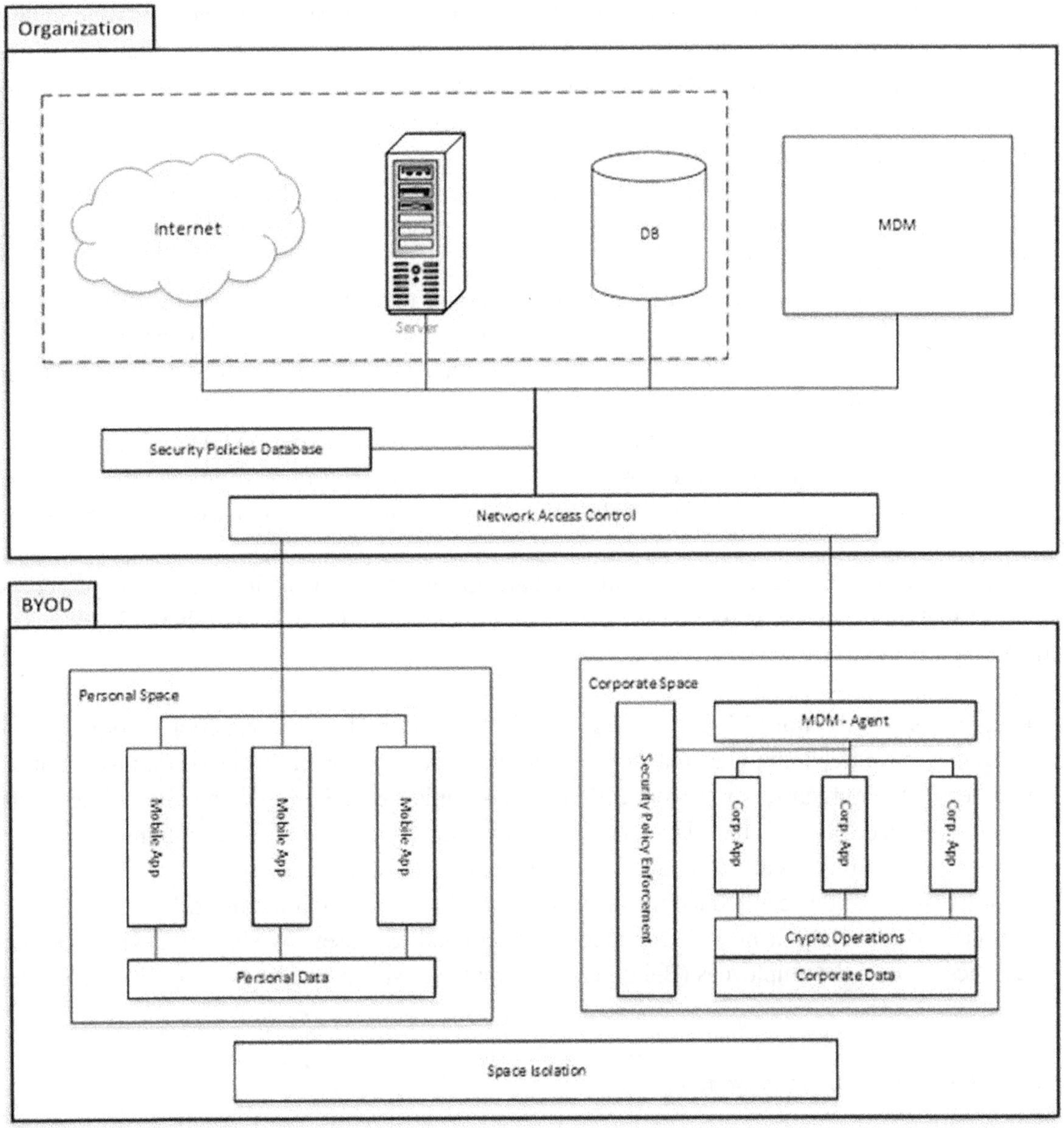

BYOD programme consists of the policies, guidelines, and tools for implementing and operationalizing BYOD in the organisation. Organisations have certain objectives and goals before applying for a new IT programme or improving an existing one. There is the necessity of defining a goal to implement BYOD programme strategically important for organisations (Bello Garba, Armarego, & Murray, 2015). Organisations have been increasing their BYOD utilisation rate, and this improvement is based on the following key factors: employee code conduct, installation of security programs, and increasingly efficient management rules. These factors are responsible for the overall performance of BYOD (Dhingra, 2016).

3.1. Benefits of BYOD in Organisation

The benefits of BYOD are clear to organisations. Collaborators are more familiar and satisfied with the usage of their own devices in the organisations. At the same time employees can save money since they do not have to pay for an expensive devices data plan. The goals of organisations with the adoption of BYOD are to increase the flexibility, coexistence, and portability of devices to meet the workflows of their employees, increasing their productivity.

The organisation directors know how the BYOD usage can be a benefit to the organisation itself. According to the study conducted by Tech Pro Research 2, about 74% of the organisations interviewed said they are using or planning to use BYOD (Dhingra, 2016).

This study concludes that 60% (blue part) of the organisation inquired are using BYOD in their activities. 26% (red part) of the organisation inquired do not use BYOD on their business, but they are planning to use it on next 12 months. Finally, the 14% (green part) of the organisation inquired do not use BYOD, and they do not plan to use it.

Organisations should provide an efficient and effective policy for using BYOD and should clearly indicate all the objectives and drawbacks regarding the BYOD usage in organisations. It is necessary to describe everything that is allowed on mobile devices when they are being used in the organisation networks.

The benefits of BYOD usage in the organisation are: employee's satisfaction, cost savings, accessibility, and flexibility, increased productivity and innovation, current devices, and others (Bruder, 2014; Kestle & Self, 2013).

- **Employees Satisfaction**: BYOD can also lead to greater employee satisfaction in organisations since they have freedom to use the devices that they have chosen and invested in, instead of was selected by their organisation (Evans, 2013). When employees are using their own mobile devices at the workplace, they fill that they have more flexibility to their work, to communicate, to solve their personal problems at the same time, and more collaboration using one single device.
- **Cost Savings**: BYOD can reduce the cost to travel, office space and facilities, labour, stationery, and printed materials. It may also reduce organisational expenses, by shifting devices and data services costs to the employees (Bello Garba, Armarego, Murray, & Kenworthy, 2015). The em-

Figure 2. BYOD usage in organisations
Source: Dhingra (2016)

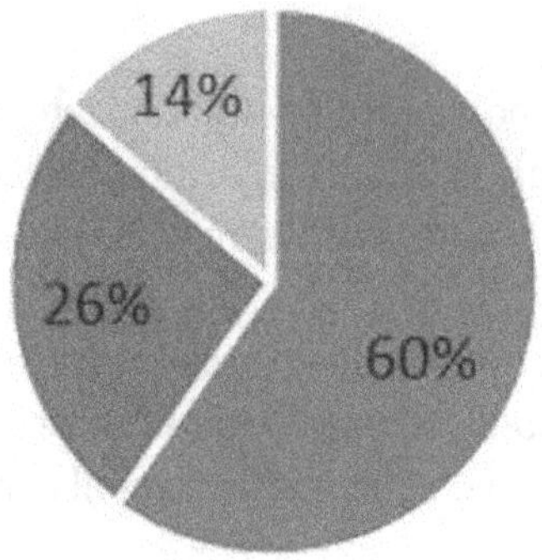

ployee can use Virtual Private Network (VPN) to connect remotely and safe to the organisation to do their job instead of going to the organisation building physically every day. In this aspect, the employee can reduce the cost of travel to the organisation building.

- **Accessibility**: BYOD allows access and retrieval of organisational resources and materials online. It allows employees to access network resources made available by their organisations, and study or work with these resources at their own desired pace. BYOD opens new windows of opportunities for organisations and employees by allowing them to work anytime and anywhere. When you are using BYOD, the knowledge and information are available to employees at any time and any moment. The availability of wireless networks and technologies reduce the physical or geographical constraints allowing them to remain productive while on the move (Bello Garba, et al., 2015). The evolution of technologies has enabled organisations employees to have access to information now at a distance of one click on their own mobile devices at any time or any location.
- **Convivence and Flexibility**: BYOD can offer a significant amount of work flexibility and convenience to employees in an organisation (Blizzard, 2015). Employees can work from remote locations, as well as take breaks during work at their own convenience. Some work environments do not require the use of sophisticated technological systems; rather the simple access to a smartphone and a network (Internet) is proven to be enough (Bello Garba et al., 2015). Employees can use remote connection (like VPN) to do their job instead of going every day to the workplace.
- **Increased Productivity and Innovation**: Since there is a prospect that employees are more satisfied and comfortable with their chosen personal devices, they swiftly become experts in using them, thus making them more productive at their jobs. Organisations could also benefit from the latest technologies since most users often have a habit of upgrading to the most recent software or hardware (Bello Garba et al., 2015). This approach allows the employees the opportunity to utilise a device they are used to and more comfortable with, they can respond to requests faster and are more comfortable working in their desired environment, thus leading to a significant increase in employee productivity (Secure Edge Networks, n.d.).
- **Up-to-Date Devices:** Technology is constantly changing, so it can be almost impossible and costly to keep up with the latest mobile device trends. Since BYOD devices are usually more updated and innovative than the IT issued devices, the company gets to reap the benefits of the most modern features, capabilities, and upgrades ("Bring Your Own Device, BYOD, BYOT | DEEPTECH," n.d.). Organisations take advantage of the new generation of mobile devices that employees acquire without having to invest in new equipment. These devices are increasingly powerful, modern with high computing capacity and data processing so that companies always benefit indirectly from the use of these powerful devices by employees.

BYOD presents numerous benefits for both the organisation itself and the organisations own employee. According to a study of a total of 2000 people, it was concluded that 61% of employees is satisfied and are more productive when using the technologies, they have chosen (Budak, 2012).

3.2. BYOD Advantage and Disadvantage

As far as we know everything that has advantages, it also has some drawbacks, and BYOD is not an exception. It is important for the organisations to identify the major's benefits and the possible disadvantage of

BYOD utilisation. There is a set of characteristics that determine the pros and cons of BYOD use and will be presented and explained in the next subsection (Bradley, 2011; Zolfo, n.d.; Nitish Kirtiraj Shah, n.d.).

3.2.1. BYOD Advantages

- **Lower Costs**: The most obvious benefit to a company using BYOD is that it means they do not have to purchase a significant amount of expensive devices for employees to be able to do eLearning. So, if you do not have to buy any devices, that represents significant savings (Bello Garba et al., 2015). Breakages and wastage are also likely to be reduced by the fact people tend to take better care of their own stuff than company-owned devices, and any repair costs are the employee's burden anyway (Advantages, 2016). Companies reduce the cost of the purchase of the devices for employees since they bring their own devices to use in the workplace.
- **Technology Familiarity**: Most people tend to be familiar with their own devices. Apple fans are right with Apple technology, and Windows fans are better with devices with Windows operating systems. Getting used to another one can be irritating for any employee. BYOD takes this issue away, as they are working on their own personalised device which is already suited to their own needs and that they are already perfectly competent on it (Advantages, 2016). When the employee uses a mobile device that is familiar, he/she is more satisfied, and this makes him/her more productive, he/she felt encouraged to work more.
- **Flexibility:** Employees will not need to travel with several devices satisfying their home and work needs, as the one device will fulfil both. Work that could normally only be done in the office will be able to be done wherever, as employees have access to all the data they need anywhere they want and finally – employees are not hindered by the usual strict rules that they have to adhere to when using company property. BYOD allows greater freedoms to your employees (Advantages, 2016; Bello Garba et al., 2015). Employees just need to have one device (both for personal utilisation and professional utilisation), to do their work, when and where they want.

3.2.2. BYOD Disadvantage

- **Security:** All organisations spend an enormous amount of money on their security systems as they know that they cannot afford for their data to be leaked or viruses to be caught. Employees, however, are unlikely to have this level of security. While the common security software for home use can cover all day to day activities; you might not trust them to be up to the job of protecting your valuable customer data. Also, "how do organisations with BYOD stop employees who are leaving the company from walking away with a significant amount of your data, available at a touch of the button on their device?" This can also be flipped for the employees – they may feel their own privacy is at risk if they do personal web surfing on a device that is linked to their company's systems (Advantages, 2016).
- **Costs for the Employee**: As mentioned before, the costs of BYOD are down to the employee. Not everybody has such a device or even want one. Factor in the increased usage and transportation of the instrument is likely leading to quicker depreciation of the device and possible accidents – repairs could also prove to be costly for the employee. They may not be happy shouldering this cost (Advantages, 2016). In this case, if the organisation has reduced costs with mobile devices, on

the other hand, employees have more costs due to the acquisition of new appliances. Often these devices have an increased cost due to the data plan that employees sign.

- **Device Disparities:** When a company buys devices for their staff they have the freedom to buy the perfect device for their need. Therefore, it will have the right technological features for the purpose they are serving. However, with BYOD, your employees are likely to have a whole plethora of devices, however, all with different capabilities and operating systems that run different software at the various levels of quality. It is hard to get software that is of high quality but it is also able to cover all platforms and realistic quality of devices, so this could cause issues. You also have to adapt your system to be able to deal with a BYOD policy (Advantages, 2016). Each employee prefers mobile devices, and in BYOD each employee takes the mobile device of their choice to the workplace. In this case, creating a unique environment of integration of all these mobile devices in organisation network is hard because these devices have different hardware and software specification and compatibility in most cases.

4. BYOD SWOT ANALYSIS

Making a SWOT analysis aims to identify the main strengths as well as determine the main weaknesses of this approach. On the other hand, it is important to determine the main opportunities and threats based on this method. This analysis aims to identify the strengths, weaknesses, opportunities, and threats of BYOD usage in organisations. Through the identification of the weaknesses and threats through SWOT analysis prevents organisations from certain situations that may be less benefit, while identifying the strengths and opportunities through SWOT analysis shows what benefits the organisations can have with this approach. Strengths need to be on the line of being stronger while weaknesses need to be analysed and treated over the time in time. The BYOD vendors should take advantage of the opportunities and be prepared for the threats.

Currently, business environment and economic competition are becoming global, customers and technology use are changing rapidly, these changes had forced the organisations to find ways to build proper strategic plans and right decisions to develop effective business and influence the competition. These business environment technology developments have a lot of risks and impact, which influence economically and affects life cycle as well as the workforce. BYOD is a phenomenon that helps the organisations to correspond their employee's demands about bringing their own devices for business purpose and the benefits of the organisation (Nitish Kirtiraj Shah, n.d.; IIPRD, 2012).

According to the SWOT analysis present in Table 1, it is possible to see the main factors that can influence BYOD success in the organisation. This analysis is important because it can support business decisions to create a proper strategy to achieve the organisation's goals. In the same way, this analysis is used to analyse the BYOD strategy in the risk and security perspective.

5. BYOD IN HEALTHCARE

The growth and adoption of the BYOD approach by organisations have also led healthcare organisations to adopt this approach. The use of mobile devices by healthcare professionals has transformed many aspects of clinical practice (Ventola, 2014). The utilisation of mobile devices in healthcare already have

Table 1. BYOD SWOT analysis

Strength	Weakness
Increase Productivity; Increase Employee Morale and satisfaction; Flexible Working Culture; Reduce IT cost of company; Simplified IT Infrastructure; Employee feel convenient while using their own devices; Bring out better efficient business tool.	Compatibility issue; Breach of Security; It affects organisation and client relationship when valuable employee exists from organisation with their own device(s); Connecting and managing and different type of application(s)/ network connectivity / operating system with an enterprise network is complex.
Opportunities	**Threats**
Gain business intelligence for new ideas; Growth in middleware and mobile device management technology; Growth in software development for BYOD devices; Huge demand for memory management, antivirus, and anti-spyware software development technology; Huge demand for unified collaborative tool for managing different type of application(s)/network connectivity/operating system with enterprise system(s) as well as employee device(s).	Data stole; Device is stolen; Habitual attitude affects productivity; Work life balance can be affected; Security Breach on Enterprise data.

Adopted from IIPRD (2012)

clear benefits, namely the reduction of short-term costs in hospital units. However, costs associated with potential risks of this utilisation, such as security breaches, theft, and hospital data loss, appear to significantly outweigh the potential benefits to healthcare professionals using their own mobile devices in the healthcare organisation.

Mobile devices in healthcare are rapidly becoming an integral part of healthcare information systems. Deployment of these devices is becoming an important IT strategy designed to assist in improving the quality of care, enhancing patient services, increasing productivity, lowering costs, improving cash flow, as well as facilitating other critical delivery processes (Meixner & Zuehlke, 2012). Healthcare professionals can use mobile devices for many purposes, that can be grouped into five categories: administration, health record maintenance and access, communications and consulting reference and information gathering, and medical education (Ventola, 2014).

Patient privacy is one of the many concerns that BYOD has in healthcare since healthcare organisation are still in the early process of adoption of BYOD, it is important to ensure that mobile devices that store and transmit patient data are HIPAA-compliant (Gaglani & Topol, 2014).

Health Insurance Portability and Accountability Act (HIPAA) is an international organisation that defines and manages the standards for the use of mobile devices in the healthcare area. According to this entity, organisations that adopt the BYOD approach must meet a set of requirements, regarding the utilisation of the devices to access. When we are talking about BYOD in healthcare, there are still some challenges that need to be overcome. These challenges are in four different areas, such as (Lund & Dunbrack, 2015):

- The healthcare regulatory environment;
- The safety of the mobile device;
- The security of access to clinical data and clinical applications;
- Updates, policy changes and support issues, such as Mobile Device Management (MDM);
- The financial costs of associated with voice and data usage.

In another hand, it is necessary to create laws that covered all the aspect of BYOD in healthcare. These laws can be about: security, data cover, information requirements, consent requirements, data retention, data transfer, and breach notification obligations.

The HIPAA Security Rule requires that healthcare providers set up physical, administrative, and technical safeguards to protect the electronic health information with safety measures such as access control to the information and encryption of the stored information (Office of Civil Rights Department of Health and Human Services, 2003). With the increased demand for mobile devices to expedite clinical practice, hospitals need to identify strategies to cost-effectively and safely incorporate such devices into HIPAA guidelines. Having healthcare providers bring their own medical devices BYOD will be time-efficient and cost-effective for hospital staff to avoid the costs associated with frequent upgrades, warranties, and other types of care.

Although the technology exists to protect mobile devices from security breaches safely, the lack of standardisation of security safeguards as well as theft and loss issues pose significant challenges for hospital privacy officials (Moyer, 2013). Since mobile devices are already being used in hospitals, an approach toward educating the users instead of trying to control the technology may be more practical in the short term.

5.1. BYOD Benefits in Healthcare

Nowadays it is already possible to identify the obvious benefits of BYOD in healthcare since the use of these devices has a strong impact on the development of activities by health professionals. Some of the identified benefits of BYOD have in healthcare are (Lund & Dunbrack, 2015):

- Cost reduction in the acquisition of new mobile devices by the organisation;
- Healthcare professionals are more satisfied as they can use the mobile devices of their choice;
- Enables healthcare professionals to access patient's clinical records using the device itself;
- Healthcare professionals will not have to register patient data on paper since mobile devices have come to suppress this type of registration. The records are made directly on these devices;
- The use of mobile devices by healthcare professionals allows them to have greater flexibility in carrying out their activities.

These benefits clearly present the importance of BYOD in healthcare currently, in an increasingly globalised and automated world, it is especially relevant that healthcare services also follow this trend.

5.2. BYOD in Healthcare SWOT Analysis

A SWOT analysis of BYOD in healthcare identifies what the strengths, the opportunities, the weaknesses, and threats inherent in the adoption of this approach in healthcare organisations are. This analysis intends to present the major concerns about BYOD in healthcare that healthcare organisations should care out when they decide to adopt it.

This analysis allows identifying the competitive advantages that healthcare organisations have when adopting BYOD in their policies. Although this analysis helps identify the biggest problems that face the internal and external adoption of this policy by the healthcare organisations.

Table 2.

Strength	Weakness
Better Control, Healthcare organisation decrease cost, Healthcare professionals more satisfied	Legal, Ethical and Privacy Laws
Opportunities	**Threats**
Better capacity to adapt to new challenges in healthcare; Reduce the potential technical support request for IT staff	Government regulations impacting mobile healthcare Privacy and Security concerns, Patient data loss or stolen

6. CONCLUSION

Concluding this article, it can be stated that BYOD in the organisation has different purposes such as employee's satisfaction and productivity, improvement, collaboration, and removing the boundary of employees working only within office premises. Some organisations must adopt BYOD because they may concede to their businesses rivals that use BYOD which results in an improved customer/employee's satisfaction, a better employees' productivity, and faster response to the customers.

On the other hand, it was possible to identify the advantages and disadvantages that BYOD has for organisations. Organisations that wish to maintain more competitive edge over their competitors should adopt this new trend, but rather should consider the risks associated with this trend. A SWOT analysis of the BYOD approach to the organisation is always a good starting point for its adoption.

As the approach is new in organisations, some risks and challenges still need to be overcome to make the best use of BYOD in organisations. Nowadays, there are already some BYOD solutions to solve the main risks and challenges that they present to organisations, but these solutions are not enough in the face of the needs of organisations in an increasingly globalised and connected world.

Although BYOD is a new approach, it is already having a strong impact on healthcare, and it is various visible fields of action of BYOD and the gains that this approach brings to the healthcare organisation.

Concluding, it is possible to affirm that BYOD has a strong impact in healthcare organisation for several reasons. That reasons are healthcare professionals that bring their own device and seek to use them in their work, as well their personal life. Healthcare providers cannot afford to give everyone who would benefit from a device a device. So, having the physician on the medical staff or an employee use their own device can provide access to mobile tools to people who might otherwise not be able to benefit from mobile tools ("The Impact of BYOD on Healthcare Providers and Hospitals," 2017).

It is important that healthcare organisations take advantage of the BYOD trend and adopt it to follow the technological development of utilisation of mobile devices at work and take better advantage of the benefits that this practice has for healthcare, more specifically with pervasive devices.

Even though the advantages of BYOD in healthcare are clearly visible, it is essential that at moment of BYOD adoption the data privacy and data security policies need to be established by HIPAA regulations.

Here it just covered a small area of BYOD in organisations including healthcare organisation, but there are many other sectors that still to investigate about BYOD in organisations like BYOD new solutions, BYOD in school, among other areas.

REFERENCES

Advantages, T. (2016). *The Advantages and Disadvantages of BYOD*. Retrieved from http://www.businesszone.co.uk/community-voice/blogs/scott-drayton/the-advantages-and-disadvantages-of-byod

Bais, A. (2016). *Security Risks associated with BYOD*. Academic Press.

Bello Garba, A., Armarego, J., & Murray, D. (2015). A Policy-Based Framework for Managing Information Security and Privacy Risks in BYOD Environments. *International Journal of Emerging Trends & Technology in Computer Science*, *4*(2), 10.

Bello Garba, A., Armarego, J., Murray, D., & Kenworthy, W. (2015). Review of the Information Security and Privacy Challenges in Bring Your Own Device (BYOD) Environments. *Journal of Information Privacy and Security*, *11*(1), 38–54. doi:10.1080/15536548.2015.1010985

Blizzard, S. (2015). Coming full circle: Are there benefits to BYOD? *Computer Fraud & Security*, *2015*(2), 18–20. doi:10.1016/S1361-3723(15)30010-5

Bradley, T. (2011). *Pros and cons of byod bring your own device*. Retrieved February 22, 2017, from http://www.pcworld.com/article/246760/pros_and_cons_of_byod_bring_your_own_device_.html

Braga, A., Portela, F., Santos, M. F., Machado, J., Abelha, A., Silva, Á., & Rua, F. (2016). *Pervasive Patient Timeline for Intensive Care Units* (pp. 527–536). Cham: Springer. doi:10.1007/978-3-319-31307-8_55

Bring Your Own Device. (n.d.). Retrieved March 22, 2017, from http://www.deeptech.com.au/solutions/byot/

Bruder, P. (2014). Gadgets Go to School: The Benefits and Risks of BYOD (Bring Your Own Device). *Education Digest*, *80*(3), 15–18. Retrieved from http://navigator-iup.passhe.edu/login?url=http://search.ebscohost.com/login.aspx?direct=true&db=eue&AN=99173566&site=ehost-live

Budak, J. (2012). Should you bring your own mobile device to work?. *Canadian Business, 85*(8), 79. Retrieved from http://www.canadianbusiness.com/lifestyle/should-you-bring-your-own-mobile-device-to-work/

Dhingra, M. (2016). Legal Issues in Secure Implementation of Bring Your Own Device (BYOD). *Procedia Computer Science, 78*, 179–184. https://doi.org/10.1016/j.procs.2016.02.030

Evans, D. (2013). *What is BYOD and why is it important?* Academic Press.

Gaglani, S. M., & Topol, E. J. (2014). iMedEd: the role of mobile health technologies in medical education. *Academic Medicine: Journal of the Association of American Medical Colleges, 89*(9), 1207–9. https://doi.org/10.1097/ACM.0000000000000361

IIPRD. (2012). *Landscape analysis - bring your own device*. IIPRD.

Kestle, R., & Self, R. (2013). IS Practices for SME Success Series. *IS Practices for SME Success Series, 1*(1), 1–148. https://doi.org/10.1093/itnow/bws010

Lund, D., & Dunbrack, L. (2015). *The Healthcare Industry: Embracing BYOD for Success.* IDC Opinion.

Media, D. H. (n.d.). In this. *Update, 21*(12).

Meixner, G., & Zuehlke, D. (2012). A new paradigm for the development of future medical software systems. *ACM SIGHIT Record, 2*(1), 20–20. https://doi.org/10.1145/2180796.2180812

Moyer, J. E. (2013). Managing Mobile Devices in Hospitals: A Literature Review of BYOD Policies and Usage. *Journal of Hospital Librarianship, 13*(3), 197–208. doi:10.1080/15323269.2013.798768

Nitish Kirtiraj Shah, B. (n.d.). *Developing a decision support framework for planning and implementing Bring Your Own Device programmes in organizations, 2013–2015.* Academic Press.

Ocano, S. G., Ramamurthy, B., & Wang, Y. (2015). Remote mobile screen (RMS): An approach for secure BYOD environments. In *2015 International Conference on Computing, Networking and Communications (ICNC)* (pp. 52–56). IEEE. https://doi.org/10.1109/ICCNC.2015.7069314

Office of Civil Rights Department of Health and Human Services. (2003). *Summary of the HIPAA Privacy Rule.* OCR Privacy Brief. https://doi.org/10.1016/j.chroma.2005.11.119

Orwat, C., Graefe, A., & Faulwasser, T. (2008). Towards pervasive computing in health care - a literature review. *BMC Medical Informatics and Decision Making*, *8*(1), 26. doi:10.1186/1472-6947-8-26 PMID:18565221

Pereira, A., Portela, F., Santos, M. F., Machado, J., & Abelha, A. (2016). ScienceDirect Pervasive Business Intelligence: A new trend in Critical Healthcare. *Procedia Computer Science, 98*(98), 362–367. https://doi.org/10.1016/j.procs.2016.09.055

Portela, F., Santos, M. F., Machado, J., Abelha, A., & Rua, F. (2017). Step Towards Pervasive Technology Assessment in Intensive Medicine. *International Journal of Reliable and Quality E-Healthcare*, *6*(2), 1–16. doi:10.4018/IJRQEH.2017040101

Scarfo, A. (2012). New security perspectives around BYOD. In *Proceedings - 2012 7th International Conference on Broadband, Wireless Computing, Communication and Applications, BWCCA 2012* (pp. 446–451). IEEE. https://doi.org/10.1109/BWCCA.2012.79

Secure Edge Networks, L. (n.d.). *7 Benefits of BYOD on Enterprise Wireless Networks.* Retrieved May 11, 2017, from http://www.securedgenetworks.com/blog/7-Benefits-of-BYOD-on-Enterprise-Wireless-Networks

Sen, J. (n.d.). Ubiquitous Computing: Applications, Challenges and Future Trends. In Embedded Systems and Wireless Technology: Theory and Practical Application. CRC Press.

Singh, N., & Phil, M. (2012). B . Y . O . D . Genie Is Out Of the Bottle – " Devil Or Angel ". *Journal of Business Management & Social Sciences Research, 1*(3), 1–12.

The Impact of BYOD on Healthcare Providers and Hospitals. (2017). Retrieved March 29, 2017, from http://mhealthintelligence.com/features/the-impact-of-byod-on-healthcare-providers-and-hospitals

Ventola, C. L. (2014). Mobile devices and apps for health care professionals: uses and benefits. *P & T, 39*(5), 356–64. Retrieved from http://www.pubmedcentral.nih.gov/articlerender.fcgi?artid=4029126&tool=pmcentrez&rendertype=abstract

Wang, Y., Wei, J., & Vangury, K. (2014). Bring your own device security issues and challenges. *2014 IEEE 11th Consumer Communications and Networking Conference (CCNC)*, 80–85. https://doi.org/10.1109/CCNC.2014.6866552

Zolfo, M. (n.d.). *How to weight BYOD benefits and risks.* Academic Press.

Chapter 4
Big Data and mHealth:
Increasing the Usability of Healthcare Through the Customization of Pinterest – Literary Perspective

Nancy Shipley
Towson University, USA

Joyram Chakraborty
Towson University, USA

ABSTRACT

Technology has greatly improved healthcare. Research has shown that improved user experience can vastly increase the volume and quality of knowledge gained from the accessible resources. Electronic medical records have been mandated by the U.S. government transitioning the medical field to computer based applications with the goal of efficiency and meaningful use. From this vast data, the end user could potentially increase their healthcare understanding through a centralized mobile-platform that brings the expertise from medical professionals, smart health and well-being best practices, alternative medicine and social media such as crowd-sourcing materials. In this chapter, we present a mHealth solution incorporating the features of Pinterest in order to provide a single portal for the dissemination of healthcare information.

INTRODUCTION

Although technology in healthcare has increased greatly over the past decade, the user experience of the combined available resources can unquestionably be improved (Blumenthal, 2009). Many Healthcare functions have been transferred to computer-based applications such as the institution of electronic health records (Jha et al., 2009). However, the end user could conceivably increase their healthcare knowledge through a platform that brings the knowledge from medical experts, smart health and wellbeing proven practices, alternative medicine and social media and crowdsourcing material (Alyass et al., 2015). In the past decade technology has also improved rapidly as cloud computing and big data have broadened the

DOI: 10.4018/978-1-5225-2851-7.ch004

scope of technical offerings increasing the ultimate experience for the end users. However, this technology has not been maximized, especially for health care uses (Bizer et al., 2012). The use of enhanced visualization could increase the user experiences for healthcare best practices and implementation. Employing a new frame work that could be quickly accessed via mobile devices could offer the patient an improved user experience with their medical information queries as they fight against diseases and sustain healthy living. Building on the discovery principal that Pinterest has established through their superior search capability and enriched user interface, customization can occur to offer a single source for patients to research, medical diagnosis, smart health and wellbeing, alternative medicine and social media solutions. A carefully designed empirical study could determine if customizing Pinterest would improve the use of Healthcare Big Data by expanding the patients' knowledge concerning their health issues via a mHealth solution. The specific contributions of this chapter are an identified solutions gap in the eHealth literature that can be addressed by using our proposed solution of customizing the Pinterest application.

The healthcare community is confronting an almost insurmountable amount of health and healthcare-related content generated from numerous patient care points of contact, highly technical medical instruments, and web-based health communities (Arunasalam, 2013). The contemporary healthcare big data areas that are taking shape are genomics-driven big data covering genotyping, gene expression, sequencing data and payer–provider big data including electronic health records, insurance records, pharmacy prescription, patient feedback and responses (Raghupathi & Raghupathi, 2014). Over the past decade, electronic health records (EHR) have been extensively implemented in hospitals and medical facilities giving way to significant clinical knowledge and a deeper understanding of patient disease patterns from such computer based collections. Using this vast healthcare data, doctors and patients alike may be more readily able to diagnosis the issues and determine treatments to remedy their health problems. Utilizing lessons learned from the immense healthcare data, the end user could increase their healthcare knowledge. Expanding on a unified mobile accessible platform, the healthcare big data could offer patients a wealth of awareness via a mHealth application. Medical professionals have been publishing their expertise in journals that can be tapped to expand the patient health understanding. In addition, there are many websites that offer smart health and wellbeing proven practices. Physical ailments can also be addressed through alternative medicine. Social media offers many remedies to health issues as those seeking wellness write blogs and effectively crowdsource to seek healthy solutions. These offerings along with many others could be bundled together to offer a superior distinct healthcare tool.

After decades of implementing computer-based applications in almost every field of study, a by-product taking shape is immense data which is now known as big data (Peters et al., 2014). This vast amount of data now collected and accessible via mobile devices via cloud computing technology allows for humans to move more deeply into the exploration of the information age. Not harnessed to its fullest, the big data technology now being researched will give way to superior growth of understanding for decision making and everyday life especially in healthcare (Jee & Kim, 2013) . Challenges are apparent in this new technology of big data on cloud computing. Although they cover all ranges, the main few areas are data capture, data storage, data analysis, and data visualization (Chen, 2014). Traditional data was mapped and placed in organized relational databases to be searched and presented in software applications for the various end users to perform their daily tasks. Unlike traditional data, big data is readily available on the internet, from sensors, and even disjointed databases with none of it organized for customary relational database viewing methods (Ma et al., 2015). The user friendly platform for searching and analyzing this great amount of big data sources is still in the beginning stages.

BACKGROUND

Presently, the process of visualization in big data projects is most often the image of dots on a map or graphical views. By enhancing the view of big data, the user experience will most likely increase and additional knowledge will be obtained. To present this information, a search for an optimal framework has occurred exposing that Pinterest can offer big data information in the most succinct manner to the end user. Not only will the user be able to access the big data platform from traditional PCs and laptops, but mobile access using smartphones and tablets will be the ultimate end goal. A potential solution is streamlining big data interface that can be accessed from anywhere allowing the end user to easily obtain healthcare information to better their lifestyle.

Through the power of cloud computing and big data, the end users can now demand more from software applications. This superior technology can be exploited for healthcare uses to more easily sift through medical data discovering greater medical solutions. Several studies have articulated the benefits of improving visualization of healthcare big data to increase the users' experience as they move toward a better understanding of healing remedies and healthy living guidelines (Zhang et al., 2008). Employing a new framework accessed by mobile devices, patients could harness this knowledge as they combat diseases and achieve healthy living. Fully utilizing the discovery principal available through Pinterest by utilizing their comprehensive search and powerful user interface, customization can occur to offer a unified software mHealth application for patients to research medical diagnosis, healthy living, alternative medicine and social media options.

A continued pursuit took place where many in the millennial generation were sought for their opinions to find popular sites. Time and time again, the young adults said they preferred Pinterest. Reviewing the About page on the Pinterest site, they classify themselves as the world's catalog of ideas. Their mission is to help people discover the things they love, and inspire their users to go do those things in their daily lives. Back in March 2010, when they co-founded Pinterest, Ben Silbermann, Evan Sharp and Paul Sciarra sought out to create a site about discovery of all the relevant and interesting information that can be found on the internet. Using the website, users discover and organize things they like. From a technology view, the company is based on big data, where the software captures rich metadata around each image and stores them for latter access. Considering users love the site and the big data search technology is powerful, the idea began of customizing Pinterest to meet patient's healthcare needs.

IMPROVING HEALTHCARE SOLUTIONS

Healthcare Information Sources

Through numerous patient care points of contact, highly technical medical instruments, health related payment systems and web-based health communities, our society now has access to a vast amounts of health and healthcare-related internet based content (Avinash et al., 2005). Many healthcare big data projects have been put in place to utilize the information including genomics-driven big data covering genotyping, gene expression (O'Driscoll, 2013); sequencing data and payer–provider big data including electronic health records (Rind et al., 2011); insurance records, pharmacy prescription, patient feedback and responses, and health and well-being best practices (Stroetmann, 2013). Still studies have shown that the end users' healthcare needs are not fully met (Harrison & Mort, 1998).

HEALTHCARE TECHNOLOGY

Electronic health records (EHR) have been widely implemented in hospitals and medical facilities allowing patients' access to their records online and opening clinical research areas increasing understanding of patients' diseases patterns from healthcare big data collections (Ludwick & Doucette, 2009). Access to this healthcare data is greatly expanding the knowledge of patients and medical professionals alike (Murdoch & Detsky, 2013). Clinical improvements are an example where analyzing patient characteristics in conjunction with the cost and outcomes of care work to identify the most clinically cost effective treatments are occurring to help doctors' aid patients (Arunasalam, 2013). Reduction of costs to identify, predict and minimize fraud is another area of interest which utilizes big data technology (Bates et al., 2014). Efficiency of processes to help patients locate providers, manage their care, and improve their health is yet another sample of healthcare technology possible improvements (Neff, 2013). Other areas that are being explored include genomics, bioinformatics (Swan, 2013), pharmacogenomics, dentistry, HIV epidemiology, cardiovascular research (Pah et al., 2015) and much more. Given the technology available and the data being collected, doctors and patients may be more readily able to diagnosis the issues and determine treatments to remedy their health problems (Vaitsis et al., 2014). The medical expertise of various professionals can now be shared through the technology offerings (Philips et al., 2004). The collection of all the medical knowledge could help patients with their health needs especially patients with chronic health issues (Wyber et al., 2015).

In addition to the typical medical advice, patients are seeking alternative medicine to address all of their health needs (Eisenberg et al., 1998). Smart health and well-being best practices can also be instituted by patients to address their health concerns outside of offerings from basic medicine offerings. While it holds true that most patients are not alone with their health problems, very often they are not able to connect with a community of people who have had the same issues. Through Social Media, patients could help each other morally, technically through suggestions for medical care, and specifically through healthy practices such as diet and exercise as they share their challenges and needs (Wen-ying et al., 2009). Another avenue of this health knowledge can be obtained from the mobile access that the user is utilizing to extract the data (Kumar et al., 2013). As the application obtains the patients geographical location, data presented can be altered based on health care needs in the area (Free et al., 2013). For example, virus breakouts can be warned to travelers, detailing of best practices to ward off diseases.

The application of technology in healthcare is increasing overtime (Yao et al., 2015). Although the rate may not be as fast as society's expectance of the digital practical applications, the health-based profession is finding usage for technology to replace their paper based systems. Driving down costs, like most other businesses, is the main factor for the adoption of technology in healthcare (Hayhurst, 2015). In health insurance claims, detecting fraud, abuse, waste, and errors, thereby reducing recurrent losses and facilitating enhanced patient care has been a main focus for healthcare technology. In addition, for medical facilities directly streamlining patient related applications such as medical records, patient registration systems, and clinical based applications has greatly increased the efficiency of hospitals and medical practices. Big data applications have been identified to assist in reducing costs in the areas of high-cost patients, readmissions, triage, decompensation, adverse events, and treatment optimization for diseases (Kuiken, 2013). For the ease of use that technology offers, medical professionals also find that the use of software applications assist in their everyday use through clinical applications, research studies of diseases, and overall trending analysis.

MEDICAL EXPERTISE

Medical professionals utilize software applications to assist their day to day operations in areas such as research of genomics, bioinformatics, pharmacogenomics, HIV epidemiology, chronic disease research and much more (Schmidt et al., 1990). For example, in the field of genomics, researchers are producing genome-wide data sets on ever-expanding study populations. Because of technology, broad access to these data, stored samples, and EMRs are accelerating society's understanding of the role of genes, environment, and behavior in health and disease. With this information, new knowledge is gained by improving diagnostics, targeting drug development, and exploration into new insights about how to prevent and treat disease (Curtis et al., 2014). As an interdisciplinary field, bioinformatics is another example of technology in healthcare where methods are developed using software tools for understanding biological data. Bioinformatics combines computer science, statistics, mathematics, and engineering to analyze and interpret biological data. Digital uses are found very important in the study of pharmacogenomics which identifies how genes affect a person's response to drugs. In addition, chronic diseases are studied and identified using technology to sort through the vast amount of data points. Patients, as the final end users of the healthcare technology implementations, have various applications that can be used to assist in their healthcare knowledge (Lin, 2015). However, as technology improves, combining all of these areas will also assist to offer more sophisticated software usages. Within a single source search area, having access to the medical expertise information would greatly help patients and doctors diagnosis issues and determine best practices to stay healthy. The big data platform is the best technology available to offer the medical expertise documentation in a single search application.

DISPERSED HEALTHCARE INFORMATION SOURCES

Patients often have many healthcare solutions available to them. However, they are located at many dispersed sources. There is healthcare technology that can offer them insight into their actual vital signs. Their medical records are now electronically stored and can be accessible to review. Medical experts have a plethora of information which is reachable at many different locations on the internet. Alternative medicine may also offer healthy solutions to address the patient's needs. Feeding into the health information sources, smart health and wellbeing regiments are available online. In addition, social media offerings can also offer peer support as others also are affected with similar diseases. Figure 1 shows how health knowledge is scattered and dispersed throughout various points of access.

Big Data and the Technical Revolution

The large swathes of data being generated through the many computer-based applications continuously can be queried and reachable through cloud computing technology (Rayport & Heyward, 2011). This big data technology has potential to offer everyone greater knowledge to improve every aspect of their lives particularly in healthcare. Building on cloud computing, the big data technology is uniquely different than previous database technology in that with only simple configuration systems can be expanded to calculate extensible algorithms on terabytes of data.

Figure 1. This diagram shows health knowledge is scattered and dispersed throughout various points of access

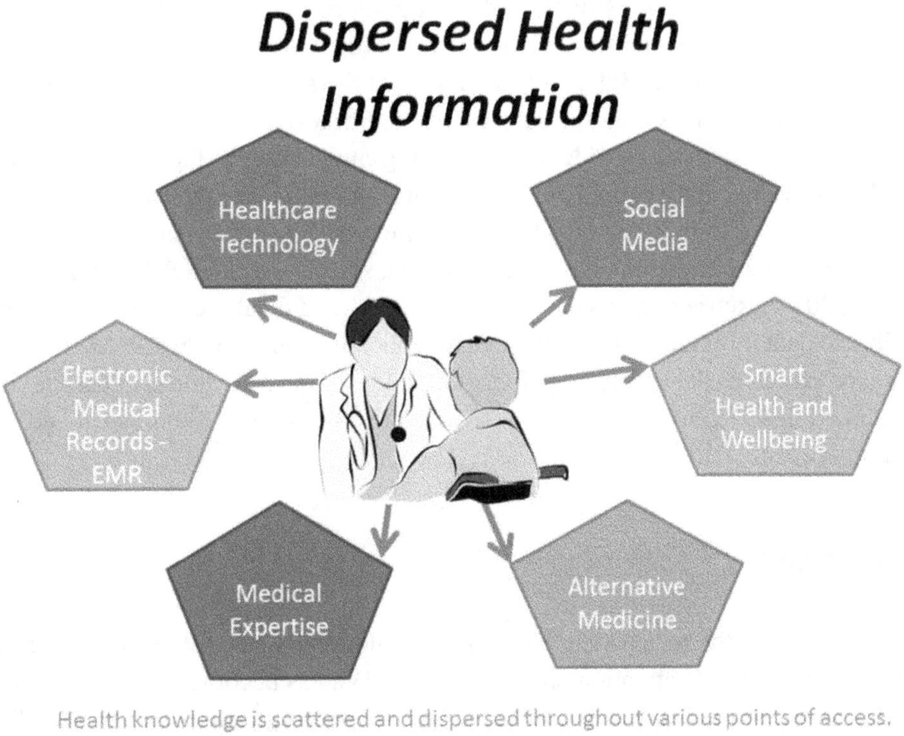

BIG DATA OVERVIEW

At any time, data is being gathered and generated across the internet (Xia et al., 2012). There is digital data that is emitted from sensors such as mobile phone usage. There is data generated from paper-based forms as processes become almost completely computer based such as Tax Forms (Emani et al., 2015). There is personal data such as address and contact information found with a quick review across the internet. There is social media data as people go online to state their opinions. The amount of data available via the internet is almost endless. The issue lies in how to present meaningful results from the data. As defined by Gartner (Gartner, 2014), big data is high-volume, high-velocity and high-variety information assets that demand cost-effective, innovative forms of information processing for enhanced insight and decision making. Taking this data and being able to create progressive decisions based off of the analytical results is the main goal of big data (Demirkan, 2013). The term "Big" is applied because traditional data processing cannot be utilized as the data is too large and it is often unstructured which makes it a challenge to organize in customary formatting (Gandomi & Haider, 2015).

BIG DATA TECHNOLOGY

Utilizing the Cloud Computing infrastructure offers a platform for the big data to finally begin to be managed and analyzed (Andreolini et al., 2015). As best defined by Hashem and his team, "Cloud computing and big data are conjoined. Big data provides users the ability to use commodity computing to process distributed queries across multiple datasets and return resultant sets in a timely manner" p. 102 (Hashem, 2015). Cloud computing provides the underlying engine through the use of Hadoop Distributed File System (HDFS) (Reyes-Ortiz et al., 2015), a class of distributed data-processing platforms (Feller et al., 2015). Large data sources from the cloud and Web are stored in a distributed fault-tolerant database and processed through a programming model for large datasets with a parallel distributed algorithm in a cluster (Hu et al., 2014). Retrieving this data, NoSQL is a type of database that allows for management of large distributed data through a scheme free, easy replication, and simple API. At the programming layer, MapReduce sanctions the processing of large amounts of datasets stored in parallel in the cluster (Darji & Waghela, 2014). From there, views of the data can be compiled and visualized for end users via APIs (Maitrey & Jha, 2015).

BIG DATA USABILITY

Big data usability was not the focus when big data technology was first established. Not implemented like most technologies with the attention on end user, big data has become a technology more because of an outcome and not just because end users made requirements (Kambatla et al., 2014). Therefore, the existing big data usability is a view of datasets in graphs and maps. There are not requirements and use cases that can be identified for the creation of big data usability (Kum et al., 2015). The data is simply there, and usability experts need to now figure out how best to use the overwhelming amount of information (Walji et al., 2013).

A good example of big data usability comes from the database designer field. To address the need for more comprehensive views of big data, Macneil & Elmqvist (MacNeil & Elmqvist, 2013) set out to create visual interfaces that could easily interrupt large data sets from a web based view. The overall concept is to make large data more readily understandable to the end user. The key feature the team determines is not the ability to represent all data in a single view, but rather the capability for the end user to be able to easily create new views and coordinate these views to support comparison and correlation. To address the viewing need, the team created a visualization mosaic which they describe as a hierarchical container structure for visual representations in tiles that present a predefined data set. The main features of mosaics are space-filling layout, visual transformations, mosaic management and formal notation. Although the team explained various applications that are similar, only their solution was built on Java for Web based solutions. Examples of their efforts are described as they built a crime scene map and rock climbing view. Each process was analyzed as the overall steps were noted on how the implementation could be executed to view a map in both scenarios of data elements of the items. Crime blots were shown in Seattle and a rock climbing map was shown for Tibetan Himalaya region. This usability allowed certain sets of data to be displayed in visual usage, related to mapping features.

BIG DATA IN HEALTHCARE

In the world of medicine, the first great revolution was the gathering of research to improve medical practices. The next great medical revolution is here with the incorporation of biomedical sciences and the data sciences (O'Driscoll, 2013). That is to say with "big data" now widely used, research can be compiled and analyzed giving way to much more accurate medical decisions with the amalgamation of the computer sciences (DJ, 2014). At Johns Hopkins Hospital, new research is moving forward incorporating big data processes into specific areas of medicine. These studies hope to improve medical practices and create better outcome for the patients (Al-Jumeily et al., 2015). Areas of focus include HIV (Young, 2015), genomics (Fan & Liu, 2013), rheumatology, radiology, and cancer research. Questions are asked that research hopes to address such as should all cancer patients be treated, can the medical staff predict how often patients will visit the doctors, and does the correlation between office visits and treatments relate to overall health (Calyam et al., 2016). Utilizing big data analytics together with the medical experts and the computer sciences professionals the goal is to enhance the usage for patients given the wealth of medical data (Marx, 2013).

The Proposed Portal Experience

The user experience for big data is in only the beginning stages. Although there are some types of views of big data and limited search availability, the overall user experience can be greatly increased. This limited user experience for big data in health care is greatly lacking. In addition, there are many areas that can offer more options for the end user (Suchanek & Weikum, 2013). Data visualization is the present most common means for the industry to access big data technology (Wright et al., 2013). Analytics transforms the data in to a visual depiction of the data offering map views or other high-level charts and graphs from the data summation. The end-user for these processes is generally upper management or decision makers trying to determine a path forward for their business or government agency (GE et al., 2014). However, big data has more to offer than simple hints towards future plans. The general public already enjoys big data searches through Google and other search engines to find knowledge to enrich their lives. Elevating these search offerings could certainly improve the user experience for big data technology. Building on an existing search framework, the user experience could be increased with only incremental changes. This framework must be available on all devices for the best user experience including desktops, laptops, smart phones and all mobile devices. Ensuring that the interface is simple and yet easy to use is extremely important for the best user experience.

VISUALIZATION

Data visualization is defined as the presentation of data in a pictorial or graphical format (Tam & Song, 2016). The objective is to enable decision makers to view data analytics presented visually with the expectation to take the data summation and understand difficult concepts or identify new patterns (Lee et al., 2013). Allowing the user to control the views, many companies employ interactive visualization tools to maneuver through the data rapidly customizing charts and graphs to gain more knowledge from the data (Liu et al., 2013). Using pictures to understand data has been utilized for centuries, using maps and graphs as early as the 1600s and then pie charts in the early 1800s (Miksch & Aigner, 2014).

Superior technology now allows for even more improvement and usage of data visualization (Tatarchuk et al., 2008). Data Servers now make it possible to process enormous amounts of data at extremely fast speed (Shvachko et al., 2010). Data visualization has become a rapidly evolving blend of science and art that feasible because of data analytics (Thorvaldsdóttir et al., 2013). These computers are processing extensive algorithms to meet the views that the users are requesting (Yang et al., 2015). With this big data technology there is potential for great opportunity; the next phases of data visualization are researching how to expand the present visual interfaces that are offered of primarily charts, maps and contextual searches (Krämer & Senner, 2015).

Visualization methods have offered increased benefits to many organizations over the past decade beginning with business intelligence and moving to full visual analytics for many subjects (Sagiroglu & Sinanc, 2013). The developing field of visual analytics concentrates on making sense of the big data through integrating human judgement using visual representations and interaction techniques in the analysis process (Keim et al., 2008). The Healthcare field is using visual analytics to extract insights from Electronic Health Records (Wang et al., 2011), gain knowledge from medical professionals (Zhang et al., 2008), and view how patients are searching for diagnosis on the web (Brownstein et al., 2009). Building on these applications of visualization and visual analytics, big data technology can move forward in its functionality and uses. Still, big data visualization has much improvement ahead to become a superior user friendly experience (Thomas & Kielman, 2009).

USER EXPERIENCE

Research into big data technology user experiences are only at the very beginning stages (Chan, 2015). In fact, research has found that the user interface of the most big data projects is an afterthought (Fisher et al., 2012). The bulk of the big data projects are centered on setting up the platform, gathering the data and then at some stage a user requests to see the data. Only at that point, the technical team discovers that the data is not as useful for true end user knowledge and have a very little view of how the users can actually benefit from the terabytes of data that is available for searching. However, for a truly good user experience of any software application, the end user requirements must be established first, and not only as an addendum.

To improve big data applications, the users need to be contacted and surveyed to determine how they could use an application and what tools would best suit their needs. The issue with the big data platforms is no one, not even the user, truly knows what they want or could even have from this new technology. Modern end users enjoy the benefits of having rich data at their hand through their mobile devices. However, improving the software interface could be improved to offer them a better view of the data (Marchionini, 1989). Search engines and some few applications such as Facebook, Instagram and Pinterest offer users some satisfaction for probing the vast array of data to meet their needs. Unfortunately, there have been few studies to truly understand how users could utilize big data and how to improve their user experience (Senkowski & Branscum, 2015). A simple incremental improvement to a modern application may offer enhancements that may meet the users' needs (Hassenzahl & Tractinsky, 2006). With true user feedback on specific application information, user experience could be improved (Kim & Chang, 2007). Design changes could be implemented with the end user as the central goal (Kopetz, 2011). Thereby, step by step the user experience of big data technology will ultimately improve.

FRAMEWORK

To make the most of the user experience, a framework to view the big data technology works best. Already users are comfortable with maneuvering through software systems that function with set features available in all screens (Cohen & Oviatt, 2000). For example, many well established applications display buttons along the top and left side for changing the views and acting on the data such as Outlook, Internet Explorer, and Microsoft Word. Having an existing framework will allow the users to more easily transition their existing interface ability to the new big data interface usages (Marchionini & Komlodi, 1998). Not only should the user interface be based on an existing framework, the architecture should be building upon best practices of solid infrastructure conventions (Ghezzi et al., 2015). Maintaining both a framework for the user interface and the technical platform will allow incremental changes that improve the big data offerings.

MOBILE TECHNOLOGY

Mobile application offerings are the most user friendly technology of the present day. It is hard to walk down the street without seeing somebody looking at their handheld devices for many of their daily tasks or for simply just socializing (Cifuentes, 2013). Thanks in part to Steve Jobs, the mobile device technology has changed the world for ever. Using a standard framework, software engineers can create software applications called "apps" that can be easily downloaded to a mobile device for almost any purpose. The application is installed on the mobile device, but primarily works off of the wireless network hooking the application up to servers in data centers (Han et al., 2015). Now with cloud computing being accessible to anyone for inexpensive monthly fees, applications can fully utilize cloud technology and big data architecture with relative low overhead (Laurila et al., 2012).

Not to be left behind, the healthcare industry has many uses for mobile applications (Strack et al., 2015). In fact, the need is growing so rapidly that there is a new word for mobile health which is entitled mHealth, meaning the practice of medicine and public health supported by mobile devices. "For the healthcare industry, mobile applications provide a new frontier in offering better care and services to patients, and a more flexible and mobile way of communicating with suppliers and patients. Mobile applications will provide important real time data for patients, physicians, insurers, and suppliers. In addition, it will revolutionize the way information is managed in the healthcare industry and redefine the doctor – patient communication." (Siau & Shen, 2006) To begin, the mobile device can be used to encourage a patient to exercise and increase their baseline of healthiness (Monroe et al., 2015). The goal, of course, would be to create an app that could assist users to manage their exercise and weight (Gowin et al., 2015). From there, mobile applications give users the knowledge they need when they are moving through their everyday life activities. Mobile users want to be able get the information they need at their fingertips, and that includes more healthcare knowledge (Miller et al., 2015). Patients are looking for answers for their medical issues such as common infectious diseases, fending off heart disease (Logan, 2013) and even researching mental health issues (Bardram et al., 2013).

There are many existing mobile device applications monitor physical activity, manage in-home care, and assist medical professionals in collecting patient data assessment to address their medical needs. For example, the software application Ginger.io (Kuiken, 2013) offers a mobile application in which diabetic patients agree to be tracked through their mobile phones and assisted with behavioral health treatments. Utilizing the sensors in smartphones, the application records location, texting, calling, and even movement in conjunction with patient surveys delivered to their smartphones. The Ginger.io application incorporates the patient's health details with public research from NIH and other public sources to create a wealth of behavioral health data for each patient. Together with their doctors the patients gain helpful insights pointing out changes in activity, food intake and general health care to improve diabetic issues (Kuiken, 2013). A patient could be traveling to another country and not able to speak the language, however, with the help of a mHealth application, finding native health care for emergencies and having warnings documented concerning local health issues could be available at the finger tips (Paul & Dredze, 2011). At some point in the future, the end user may find this technology invaluable.

SOLUTIONS AND RECOMMENDATIONS

Solutions are few to meet this mHealth single search solution. The literature review suggests there is a gap where end users are lost as they try to meet their healthcare needs. The use of Google is one of the best most utilized search engines to answer health related questions. Patients presently utilize the superior search of big data offerings to sort through the vast internet to try to answer their health concerns. The issue that occurs is easily sorting and categorizing the new information for easy retrieval at another time. Accessing the big data easily allows the user to transition from simple data information to knowledge. Therefore, the examination continued to increase the user experience of the resulting set offered.

With the goal of a superior mobile platform for big data searching that already has a satisfied user-base; Pinterest was selected as the best option to improve a big data offering for the healthcare industry. Pinterest can be customized to meet the needs of the ever growing user base offering a superior mHealth solution. Easily searchable and retrievable big data offerings can now be accessed routinely. As shown in Figure 2, the mHealth Pinterest App can be the Portal for the various healthcare software offerings. A customized Pinterest application can offer end users the ability to research the various healthcare technology solutions available, view their own medical diagnosis via Electronic Medical Records, search the assessments of medical professionals, review alternative medicine, research healthy living possibilities, and explore social media options.

Many users simply enjoy Pinterest to share ideas such as home improvements, food and recipes or crafts. However, the user profile can be customized to present topics that have specific interests such as exercise, healthcare, and healthy living. With specific health related topics established and reputable health content "Pinned", the Pinterest interface can offer a superior search engine for reviewing healthy topics that could help injured or sick patients find solutions to their illnesses and even the everyday person find methods to staying healthy longer by extending fit habits. Patients could use Pinterest to research any health issues that they are facing such as the good recipes for the common flu, how to ward off malaria when traveling aboard, or treatments and social support for Chronic Obstructive Pulmonary Disease (Paige et al., 2015). For the reasons of big data usage, superior search capability, an easy to use mobile platform, and high end user acceptance, Pinterest is a good big data solution from which to build upon to offer a mHealth solution.

Although there are many ways to address healthcare needs, one possible solution worthy of study is to implement the popular big data search engine Pinterest to determine if it can be customized to improve the patients' understanding of their healthcare issues. There is very little research performed on the Pinterest application especially in the field of healthcare. Therefore, it may be that only minor

Figure 2. This diagram shows how dispersed health knowledge solutions in various software applications can be brought together through a big data mHealth Portal app

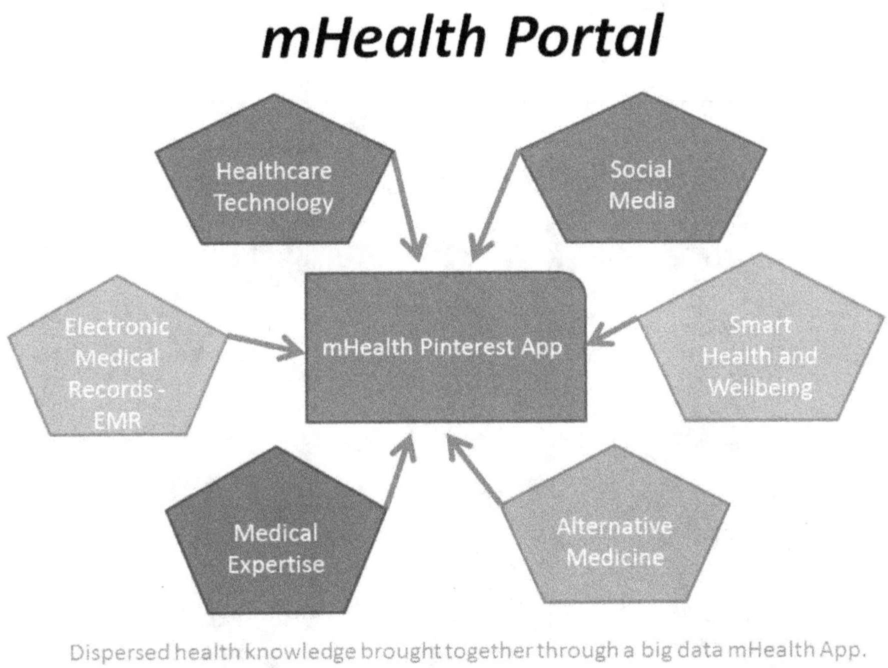

changes to Pinterest could address the needs of the patients' population. Figure 3 shows a view of the proposed Portal Screenshot. Using a healthcare Pinterest application as their source of greater knowledge, patients may find their ideas moving them forward in healthcare remedies and smart wellbeing choices.

FUTURE RESEARCH DIRECTIONS

There is an increasing need for universally accessible initiative in healthcare technology, especially in healthcare. Big data in healthcare is rapidly evolving and has much to offer even the older population and accessibility should be considered in the design stages of every visualization application project to enhance the usability for all. Further research is needed to understand the outcomes of improvements in big data software usage. This research offers a first step in understanding how incremental changes to an interface can offer much greater satisfaction to the patients and health seekers. Beginning with the Pinterest application, small changes could be implemented to make the vast amount of data useful to all. Decisions could be made more rapidly once the patient has full access to the insight the data can foretell.

CONCLUSION

The user experience of viewing healthcare big data can be greatly improved gaining superior knowledge from the vast array of information readily available (Raghupathi & Raghupathi, 2014). With the expan-

Figure 3. This image is a view of the proposed Portal Screenshot to address the big data mHealth Portal app solution

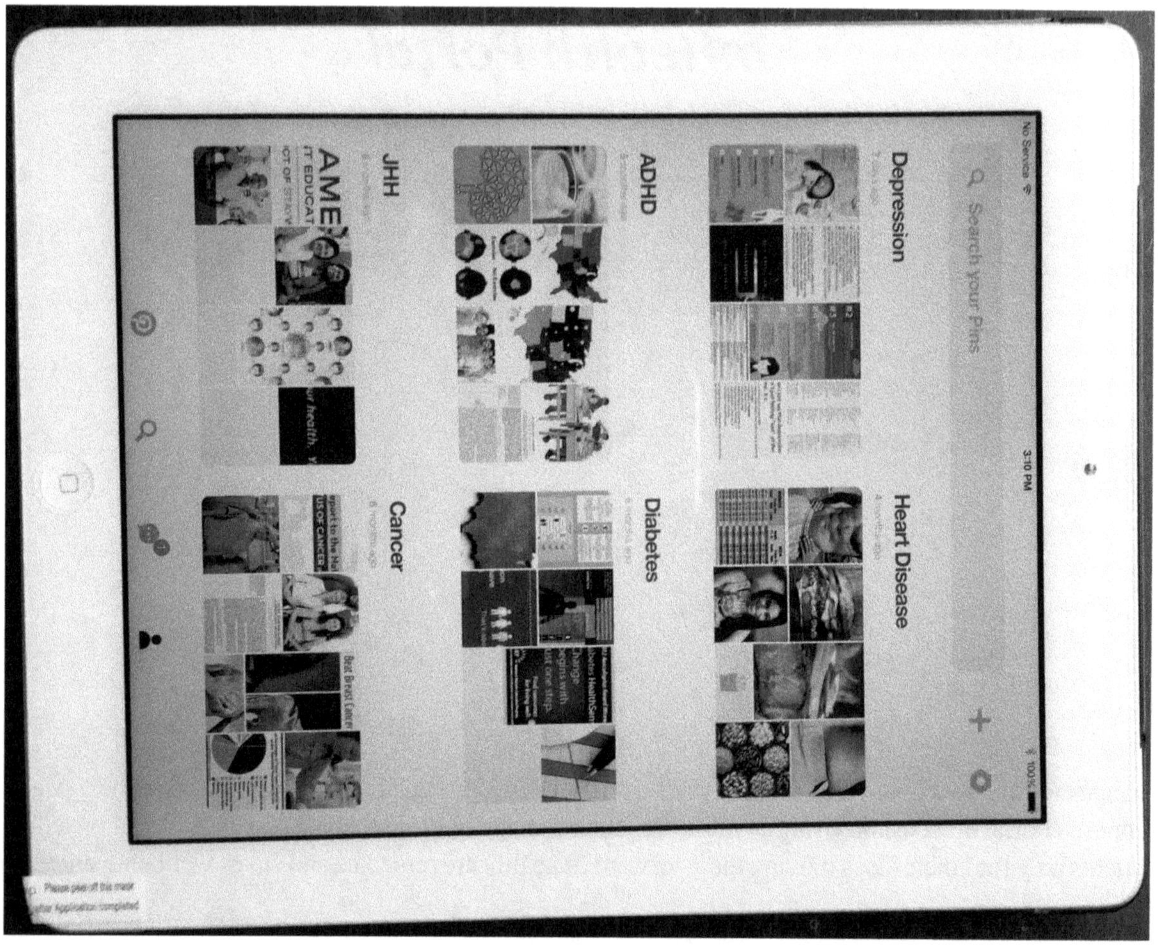

sion of electronic medical records and much of the medical industry digitized, boundless information is at the patient's finger tips. From this immense data, a platform that brings the expertise from medical professionals, smart health and wellbeing proven practices, alternative medicine and social media could increase the end user's healthcare understanding. With a technological breakthrough in cloud computing and big data, mHealth software applications can offer substantially more information to the end users. This innovative technology can be utilized for healthcare uses to more easily search medical related information discovering greater medical solutions. Cultivating healthcare big data visualization could intensify the user experience gaining a better understanding of healing remedies and healthy living guidelines leading toward longevity. This original framework could be accessed using mobile devise such as tablets in assisting patients to attain healthy living. This research study may prove that employing the discovery principals available through a customized Pinterest application can offer patients the ability to research their own medical diagnosis, healthy living, alternative medicine and social media options.

REFERENCES

Al-Jumeily, D., Hussain, A., Mallucci, C., & Oliver, C. (2015). *Applied Computing in Medicine and Health*. Morgan Kaufmann.

Alyass, A., Turcotte, M., & Meyre, D. (2015). From big data analysis to personalized medicine for all: Challenges and opportunities. *BMC Medical Genomics*, *8*(1), 33. doi:10.1186/s12920-015-0108-y PMID:26112054

Andreolini, M., Colajanni, M., Pietri, M., & Tosi, S. (2015). Adaptive, scalable and reliable monitoring of big data on clouds. *Journal of Parallel and Distributed Computing*, *79*, 67–79. doi:10.1016/j.jpdc.2014.08.007

Arunasalam, U. S. a. B. (2013). Leveraging Big Data Analytics to Reduce Healthcare Costs. *IT Pro*, 21-28.

Avinash, G., Liu, R., & Roehm, S. (2005). *System and method for integrated learning and understanding of healthcare informatics*. Google Patents.

Bardram, J. E., Frost, M., Szántó, K., Faurholt-Jepsen, M., Vinberg, M., & Kessing, L. V. (2013). Designing mobile health technology for bipolar disorder: a field trial of the monarca system. *Proceedings of the SIGCHI Conference on Human Factors in Computing Systems*. doi:10.1145/2470654.2481364

Bates, D. W., Saria, S., Ohno-Machado, L., Shah, A., & Escobar, G. (2014). Big data in health care: Using analytics to identify and manage high-risk and high-cost patients. *Health Affairs*, *33*(7), 1123–1131. doi:10.1377/hlthaff.2014.0041 PMID:25006137

Bizer, C., Boncz, P., Brodie, M. L., & Erling, O. (2012). The meaningful use of big data: Four perspectivesfour challenges. *SIGMOD Record*, *40*(4), 56–60. doi:10.1145/2094114.2094129

Blumenthal, D. (2009). Stimulating the adoption of health information technology. *The New England Journal of Medicine*, *360*(15), 1477–1479. doi:10.1056/NEJMp0901592 PMID:19321856

Brownstein, J. S., Freifeld, C. C., & Madoff, L. C. (2009). Digital disease detection—harnessing the Web for public health surveillance. *The New England Journal of Medicine*, *360*(21), 2153–2157. doi:10.1056/NEJMp0900702 PMID:19423867

Calyam, P., Mishra, A., Antequera, R. B., Chemodanov, D., Berryman, A., Zhu, K., & Skubic, M. et al. (2016). Synchronous Big Data analytics for personalized and remote physical therapy. *Pervasive and Mobile Computing*, *28*, 3–20. doi:10.1016/j.pmcj.2015.09.004

Chan, A. (2015). Big data interfaces and the problem of inclusion. *Media Culture & Society*, *37*(7), 1078–1083. doi:10.1177/0163443715594106

Chen, C., & Zhang, C.-Y. (2014). Data-intensive applications, challenges, techniques and technologies: A survey on Big Data. *Information Sciences*, *275*, 314–347. doi:10.1016/j.ins.2014.01.015

Cifuentes, J. D. M. (2013). Context modelling for serendipitous discoveries in exploratory mobile search over social media. *Fifth BCS-IRSG Symposium on Future Directions in Information Access (FDIA 2013)*.

Kum, H.-C., Stewart, C. J., Rose, R. A., & Duncan, D. F. (2015). Using big data for evidence based governance in child welfare. *Children and Youth Services Review*, *58*, 127–136. doi:10.1016/j.childyouth.2015.09.014

Kumar, S., Nilsen, W. J., Abernethy, A., Atienza, A., Patrick, K., Pavel, M., & Spruijt-Metz, D. et al. (2013). Mobile health technology evaluation: The mHealth evidence workshop. *American Journal of Preventive Medicine*, *45*(2), 228–236. doi:10.1016/j.amepre.2013.03.017 PMID:23867031

Laurila, J. K., Gatica-Perez, D., Aad, I., Bornet, O., Do, T.-M.-T., Dousse, O., . . . Miettinen, M. (2012). *The mobile data challenge: Big data for mobile computing research.* Paper presented at the Pervasive Computing.

Lee, T.-Y., Tong, X., Shen, H.-W., Wong, P. C., Hagos, S., & Leung, L. R. (2013). Feature tracking and visualization of the Madden-Julian Oscillation in climate simulation. *IEEE Computer Graphics and Applications*, *33*(4), 29–37. doi:10.1109/MCG.2013.36 PMID:24808057

Lin, W., Dou, W., Zhou, Z., & Liu, C. (2015). A cloud-based framework for Home-diagnosis service over big medical data. *Journal of Systems and Software*, *102*, 192–206. doi:10.1016/j.jss.2014.05.068

Liu, Z., Jiang, B., & Heer, J. (2013). *imMens: Real-time Visual Querying of Big Data.* Paper presented at the Computer Graphics Forum. doi:10.1111/cgf.12129

Logan, A. G. (2013). Transforming hypertension management using mobile health technology for telemonitoring and self-care support. *The Canadian Journal of Cardiology*, *29*(5), 579–585. doi:10.1016/j.cjca.2013.02.024 PMID:23618506

Ludwick, D. A., & Doucette, J. (2009). Adopting electronic medical records in primary care: Lessons learned from health information systems implementation experience in seven countries. *International Journal of Medical Informatics*, *78*(1), 22–31. doi:10.1016/j.ijmedinf.2008.06.005 PMID:18644745

Ma, Y., Wang, L., Liu, P., & Ranjan, R. (2015). Towards building a data-intensive index for big data computing–A case study of Remote Sensing data processing. *Information Sciences*, *319*, 171–188. doi:10.1016/j.ins.2014.10.006

MacNeil, S., & Elmqvist, N. (2013). *Visualization mosaics for multivariate visual exploration.* Paper presented at the Computer Graphics Forum.

Maitrey, S., & Jha, C. (2015). MapReduce: Simplified Data Analysis of Big Data. *Procedia Computer Science*, *57*, 563–571. doi:10.1016/j.procs.2015.07.392

Marchionini, G. (1989). Information-seeking strategies of novices using a full-text electronic encyclopedia. *Journal of the American Society for Information Science*, *40*(1), 54–66. doi:10.1002/(SICI)1097-4571(198901)40:1<54::AID-ASI6>3.0.CO;2-R

Marchionini, G., & Komlodi, A. (1998). Design of interfaces for information seeking. *Annual Review of Information Science & Technology*, *33*, 89–130.

Marx, V. (2013). Biology: The big challenges of big data. *Nature*, *498*(7453), 255–260. doi:10.1038/498255a PMID:23765498

Miksch, S., & Aigner, W. (2014). A matter of time: Applying a data–users–tasks design triangle to visual analytics of time-oriented data. *Computers & Graphics*, *38*, 286–290. doi:10.1016/j.cag.2013.11.002

Miller, T., Chandler, L., & Mouttapa, M. (2015). A needs assessment, development, and formative evaluation of a health promotion smartphone application for college students. *American Journal of Health Education*, *46*(4), 207–215. doi:10.1080/19325037.2015.1044138

Monroe, C. M., Thompson, D. L., Bassett, D. R. Jr, Fitzhugh, E. C., & Raynor, H. A. (2015). Usability of Mobile Phones in Physical Activity–Related Research: A Systematic Review. *American Journal of Health Education*, *46*(4), 196–206. doi:10.1080/19325037.2015.1044141

Murdoch, T. B., & Detsky, A. S. (2013). The inevitable application of big data to health care. *Journal of the American Medical Association*, *309*(13), 1351–1352. doi:10.1001/jama.2013.393 PMID:23549579

Neff, G. (2013). Why big data won't cure us. *Big Data, 1*(3), 117-123.

ODriscoll, A., Daugelaite, J., & Sleator, R. D. (2013). Big data, Hadoop and cloud computing in genomics. *Journal of Biomedical Informatics*, *46*(5), 774–781. doi:10.1016/j.jbi.2013.07.001 PMID:23872175

Pah, A., Rasmussen-Torvik, L., Goel, S., Greenland, P., & Kho, A. (2015). Big data: What is it and what does it mean for cardiovascular research and prevention policy. *Current Cardiovascular Risk Reports*, *9*(1), 1–9. doi:10.1007/s12170-014-0424-3

Paige, S. R., Stellefson, M., Chaney, B. H., & Alber, J. M. (2015). Pinterest as a resource for health information on Chronic Obstructive Pulmonary Disease (COPD): A social media content analysis. *American Journal of Health Education*, *46*(4), 241–251. doi:10.1080/19325037.2015.1044586

Paul, M. J., & Dredze, M. (2011). You are what you Tweet: Analyzing Twitter for public health. *ICWSM*, *20*, 265–272.

Peters, D. P., Havstad, K. M., Cushing, J., Tweedie, C., Fuentes, O., & Villanueva-Rosales, N. (2014). Harnessing the power of big data: Infusing the scientific method with machine learning to transform ecology. *Ecosphere*, *5*(6), 1–15. doi:10.1890/ES13-00359.1

Philips, Z., Ginnelly, L., Sculpher, M., Claxton, K., Golder, S., Riemsma, R., . . . Glanville, J. (2004). *Review of guidelines for good practice in decision-analytic modelling in health technology assessment*. Academic Press.

Raghupathi, W., & Raghupathi, V. (2014). Big data analytics in healthcare: Promise and potential. *Health Information Science and Systems*, *2*(1), 1. doi:10.1186/2047-2501-2-3 PMID:25825667

Rayport, J., & Heyward, A. (2011). *Envisioning the cloud: The next computing paradigm and its implication for technology policy*. Accessed May.

Reyes-Ortiz, J. L., Oneto, L., & Anguita, D. (2015). Big data analytics in the cloud: Spark on hadoop vs mpi/openmp on beowulf. *Procedia Computer Science*, *53*, 121–130. doi:10.1016/j.procs.2015.07.286

Rind, A., Wang, T. D., Aigner, W., Miksch, S., Wongsuphasawat, K., Plaisant, C., & Shneiderman, B. (2011). Interactive information visualization to explore and query electronic health records. *Foundations and Trends in Human-Computer Interaction*, *5*(3), 207–298. doi:10.1561/1100000039

REFERENCES

Agarwal, S., Perry, H. B., Long, L. A., & Labrique, A. B. (2015). Evidence on feasibility and effective use of mHealth strategies by frontline health workers in developing countries: Systematic review. *Tropical Medicine & International Health, 20*(8), 1003–1014. doi:10.1111/tmi.12525 PMID:25881735

Almunawar, M. N., Anshari, M., & Younis, M. Z. (2015). Incorporating customer empowerment in mobile health. *Health Policy and Technology, 4*(4), 312–319. doi:10.1016/j.hlpt.2015.08.008

Angelidis, P. (2009). Mobile telemonitoring insights. In J. Tan (Ed.), *Medical informatics: Concepts, methodologies, tools, and applications* (pp. 107–112). Hershey, PA: IGI Global. doi:10.4018/978-1-60566-050-9.ch010

Anshari, M., & Almunawar, M. N. (2015). Mobile health (mHealth). In M. Khosrow-Pour (Ed.), *Encyclopedia of information science and technology* (3rd ed.; pp. 5607–5614). Hershey, PA: IGI Global. doi:10.4018/978-1-4666-5888-2.ch553

Archer, N. (2010). Mobile e-health: Making the case. In K. Khoumbati, Y. Dwivedi, A. Srivastava, & B. Lal (Eds.), *Handbook of research on advances in health informatics and electronic healthcare applications: Global adoption and impact of information communication technologies* (pp. 446–457). Hershey, PA: IGI Global. doi:10.4018/978-1-60566-030-1.ch027

Bamigboye, A. (2012). Mobile healthcare: Challenges and opportunities. In B. Ciaramitaro (Ed.), *Mobile technology consumption: Opportunities and challenges* (pp. 77–98). Hershey, PA: IGI Global. doi:10.4018/978-1-61350-150-4.ch006

Ben-Zeev, D., Kaiser, S. M., Brenner, C. J., Begale, M., Duffecy, J., & Mohr, D. C. (2013). Development and usability testing of FOCUS: A smartphone system for self-management of schizophrenia. *Psychiatric Rehabilitation Journal, 36*(4), 289–296. doi:10.1037/prj0000019 PMID:24015913

Bhuyan, S. S., Zhu, H., Chandak, A., Kim, J., & Stimpson, J. P. (2014). Do service innovations influence the adoption of electronic health records in long-term care organizations? Results from the U.S. national survey of residential care facilities. *International Journal of Medical Informatics, 83*(12), 975–982. doi:10.1016/j.ijmedinf.2014.09.007 PMID:25453201

Broberg, C. S., Mitchell, J., Rehel, S., Grant, A., Gianola, A., Beninato, P., & Sahn, D. J. et al. (2015). Electronic medical record integration with a database for adult congenital heart disease: Early experience and progress in automating multicenter data collection. *International Journal of Cardiology, 196*, 178–182. doi:10.1016/j.ijcard.2015.05.140 PMID:26142077

Ceruti, M., Geninatti, S., & Siliquini, R. (2016). Use and reuse of electronic health records: Building information systems for improvement of health services. In *E-health and telemedicine: Concepts, methodologies, tools, and applications* (pp. 961–975). Hershey, PA: IGI Global. doi:10.4018/978-1-4666-8756-1.ch049

Chen, Y., Lorenzi, N., Nyemba, S., Schildcrout, J. S., & Malin, B. (2014). We work with them? Health workers interpretation of organizational relations mined from electronic health records. *International Journal of Medical Informatics, 83*(7), 495–506. doi:10.1016/j.ijmedinf.2014.04.006 PMID:24845147

Chib, A. (2010). The Aceh Besar midwives with mobile phones project: Design and evaluation perspectives using the information and communication technologies for healthcare development model. *Journal of Computer-Mediated Communication, 15*(3), 500–525. doi:10.1111/j.1083-6101.2010.01515.x

Ciaramitaro, B. L., & Skrocki, M. (2012). mHealth: Mobile healthcare. In B. Ciaramitaro (Ed.), Mobile technology consumption: Opportunities and challenges (pp. 99–109). Hershey, PA: IGI Global. doi:10.4018/978-1-61350-150-4.ch007

Cinque, M., Coronato, A., & Testa, A. (2012). Dependable services for mobile health monitoring systems. *International Journal of Ambient Computing and Intelligence, 4*(1), 1–15. doi:10.4018/jaci.2012010101

D'Abundo, M. L. (2013). Electronic health record implementation in the United States healthcare industry: Making the process of change manageable. In V. Wang (Ed.), *Handbook of research on technologies for improving the 21st century workforce: Tools for lifelong learning* (pp. 272–286). Hershey, PA: IGI Global. doi:10.4018/978-1-4666-2181-7.ch018

de la Torre Díez, I., Sánchez, R. H., Coronado, M. L., & López Gálvez, M. I. (2010). Electronic health records in a tele-ophthalmologic application with Oracle 10g. In A. Lazakidou (Ed.), *Biocomputation and biomedical informatics: Case studies and applications* (pp. 89–105). Hershey, PA: IGI Global. doi:10.4018/978-1-60566-768-3.ch005

Deng, Z., Mo, X., & Liu, S. (2014). Comparison of the middle-aged and older users' adoption of mobile health services in China. *International Journal of Medical Informatics, 83*(3), 210–224. doi:10.1016/j.ijmedinf.2013.12.002 PMID:24388129

DeRenzi, B., Borriello, G., Jackson, J., Kumar, V. S., Parikh, T. S., Virk, P., & Lesh, N. (2011). Mobile phone tools for field-based health care workers in low-income countries. *Mount Sinai Journal of Medicine: A Journal of Translational and Personalized Medicine, 78*(3), 406–418. doi:10.1002/msj.20256

Dias, C. M., Ribeiro, A. G., & Furtado, S. F. (2016). An overview about the use of healthcare applications on mobile devices. In M. Cruz-Cunha, I. Miranda, R. Martinho, & R. Rijo (Eds.), *Encyclopedia of e-health and telemedicine* (pp. 285–298). Hershey, PA: IGI Global. doi:10.4018/978-1-4666-9978-6.ch024

Dwivedi, Y. K., Shareef, M. A., Simintiras, A. C., Lal, B., & Weerakkody, V. (2016). A generalised adoption model for services: A cross-country comparison of mobile health (m-health). *Government Information Quarterly, 33*(1), 174–187. doi:10.1016/j.giq.2015.06.003

Edirisinghe, R., Stranieri, A., & Wickramasinghe, N. (2017). A taxonomy for mHealth. In N. Wickramasinghe (Ed.), *Handbook of research on healthcare administration and management* (pp. 596–615). Hershey, PA: IGI Global. doi:10.4018/978-1-5225-0920-2.ch036

Effler, P., Ching-Lee, M., Bogard, A., Ieong, M. C., Nekomoto, T., & Jernigan, D. (1999). Statewide system of electronic notifiable disease reporting from clinical laboratories: Comparing automated reporting with conventional methods. *Journal of the American Medical Association, 282*(19), 1845–1850. doi:10.1001/jama.282.19.1845 PMID:10573276

Etheredge, L. M. (2014). Rapid learning: A breakthrough agenda. *Health Affairs, 33*(7), 1155–1162. doi:10.1377/hlthaff.2014.0043 PMID:25006141

Lan, T., Zhang, J., & Lu, Y. (2016). Transforming the blood glucose meter into a general healthcare meter for in vitro diagnostics in mobile health. *Biotechnology Advances*, *34*(3), 331–341. doi:10.1016/j.biotechadv.2016.03.002 PMID:26946282

Lang, M., Burkle, T., Laumann, S., & Prokosch, H. U. (2008). Process mining for clinical workflows: Challenges and current limitations. *Studies in Health Technology and Informatics*, *136*, 229–334. PMID:18487736

Lee, T. (2016). Mobile healthcare computing in the cloud. In *Mobile computing and wireless networks: Concepts, methodologies, tools, and applications* (pp. 1412–1432). Hershey, PA: IGI Global. doi:10.4018/978-1-4666-8751-6.ch061

Mayora, O., Frost, M., Arnrich, B., Gravenhorst, F., Grunerbl, A., & Muaremi, A. et al.. (2016). Mobile health systems for bipolar disorder: The relevance of non-functional requirements in MONARCA project. In *E-health and telemedicine: Concepts, methodologies, tools, and applications* (pp. 1395–1405). Hershey, PA: IGI Global. doi:10.4018/978-1-4666-8756-1.ch070

Mechael, P. (2010). Opportunities and challenges of integrating mHealth applications into rural health initiatives in Africa. In M. Cruz-Cunha, A. Tavares, & R. Simoes (Eds.), *Handbook of research on developments in e-health and telemedicine: Technological and social perspectives* (pp. 704–727). Hershey, PA: IGI Global. doi:10.4018/978-1-61520-670-4.ch034

Misra, R. (2016). The benefits and challenges of using mobile-based tools in self-management and care. In A. Dwivedi (Ed.), *Reshaping medical practice and care with health information systems* (pp. 1–13). Hershey, PA: IGI Global. doi:10.4018/978-1-4666-9870-3.ch001

Mitra, S., & Padman, R. (2014). Engagement with social media platforms via mobile apps for improving quality of personal health management: A healthcare analytics case study. *Journal of Cases on Information Technology*, *16*(1), 73–89. doi:10.4018/jcit.2014010107

Moghimi, H., & Wickramasinghe, N. (2017). The development of a secure hospital messaging and communication platform. In N. Wickramasinghe (Ed.), *Handbook of research on healthcare administration and management* (pp. 243–267). Hershey, PA: IGI Global. doi:10.4018/978-1-5225-0920-2.ch015

Moumtzoglou, A. S. (2016). The nexus of m-health and self-efficacy. In A. Moumtzoglou (Ed.), *M-health innovations for patient-centered care* (pp. 341–365). Hershey, PA: IGI Global. doi:10.4018/978-1-4666-9861-1.ch017

Muranaga, F., Kumamoto, I., & Uto, Y. (2007). Development of site data warehouse for cost analysis of DPC based on medical costs. *Methods of Information in Medicine*, *46*(6), 679–685. PMID:18066419

Nassar, D. A., Othman, M., Hayajneh, J. A., & Ali, N. (2015). An integrated success model for an electronic health record: A case study of Hakeem Jordan. *Procedia Economics and Finance*, *23*, 95–103. doi:10.1016/S2212-5671(15)00526-2

Nguyen, L., Bellucci, E., & Nguyen, L. T. (2014). Electronic health records implementation: An evaluation of information system impact and contingency factors. *International Journal of Medical Informatics*, *83*(11), 779–796. doi:10.1016/j.ijmedinf.2014.06.011 PMID:25085286

Nikou, S. (2015). Mobile technology and forgotten consumers: The young-elderly. *International Journal of Consumer Studies, 39*(4), 294–304. doi:10.1111/ijcs.12187

Nisha, N., Iqbal, M., Rifat, A., & Idrish, S. (2016). Mobile health services: A new paradigm for health care systems. In *E-health and telemedicine: Concepts, methodologies, tools, and applications* (pp. 1551–1567). Hershey, PA: IGI Global. doi:10.4018/978-1-4666-8756-1.ch078

Oddershede, A. M., & Carrasco, R. A. (2008). Perception of mobile technology provision in health service. In W. Huang, Y. Wang, & J. Day (Eds.), *Global mobile commerce: Strategies, implementation and case studies* (pp. 345–364). Hershey, PA: IGI Global. doi:10.4018/978-1-59904-558-0.ch019

Okuda, Y., Bryson, E. O., DeMaria, S., Jr., Jacobson, L., Quinones, J., Shen, B., & Levine, A. I. (2009). The utility of simulation in medical education: What is the evidence?. *Mount Sinai Journal of Medicine: A Journal of Translational and Personalized Medicine, 76*(4), 330–343. doi:10.1002/msj.20127

Olla, P., & Tan, J. (2009). *Mobile health solutions for biomedical applications*. Hershey, PA: IGI Global. doi:10.4018/978-1-60566-332-6

Patterson, E. S., Zhang, J., Abbott, P., Gibbons, M. C., Lowry, Z. S., Quinn, T. M., & Brick, D. et al. (2013). Enhancing electronic health record usability in pediatric patient care: A scenario-based approach. *Joint Commission Journal on Quality and Patient Safety, 39*(3), 129–135. doi:10.1016/S1553-7250(13)39019-9 PMID:23516763

Pfeiffer, P. N., Bohnert, K. M., Zivin, K., Yosef, M., Valenstein, M., Aikens, J. E., & Piette, J. D. (2015). Mobile health monitoring to characterize depression symptom trajectories in primary care. *Journal of Affective Disorders, 174*, 281–286. doi:10.1016/j.jad.2014.11.040 PMID:25527999

Prokosch, H. U., & Ganslandt, T. (2009). Perspectives for medical informatics: Reusing the electronic medical record for clinical research. *Methods of Information in Medicine, 48*(1), 38–44. PMID:19151882

Protti, D. (2008). A comparison of how Canada, England, and Denmark are managing their electronic health record journeys. In A. Kushniruk & E. Borycki (Eds.), *Human, social, and organizational aspects of health information systems* (pp. 203–218). Hershey, PA: IGI Global. doi:10.4018/978-1-59904-792-8.ch012

Pullen, T., & Al-Hakim, L. (2016). Shared electronic health records as innovation: An Australian case. In L. Al-Hakim, X. Wu, A. Koronios, & Y. Shou (Eds.), *Handbook of research on driving competitive advantage through sustainable, lean, and disruptive innovation* (pp. 500–533). Hershey, PA: IGI Global. doi:10.4018/978-1-5225-0135-0.ch021

Queirós, A., Silva, A. G., Ferreira, A., Caravau, H., Cerqueira, M., & Rocha, N. P. (2016). Assessing mobile applications considered medical devices. In M. Cruz-Cunha, I. Miranda, R. Martinho, & R. Rijo (Eds.), *Encyclopedia of e-health and telemedicine* (pp. 111–127). Hershey, PA: IGI Global. doi:10.4018/978-1-4666-9978-6.ch010

Redha, W., Hartwick, K., & Sikka, N. (2015). Mobile health in emergency care. In Z. Yan (Ed.), *Encyclopedia of mobile phone behavior* (pp. 825–838). Hershey, PA: IGI Global. doi:10.4018/978-1-4666-8239-9.ch068

Chapter 6
Pervasive Computing in Supporting Pediatric and Neonatology Care Unit Decision Process

Bia Martins
University of Minho, Portugal

Tiago André Saraiva Guimarães
University of Minho, Portugal

Mariana Santos
Unidade Local de Saúde do Alto Minho, Portugal

Simão Frutuoso
Centro Materno Infantil do Norte, Portugal

Filipe Portela
University of Minho, Portugal

Manuel Filipe Santos
University of Minho, Portugal

ABSTRACT

Neonatal units, and especially the sections devoted to intensive care require an individualized medical prescription, based on body weight and gestational age making them among the hospital settings where treatment errors are most likely to occur. These errors may harm patients and their families, as well as increase the duration of hospital stay and its costs. Tools such as Sabichão have sought, over the last years, to aid clinical decision-making to reduce clinical error. However, with the increased use and dissemination of mobile platforms, it's now possible and essential to bring the available assistance closer to the health providers and their practice. This paper describes a Framework that seeks to present itself as a more efficient and ubiquitous alternative to an existing Clinical decision support system.

DOI: 10.4018/978-1-5225-2851-7.ch006

INTRODUCTION

Neonatal and pediatric services need more attention in clinical care once children and babies are more vulnerable than adults to medical errors. It is increasingly important that electronic clinical information systems ensure an improvement in the safety and quality of pediatric patient care. Due to the specific requirements of these patients it is necessary to guide Information Technology to their needs (Peverini, 2000; Technology, 2015; Lerner, 2008; Ruiz et al., 2015).

Neonatal and pediatric patients have particular guidelines for the administration of parenteral nutrition (PN) solutions. Prescribing a PN solution requires several calculations, consulting multiple tables, and considerations about the weight and clinical status of the baby / child. Thus, errors in drug dosing are the most common errors in hospital facilities and potentially the most harmful, with a higher incidence rate in the pediatric population than in the adult population. Therefore, the practice of safe medication becomes essential to improve patient safety which can be achieved by a continuous evolution of health care systems. The automation of prescriptions through the ease of calculation or query of tables aims at reducing this medical error (Peverini, 2000; Gonzales, 2010).

The neonatology or pediatrics appointments involve drug dosing and preparation of PN solutions, anthropometric analysis, specialized growth charts, recording of emergency occurrences and the evaluation of several clinical indicators. If the health professional is unable to effectively and efficiently interconnect all patient information (e.g., identification, weight, requests and administration of medications, reports, age-specific care, etc.), the medical appointment will be more time-consuming and may lead to increase the occurrence of errors (Technology, 2015).

This demand for a system that assists health professionals in the execution of their daily tasks has made Sabichão to be implemented in these services. Sabichão is a pervasive decision support system that allows interoperability between different information systems and helps physicians providing better care (Orwat, 2008).

This system provides a set of functionalities capable to overcome several obstacles that doctors face during an appointment of neonatology and pediatrics. The ease of understanding and utility of the application makes it useful and widely adopted in the centers where it was installed. Sabichão is being used and tested in the Intensive Care Units of Pediatric and Neonatology of the *Centro Hospitalar do Porto*, the *Centro Materno-Infantil do Norte* and the *Centro Hospitalar Tâmega e Sousa*.

The amount of data obtained in the information systems and the advantages related with applications such as Sabichão allow the access of vast functionalities and data driven perspectives in order to improve the provided health care (Orwat, 2008; Kovalchuk, 2015).

In this sense, this work is being done in order to facilitate this access in a web platform available for several users inside and outside the aforementioned healthcare units.

This paper is divided in five sections. The first one introduces the paper and the work and the second section refers to related works. The third intrudes important concepts and methodologies adopted. The four section indicates the architecture used and the functionalities associated with the platform. The last section, section five, presents the conclusions and future work.

While SOAP only allows data in XML format, REST is easy to understand and can be used by any client or server with HTTP / HTTPS support, allowing the use of different data formats. REST allows better support for web clients because of their support for JSON. In addition, REST has better performance and scalability, and its data can be cached, while SOAP does not. However, because SOAP always uses the same language, it is divided as follows: the envelope, which defines the content of the message and tells how to process it; A set of encoding rules for the data types; And layout for call and answer procedures. This "envelope" is sent via (for example) HTTP / HTTPS and a Remote Procedure Call (RPC) is run, and the envelope returns with the information from the formatted XML document. In this way, the main advantage of SOAP is its "generic" transport.

REST is easier to use, more flexible and has great efficiency. As it does not require extensive processing as in SOAP it becomes faster and better functioning in Web applications (Pautasso, 2009; Liu, 2015).

SABICHÃO

Sabichão e Sabipharma

The Sabichão, based on the original excel application, is a Decision Support System currently in the testing phase in Pediatric and Neonatology services. This new version aims to improve existing features in the initial prototype, namely, ease of access to information, availability, data sharing and interoperability.

In order to support the operation of this System, two databases were created where it is possible to store the information coming from the Sabichão, and in this way, make it possible to access at any time a platform implemented in the hospital pharmacy that allows the management of prescriptions, and a Web Service responsible for communication between all the components.

The Sabipharma was another application designed to improve the architecture of this system. This application followed the principles of the methodology used in Sabichão, with an easy-to-understand interface and implemented in Java in the pharmacy services of CHP.

After an initial testing phase the structure adopted for the application is represented in Figure 1.

As it is possible to verify, the architecture of this system is divided in:

1. Sabichão Application

Sabichão is an application developed in Java of easy use implemented in the services of pediatrics and neonatology where the health professionals have access to a variety of functionalities useful in their daily work. This application allows the prescription of PN solutions, anthropometric consultations, emergency recordings, scaling calculations, unit converters, monitoring tables, medication dosage ...

Users of this system can also contact the pharmacy service available at the hospital for prescription nutrition bags. In this way, they have a direct contact with the production of the patient's medication and can consult, edit or cancel requests made to the pharmacy.

2. SabiPharma Application

Physicians when prescribing a PN solution send this data to the hospital pharmacy. In order to enable the elaboration of these efficiently, an application was implemented in these services, Sabipharma,

Figure 1. Architecture used in the Sabichão application

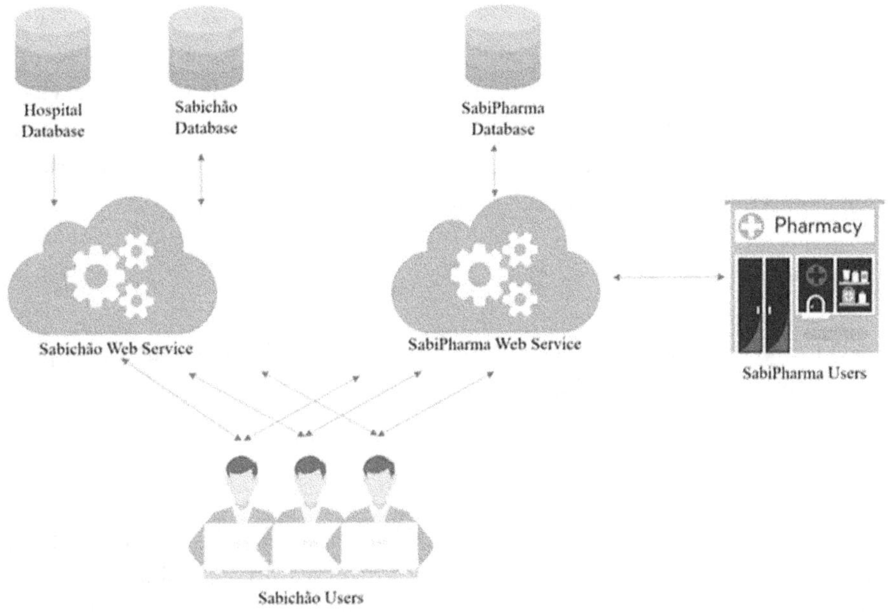

where all the orders made are registered. Health professionals access the application that is constantly updated and check the requests that were introduced in the system or that have already been elaborated.

3. Hospital Database

This database provides inpatient data to the Sabichao application. This process avoids the need to routinely query patient data, avoiding information transfer errors.

4. Sabichao Database

This database stores activities and queries performed on Sabichão. Here it is possible to carry out emergency records, anthropometric data, save medical scales data, namely, save the information registered in the application. In addition, it allows physicians to have constant access to this data and thus to consult historical and to create an evolution of the clinical state of the patient.

In addition, prescriptions of PN solutions can be stored for later shipment to the pharmacy or for treatment consultation.

5. SabiPharma Database

When a request for a PN solution is made, and sent to the Pharmacy, this application is registered here to be prepared and administered. These requests can be queried, deleted, or updated. It is thus possible for the pharmacy to be in constant contact with the needs of patients and doctors.

6. Sabichão Web Service

This Web Service is used to perform the communication between the interfaces accessed by the user and the databases of the Sabichão application and the Hospital. To enable the web service in the hospital it was necessary to configure the Apache Tomcat server, one of the most used application servers on the internet. These servers are characterized by their performance and stability, characteristics necessary to prevent failures in communication within the system.

7. SabiPharma Web service

This web service, in turn, allows a link between the pharmacy database and the applications that use this database, namely the Sabichão and the Sabipharma.

Web Sabichão

While the application mentioned above was installed and tested in CHP, a new Web application has been developed. This new application brings countless advantages to users since it contributes to system interoperability, improved clinical service delivery, decreased medical error, ease of access to functionality, and to achieve a ubiquitous application for Sabichão.

In order to enhance the current application to grant the access of some specific health professionals, it was necessary to create a Web application that would allow management of users, provide tools publicly and even expose doubts. Therefore, this platform has been developed with aim to fulfill those requirements.

The architecture used is shown in the Figure 2. Since this is a Web application, the Web Service used was REST.

Figure 2. Architecture of the Sabichão Web

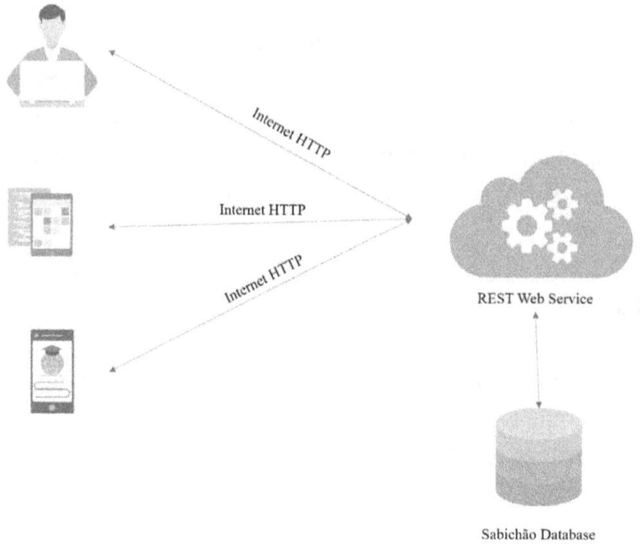

This Web application is divided into several areas in order to cover the greatest number of needs:

- **Administrator:** The application administrator is responsible for the management of platform users. These users need to be registered to query private data. The password entered by those users is never accessed by the administrator because it is encrypted. The administrator, therefore, only has access to the necessary information of the users for the correct management of them.
- **User:** Make a new record, or log in. In this area, the user can also edit their access data and personal information.
- **Public:** In this area is shown some of the features available in the Sabichão's application, such as elaboration of PN solutions, drug dosages, emergency sheets, basic acid balance verification, among others that are useful and easy to understand by users.

These components are of great interest to the general public since they can be accessed by medical students to consolidate concepts and to have a closer contact with these subjects.

In this area, patient reports and useful information may also be made available by prior identification.

- **BI:** Area dedicated to Business Intelligence (BI) on the most (or least) used modules of the Sabichão, time needed to make a PN request, collected pediatric data ...
- **Download:** Here you can download the application Sabichão or Sabipharma.
- **Discussion Forum:** In this area it will be possible for any user to present doubts about the platform, suggestions for improvement.

With this Web application it is possible to make the Sabichão available anywhere, as well as to enable access to various functionalities in any device (Yoo, 2002).

CONCLUSION AND FUTURE WORK

This new and updated application allows a new way of collecting and analyzing data for clinical decision making. This platform assists pediatricians in the exercise of their daily duties by facilitating a high set of tools that meet their needs.

This pervasive system allows the interoperability of some hospital systems that was non-existent previously. The possibility of continuous communication between the pediatric and neonatology services and the pharmacy contributes to an improvement in the delivery of quality care. The user-friendly interfaces available and the speed of processing allows an increase in speed response of health professionals and consequently better health care for patients.

Since this application allows you to save and access past data, doctors can create clinical histories and consult information useful for a patient's consultation. Situations experienced with previous users may serve as a basis for a more appropriate treatment of a new patient. At every moment, the doctor can consult the new inpatients and thus provide a fast and effective personalized service.

The availability of features of the Sabichão in an application makes it reach a large number of users contributing to an improvement in the quality of health services provided and consequently improving the quality of life of patients. The information is shared in an updated way in the web application where it is possible to download the complete application by any user.

ACKNOWLEDGMENT

This work has been supported by COMPETE: POCI-01-0145-FEDER-007043 and FCT – Fundação para a Ciência e Tecnologia within the Project Scope: UID/CEC/00319/2013.

REFERENCES

Gonzales, K. (2010). Medication administration errors and the pediatric population: A systematic search of the literature. *Journal of Pediatric Nursing*, *25*(6), 555–565. doi:10.1016/j.pedn.2010.04.002 PMID:21035020

Guimarães, T., Coimbra, C., Portela, F., Santos, F., Machado, J., & Abelha, A. (2015). Step towards Multiplatform Framework for supporting Pediatric and Neonatology Care Unit decision process. *Procedia Computer Science*, *63*, 561–568.

Kovalchuk, S. V. (2015). *Personalized Clinical Decision Support with Complex Hospital-Level Modelling*. Elsevier Masson SAS.

Lerner, R. L. (2008). *Medication errors in a neonatal intensive care unit*. Jornal de Pediatria, Sociedade Brasileira de Pediatria.

Liu, Y. X. L. (2015). Characterizing RESTful Web Services Usage on Smartphones: A Tale of Native Apps and Web Apps. *Proc. - 2015 IEEE Int. Conf. Web Serv. ICWS 2015*, 337–344. doi:10.1109/ICWS.2015.53

Orwat, C., Graefe, A., & Faulwasser, T. (2008). Towards pervasive computing in health care - a literature review. *BMC Medical Informatics and Decision Making*, *8*(1), 26. doi:10.1186/1472-6947-8-26 PMID:18565221

Pautasso, C. (2009). RESTful Web service composition with BPEL for REST. *Data & Knowledge Engineering*, *68*(9), 851–866. doi:10.1016/j.datak.2009.02.016

Peverini, . (2000). Graphical user interface for a neonatal parenteral nutrition decision support system. *Proc. AMIA Symp.*, 650–654. PMID:11079964

Portela, F., Gago, P., Santos, M. F., Machado, J., Abelha, A., Silva, Á., & Rua, F. (2013). Implementing a pervasive real-time intelligent system for tracking critical events with intensive care patients. *International Journal of Healthcare Information Systems and Informatics*, *8*(4), 1–16. doi:10.4018/ijhisi.2013100101

Ruiz, M. E., Suñol, M. M., Miguélez, J. R., Ortiz, E. S., Urroz, M. I., Camino, M. d., & Aloy, J. F. (2015). *Medication errors in a neonatal unit: One of the main adverse events. Anales de Pediatría.*

Technology, C. U. (2015). Pediatric Aspects of Inpatient Health Information Technology Systems. *Pediatrics, 135*(3), 756–768.

Varshney, U. (2007). Pervasive healthcare and wireless health monitoring. *Mobile Networks and Applications*, *12*(2–3), 113–127. doi:10.1007/s11036-007-0017-1

Yoo, K. L. (2002). Issues and challenges in ubiquitous computing. *Introduction. Commun. ACM*, *45*(12), 62–65.

Chapter 7
Augmented Reality in Surgery:
A New Approach to Enhance the Surgeon's Experience

José Inácio
University of Minho, Portugal

João Ribeiro
Peek Health S.A., Portugal

Jaime Campos
Peek Health S.A., Portugal

Sara Silva
Peek Health S.A., Portugal

Victor Alves
University of Minho, Portugal

ABSTRACT

In the surgical field, the patient's needs and requirements increasingly follow the newest technological developments. Nowadays it is still problematic to implement different types of technologies in operating environments due to the drawbacks that these can bring to their users and their longstanding learning process. A research was carried out with the objective of clarifying concepts and gathering some existing approaches to the solution of these problems as well as the respective technologies used. This chapter addresses a new concept of mobile applications for surgical planning using augmented reality technologies. The proposed solution aims to help the surgeon from the planning stage to the surgery intervention itself. In addition to some examples and practical demonstrations of the solution, its implementation process and system architecture are described and explained. Based on the developed prototype, the advantages of its use in a surgical context are discussed, being pointed out some improvements to be made.

DOI: 10.4018/978-1-5225-2851-7.ch007

INTRODUCTION

Nowadays the patient is more a customer than a real patient, who wants to be treated by a medical team specialized in his condition and which uses state-of-the-art technologies to address his problem.

Most surgeries are preceded by a planning phase and its success is intimately related with it. This phase consists in the patient's pre-evaluation and it is supported by its existing clinical information and other studies, which will establish a surgical procedure suitable to him. One of the current major problems is the lack of solutions which help surgeons to better reproduce what they did in the planning stage inside the operating room. Solutions such as the Surgery Navigation Systems (SNS) appeared. Initially, these systems have been implemented only with the purpose of helping and increasing the surgeon's field of view through micro cameras, microscopes and tracking screens during surgeries. The technological advances and another facts such as the increasing interaction, manipulation and visualization of information, were the main triggers for the development of Augmented Reality (AR) technologies (Pelargos et al., 2016) and for their implementation in SNS systems. At the same time, mobile technologies have followed this evolution assuming an increasing role in multiple domains of society. However, one of the less explored field has been their use for practical medical solutions.

Despite of the initial success of SNS solutions, some limitations were detected and pointed over time, many of them associated with mobility and portability issues. The extensive configuration process, the complexity of devices' manipulation (not users' friendly) and the slow learning process are some of the described disadvantages along with the high investment they require.

In this chapter the authors present an approach which combines the potential that AR technologies bring to their users along with the issue of mobility and remote access to graphic information and data sources. The designed solution may have the possibility to acquire an important and useful status in the clinical procedures in which it would be apply by solving the above pointed limitations in an intuitive, simple, viable and inexpensive way. The importance of this work is reflected on the enlargement and improvement use of the current technological resources for medical surgery area in order to enhance the quality of clinical interventions as well as the experience between patient and physician.

The presented work in this chapter started with a research on the AR techniques already implemented on surgical level and a survey of their users' requirements. Meanwhile, the authors analysed some existent literature associated with these technologies in order to clarify some concepts and know the development state of another existing projects related to them. Then, image process studies were performed to find an efficient and easy way to execute the calibration process of the tracking device, a fundamental process for any AR application (developed and explained in the "Augmented Reality Process" section). Afterwards, was designed the application workflow and conceptualized its implementation architecture. At the same time, a survey of the necessary tools and software that fit the project requirements was made. A prototype application and a web server were developed in order to test and verify the efficiency and usability of the proposed solution. Finally, after the tests and simulations were carried out an evaluation of the presented solution was made in conjunction with a survey of directions and improvements to be considered in the future.

The next section of this chapter explains briefly some important concepts needed to know the state and evolution of the existing technologies in the field as well as clarify and describe the target users and implementation environment. Issues and problems are summarized in the following section and the existing solutions are reviewed. The authors proposed solution, called by ARPEEK, is presented and in its own section and all the development's stages are also described. Finally, the conclusion and discussion are made covering the whole chapter.

BACKGROUND

Surgical planning has been linked to and associated with many successful cases in different medical specialties. Besides that, surgeons are continually looking for ways and tools to increase their accuracy and improve their performance (Herford et al., 2017).

Currently, all surgeries are preceded by a pre-operative planning phase, which consists in the definition and projection of appropriate guidelines supported by patient information or external data from other health specialties. This consists in defining several parameters to ensure a successful and simple intervention, not only for the surgeon, but also for the patient.

In this scenario, the patient's situation can be previously and meticulously analysed with time and without decision-making pressure. Thus, during surgery all those issues are eased and the surgeon may focus on his rigor and effectiveness.

Despite the unquestioned usefulness of this process, it is still difficult for the surgeon to have a perception of what impact it will have on the patient during and after intervention. This takes on an even more important role in surgeries that involve implants such as orthopaedic surgery (Ribeiro, Alves, Silva, & Campos, 2015). It would be extremely important for the surgeon to analyse the placement of the implant in the patient's body and note the actual position / location of the implant in it, which currently is only possible in real time, i.e. during surgery.

AR is defined by the integration and overlapping of virtual information over a perceptive environment and in real time allowing the user to manipulate and view information in a practical, intuitive and even exciting way (Helie, 2017). The user's perception of the combination between virtual and real content can be achieve using mobile devices, screens, see-through optical devices, monitors, headphones and fictitious windows that can interact with each other or separately.

In the surgical environment, the needed information comes from multiple medical modalities, mostly Medical Imaging, and can assume graphical or textual formats. For a medical AR application these can be anatomical models computationally generated such as soft tissues, blood vessels, nerves or solid structures, like bones or even surgical instruments (Chen et al., 2015; Fischer, Neff, Freudenstein, & Bartz, 2004). An AR application has to measure in real-time the spatial position of the camera in the user's field of view. This can be achieved using marker tracking which is a video-based method that analyses intended and pre-known elements (e.g. fiducial, magnetic or optical markers) in the video stream. (Siltanen, 2012; Conrad et al., 2016).

Allied to these technologies, mobile devices bring mobility, interaction and convenience to its user. They also potentiate graphics quality, processing power, software durability, dynamic object tracking and remote access to critical information which could solve some problems in the current existing solutions (Thomas, 2016).

Computer-aided navigation systems that use AR technologies have experienced tremendous development for minimizing the risks and improving the precision of the surgery such as in preoperative procedures for patient diagnosis.

Badiali et al. (2014) describes an AR solution that aims to aid maxillofacial surgeries. This system is composed by an optical device, the tracker of the navigation system, physical markers and a software for 3D construction models from medical images (Badiali et al., 2014). The optical device is composed by two cameras simulating human vision, which are responsible for capturing the real environment image, the sphere markers and the tracker device relative positioning for the calibration process. The system they propose performs a matching between the points previously marked in the 3D model and the ones in the patient. Thus, the surgeon is capable of using the optical device while performing the intervention without losing the three-dimensional relationship between the real scene and the virtual planning displays.

AR technologies are proposed as a helpful solution for performing tailored craniotomies by Cabrilo, Schaller, and Bijlenga (2014) with the aim of identifying and locating specific vessels for donation or surgical processes. Through the 3D angio-CT and 3D angio-MRI image modalities, the characterization of the patients external and internal carotids was done. Using face surfacing-matching systems the patient head is located and referenced to the navigation station. An operating microscope is connected to the navigation system and the microscope's real-time location, focus, and zoom parameters are defined. This allows the injection of the computer generated images in the navigated patient (Cabrilo, Schaller, & Bijlenga, 2014). Thus, this system can optimize the procedures of extracranial-to-intracranial bypass intervention providing useful anatomical information.

Hallet et al. (2015) depicts an AR guided system for minimally invasive hepatectomy resection. The 3D models are obtained in the same way of the above-described solutions and then are applied segmentation process to the original images to obtain the wanted tissues. The video camera display is connected to two cameras: an exoscopic and a laparoscopic. Then, the 3D model images are manually superimposed onto the real-time operative ones captured by each camera using the visible landmarks (Hallet et al., 2015).

An AR mobile application for basal ganglia localization is described by Hou, Ma, Zhu, and Chen (2016). Mobile Augmented Reality (MAR) applications are the integration of AR technologies into mobile devices for medical use. Combining these with a simple and effective marker tracking process, the health professional would not need to resort to any physical resource besides a mobile device and an easily detectable surface. Similarly, to the previously presented applications the computational 3D models are overlapped to the patient's body. With an image segmentation software, the tumour's centroid is calculated and an outline of the incision features to be drawn on the patient is made. The calibration between the camera and the real image is made using the gyroscope of the device and also manually. Thus, the operator performs a manual matching process in order to overlap the virtual image with the real one (Hou, Ma, Zhu, & Chen, 2016).

AUGMENTED REALITY SOLUTION TO ENHANCE THE SURGEON'S EXPERIENCE

In a near future it will be necessary to respond as quickly and qualitatively as possible to both patient needs and health professional's requirements. More than ever, it is extremely important to provide surgeons with tools to improve their interventions and procedures to make them more reliable and efficient. The guidance tools for surgery are a possible solution to this proposal. However, they do not currently gather all the state-of-art technologies potentialities.

Despite the existence of some AR solutions in this field, the current ones for surgical application require extensive investments and long configuration processes, not only because of the complexity of the tracking markers used, but also because of the expensive value of the digital motion capture devices implemented in these systems. Tracking markers, such as magnetic or optical ones, generally result in more investments and concerns about their maintenance and configuration. Despite Hou, Ma, Zhu, and Chen (2016) have presented a cheap and simple solution, the system requires some extra caution and time to the calibration process. Another disadvantage is that errors can occur due to user's manual inaccuracy.

Moreover, the few inaccuracies in the computational reconstruction of the structures, incorrect alignment with the respective real scenario and the small temporal delays are some other problems pointed to these technologies. Thus, the immersion of the user to the experience and even his total dedication to the clinical intervention are diminished by the action of these external and exhaustive factors.

The main focus of the authors in this chapter was to present and develop a solution that would improve orthopaedic surgical procedures, from its planning to its development, in a simple and viable way. With it, the surgeon would be provided with a tool that integrates the possibility to simulate and define the orthopaedic intervention guidelines with the ability to visualize them during it in an augmented way. This would be possible by overlaying the planning virtual data over the operative environment in real time. The planned 3D model visualization would help and provide support to the surgeon in certain surgery details without him to lose the perception of the environment and the patients' body.

ARPEEK: A SOLUTION FOR AN AUGMENTED REALITY EXPERIENCE

The ARPEEK solution (Figure 1) was designed and developed in order to increase and improve the interaction between health professionals and their patients, providing to the first one a tool that can supply the medical diagnosis, help performing a complete preoperative study and establish guidelines for orthopaedic surgery. Furthermore, ARPEEK combines the potential of AR technologies along with the issue of mobility and remote access to information aiming the solution to most usability problems identified to date for this kind of technologies such as visualizing and exploring the preoperative information during surgical intervention itself.

The image processing studies were developed and performed in C ++ using the OpenCV libraries. The tri-dimensional models of the human body tissues were constructed using Peek Health S.A's software (Ribeiro et al., 2015). This software application generates the 3D models after a simple upload of the respective DICOM images. This software is also responsible for all the computational planning procedures. Using this tool, the surgical team has access to multiple functions such as: perform measurements and calculations, simulate and plan the surgical procedure using templates and manipulate the graphical content to a better and complete diagnosis.

In order to submit the AR application for testing so that results of its implementation can be obtained a web server prototype was developed in Laravel using PHP associated with MySQLWorkbench tool for database architecture and development. For practical reasons this was used to simulate a platform where the physician could upload the 3D models' files associated with the patient's information. The AR mobile application communicates with this server to obtain all this data.

The mobile application was created in Unity using C#. This tool was chosen due to the easiness of developing a mobile application capable of using AR technology and also because allows the creation of a multiplatform application, i.e., hybrid type. Another favourable point of using Unity was the possibility to develop in parallel the application's layout and flow combining them with the computational vision functions for image processing requirements. Additionally, this tool allows an intuitive and dynamic interaction with graphic data (in this case tri-dimensional body tissues models) with all the possible features available.

ARPEEK (Figure 1) was developed by the authors to complement an existing solution for orthopaedic surgical planning, but the same can be valid for other situations since it is independent of the three-dimensional information used as well as its origin. The solution's system consists of six main steps (represented by the letters *a, b, c, d, e* and *f* in Figure 1). The first one is the medical imaging acquisition, from several medical modalities such as CT (Figure 1a). Those images are stored as Digital Imaging and Communications in Medicine (DICOM) standard in the Picture Archiving and Communication System (PACS) of the respective hospitals. After the registration and login process in the ARPEEK's application, the surgeon can query/retrieve the PACS's for the wanted DICOM's files. Through Peek Health S.A's software, as said above, it is possible to automatically generate the 3D models of various tissues type and then save them in several file formats, such as OBJ, which makes them available for the computational planning phase (Figure 1b).

There are some rendering techniques to generate a 3D model from a CT scan, being one of them the Surface Rendering (SR). This is defined as the visualization of a 3D object from a set of isosurfaces. These isosurfaces are generated only with points which have the same intensity. In this case, this value refers to the radiation attenuation value using the Hounsfield's scale.

There are two ways to generate isosurfaces: by using contours that are extracted from each slice in order to create a surface based on its volume or by relying on voxels with a predefined value from the Hounsfield's scale. This reconstruction can be performed by multiple algorithms being one the Marching Cubes (MC) (Ribeiro et al., 2015).

A DICOM file is composed by two parts: the pixel data and a header with the image associated metadata. The last one is organized by tags with the whole volume information for each image (CT scan's slice). This metadata refers to information not only about the patient but also about the respective series. All the information needed to implement MC's algorithm, such as thickness and position, can be obtained from the existing information in those tags, as slice thickness (0018,0050), slice location (0020,1041), number of slices (0054,0081) and space between slices (0018,0088). For further information, please refer to Ribeiro, Alves, Silva, & Campos (2015).

After the computational models generation, the surgeon can also associate to them all the needed information for the planning process such as patient personal information, medical exams' results and other physicians' opinions. An important aspect that is worth noticing is the fact that it is in this step that the remote access to all this information and to the rendered models are guaranteed. By this users abstraction approach, the surgeon and his team are now able to study and visualize all the surgical planning material in any workstation or even at home, while the entire process and changes made are also saved and updated.

The whole surgical procedure can be discussed during the planning step. At this stage, both anaesthesiologists and nurses can be informed of the surgery's goals and security's norms as well as making contributions to it. At the planning step, using this software, it is also possible to evaluate which kind of implants will be needed (e.g. plates, screws, prosthesis) and their exact dimension. By doing this, the surgeon can decrease surgical times since he knows beforehand all the surgical steps and materials needed. (Figure 1c). The next step is the operating room preparation by gathering all necessary surgical material.

For step four a mobile device running the AR application (Figure 2) and a printed landmark are necessary for the surgical assistance approach proposed (Figure 1d). These will be fundamental for implement the AR application during the surgical procedure.

At this point some of ARPEEK's advantages are beginning to be noticed since there is no need of any extra operating room preparation or devices' settings. Holding on the mobile device an attending physician or the surgeon himself it is possible, through its screen, to monitor and view the planning's studies in real time by mixing the digital content with the real environment.

Figure 1. Solution description and planning: a) image acquisition through medical image modalities; b) three dimensional models' generation; c) study and planning phase; d) settings and materials needed for intervention; e) the augmented reality solution; f) surgery final result

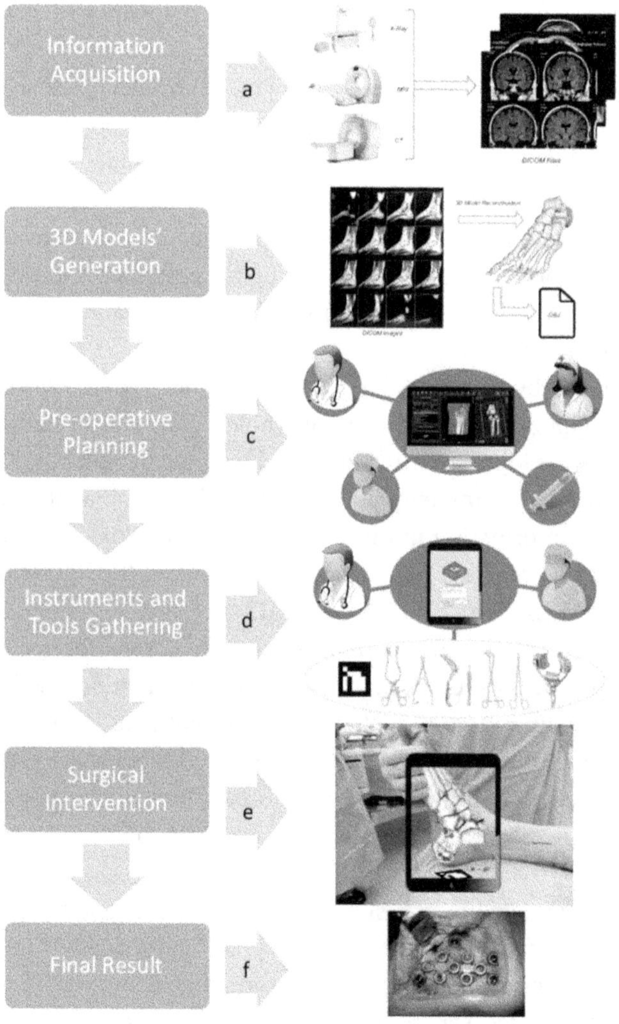

Figure 2. ARPEEK's mobile application workflow and layout: a) the login interface; b) a welcome and description interface; c) fiducial marker settings interface; d) page where the user can browse their imported models and choose one to dispose; e) AR visualization page where you can view 3D models overlapped to real environment

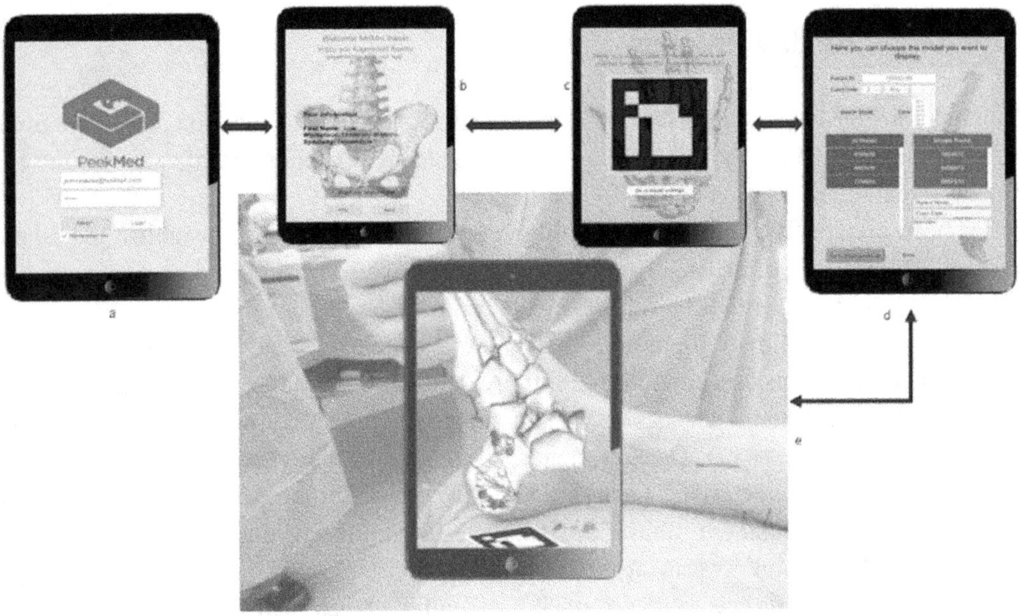

Through the landmark, the application will estimate the mobile device's position and will project the resized 3D model over the landmark as if it was the space origin. It should be noted that the model is not fixedly visualized but its size and positioning in space never varies. This means that the doctor can zoom in/out, rotate and move the device sideways without moving the 3D model. At this step and with the images mixed on the mobile device's monitor, the camera will work as the surgeon's eye, but capable of seeing beyond the actual tissues of the patient. This approach will enable the professional to interact with the graphical content so as to derive the utmost usefulness and detail from it in an extremely practical and immersive experience. (Figure 1e). As it is possible to see from Figure 1f, the final result of the surgery can be previously evaluated. This will allow the team to check and correct imperfections, suggest new approaches, increase their efficiency and accuracy and monitor all the procedure steps much better. Last but not least, this global surgical planning solution will help to turn the surgical procedure much more predictable, with higher quality, in less time and eventually with better results.

The mobile application consists in six intuitive and interactive interfaces. When the user starts running ARPEEK's application, first he needs to performs his login validating his username and password (Figure 2a). After the validation process being completed it is displayed an introduction's interface with a brief description of the system and some personal user information (Figure 2b). Here the user has the possibility to start his AR experience or go to a more descriptive interface where all the procedures and steps to be performed for using the application are described. If the "Start AR Experience" button was actioned, then it is provided to user the possibility to choose and set his favourite fiducial landmark (Figure 2c). After completing this step, the user can visualize an interface where he can search and select the wanted tri-dimensional model for AR visualization which he has previously generated and saved in his workstation (Figure 2d). Also in this moment it is presented some planning information associated with the model such as some patient information or surgery guidelines. Finally, through the button "Go to Webcam mode" it is possible to visualize the computational planning images overlapped to the real situation (Figure 2e).

The Augmented Reality Process

An AR application consists first in discovering the visualization device's location and orientation (usually a camera) and only then in the overlapping of the wanted and existing virtual data over the captured environment in real time.

As it has been previously mentioned, the calibration step is mandatory to establish the relation between the real environment dimensions and the virtual ones. This is a required parameter to correctly resize and display virtual information over the actual captured image.

In order to make the calibration possible it is necessary the existence of an image capture device associated with computer vision functions. Additionally, it has to be able to detect strategic and pre-defined points where the actual distances between them are previously known and given as input to the calibration system (Siltanen, 2012). These computer vision algorithms are basically divided in two main steps: the first one is the characteristic's extraction of the captured image, followed by the second step which is responsible for the camera calibration, i.e., the estimation of its positioning and orientation on real environment (Khandelwal, Swarnalatha, Bisht, & Prabu, 2015).

Different tracking methods have been developed for multiple areas such as computer vision, robotics or even photogrammetry (Siltanen, 2012). These methods can be differentiated based on the equipment used: sensor tracking methods, visual tracking methods and hybrid methods. Since in most augmented reality systems the camera is an implemented common device, the visual tracking methods assume an important role in AR and were the chosen ones for the presented solution.

The following procedures were performed using lower level image-processing functions included in OpenCV libraries.

From the existing tracking approaches based on computer vision, the authors in this chapter opted for those that use fiducial markers. This is due to the fact that they have shown good practical results and with execution and configuration times acceptable for real-time and clinical applications. Thus, for the marker detection the authors resorted to the descripted procedures in Figure 3.

After the image acquisition (Figure 3a) and before the actual detection of the landmark, the pre-processing phase (Figure 3b) is performed which is crucial for its success. This can be described by Program 1 which is applied to every captured frame.

After the processing phase, the contour detection process in the binary image is performed (Figure 3c). Then, the contours candidates for the desired marker, are selected considering that the fiducial marker is pre-defined and well known. Then, the contours candidates for the desired marker, are selected considering that the fiducial marker is pre-defined and well known. The selection process is performed by Program 2 which was developed according to the marker's characteristics, mainly because it is a square.

The next step of the AR development is the landmark recognition (Figure 3d). First, the perspective transformation that brings the current marker to the rectangular form is calculated. Then, with the previously calculated matrix it is applied to the chosen contour a function that outputs its representation in two-dimensional space (canonical marker image) allowing its identification.

Figure 3. Description of marker detection steps

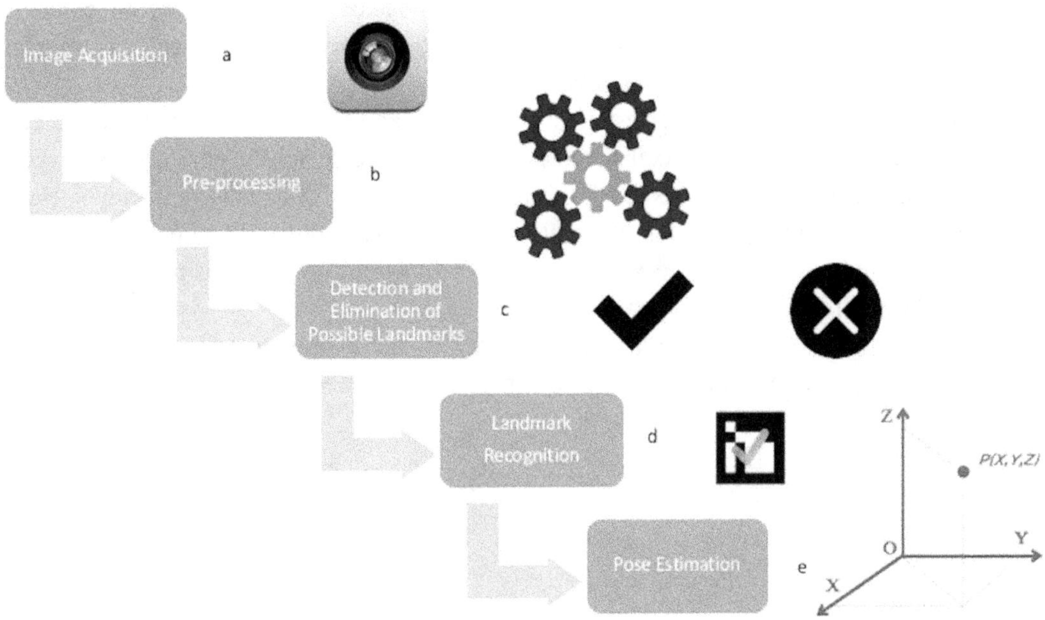

Program 1. Image pre-processing steps

```
if Camera Updated then
for each frame do
smooth the image (reduce noise);
convert image to greyscale (intensity image);
threshold image (binary image);
```

Program 2. The specifications for landmark's detection of the captured image

```
if (number of points is 4) and (points describe a convex polygon) then
check the distance between consecutive points;
if (distance is similar) and (large enough) then
calculate perimeter;
if perimeter is acceptable then
sort the contour's points in anti-clockwise order;
save the reordered contour's point as possible marker;
else
save contour as rejected;
else
save contour as rejected;
else
save contour as rejected;
```

Hereupon the supposed marker is divided in 7x7 regions which the inner 5x5 represent the real information about its id. An algorithm analyses these regions one by one and identify the colour of the same ones, which can be black or white. According to this, the contour's image matrix is transformed into binary and this value will match to the marker's id.

After sorting the points according to an established pattern regardless of the orientation of the camera, the contour corners are refined to sub pixel accuracy and they are ready for the pose estimation process.

So, at this point, the bi dimensional position of the interest contour's points is well known. However, it is necessary to estimate their position in the real world coordinate so the 3D model can be displayed according to the wanted position (Figure 3e). The OpenCV functions used for this problem are based in the so-called pinhole camera model (Figure 4).

For this model (Figure 4), the scene display is formed by the 3D points projection into the image plane using a previous calculated perspective transformation by this equation (docs.opencv.org):

$$sm' = A[R \mid t]M'$$

or

$$s\begin{bmatrix} u \\ v \\ l \end{bmatrix} = \begin{bmatrix} f_x & 0 & c_x \\ 0 & f_y & c_y \\ 0 & 0 & 1 \end{bmatrix} \begin{bmatrix} r_{11} & r_{12} & r_{13} & t_1 \\ r_{21} & r_{22} & r_{23} & t_2 \\ r_{31} & r_{32} & r_{33} & t_3 \end{bmatrix} \begin{bmatrix} X \\ Y \\ Z \\ l \end{bmatrix}$$

where:

- (X,Y,Z) are the coordinates of a 3D point in the world coordinate space;
- (u,v) are the coordinates of the projection point in pixels;
- (c_x,c_y) is a principal point that is usually at the image centre;
- f_x, f_y are the focal lengths expressed in pixel units.

With the calculation of these parameters through other OpenCV functions it is possible to estimate all the contour's points position and estimate the relative model position to them. It's important to refer that some of these equation parameters are known and pre-defined such as the landmark's dimensions. Another extremely important consideration is that, after calibration process, the landmark centre will be considered the coordinates origin, i.e., the $(0,0,0)$ point in the real world.

Therefore, it is then possible to display the three-dimensional model fully scaled by the mobile device's camera relative position to the marker and thus obtain the AR immersion.

Figure 4. Camera calibration and 3D reconstruction using pinhole camera model
Source: docs.opencv.org

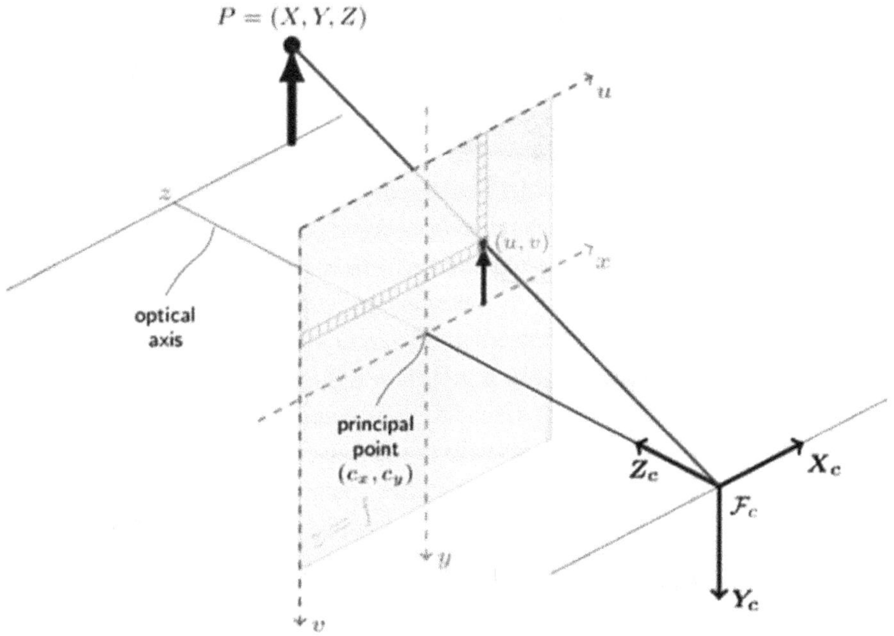

The original model will be changed and recalibrated, point by point, depending on the output parameters resulting from Unity tool´s functions for object motion which received as input some values of the previously described matrix.

The Implementation Architecture

The architecture of the implemented solution is shown in Figure 5. Integration of the main application with the hospital network and PACS system allows quick and easy access to DICOM images. At the surgeon's workstation, using Peek Health S.A's preoperative planning system, the team has the possibility to generate the 3D models and evaluate the entire surgical planning process.

The frontend server is responsible for security requirements (e.g., user access privileges, data encryption), and user interface generation. The backend is responsible for validation tasks and database accesses.

After making the necessary changes on the initial model for the study of the surgical intervention, the files are recorded through the back-end server. Thus, the surgeon will have remote access, via mobile device running the application, to all the planning work done previously.

This approach allows the user to organize and plan clinical procedures using his mobile device and what he planned with his team in the preoperative stage. With this tool, the professional can visualize through the camera of the mobile device a digital representation of the patient's structure with procedures guidelines on the real scene in a simple and intuitive way. From diagnosis to surgery, a much more immersive, efficient and complete experience is enabled for health professionals and patients.

Conrad, C., Fusaglia, M., Peterhans, M., Lu, H., Weber, S., & Gayet, B. (2016). Augmented Reality Navigation Surgery Facilitates Laparoscopic Rescue of Failed Portal Vein Embolization. *Journal of the American College of Surgeons, 223*(4), e31–e34. doi:10.1016/j.jamcollsurg.2016.06.392 PMID:27450989

Fischer, J., Neff, M., Freudenstein, D., & Bartz, D. (2004). Medical Augmented Reality based on Commercial Image Guided Surgery. *EGVE'04 Proceedings of the Tenth Eurographics Conference on Virtual Environments*, 83–86. https://doi.org/10.2312/EGVE/EGVE04/083-086

Hallet, J., Soler, L., Diana, M., Mutter, D., Baumert, T. F., Habersetzer, F., … Pessaux, P. (2015). Transthoracic minimally invasive liver resection guided by augmented reality. *Journal of the American College of Surgeons, 220*(5), e55–e60. https://doi.org/10.1016/j.jamcollsurg.2014.12.053

Helie, S. (2017). ScienceDirect Augmented reality: An ecological blend. *Cognitive Systems Research, 42*, 58–72. doi:10.1016/j.cogsys.2016.11.009

Herford, A. S., Miller, M., Lauritano, F., Cervino, G., Signorino, F., & Maiorana, C. (2017). The use of virtual surgical planning and navigation in the treatment of orbital trauma. *Chinese Journal of Traumatology, 20*(1), 9–13. doi:10.1016/j.cjtee.2016.11.002 PMID:28202368

Hou, Y. Z., Ma, L. C., Zhu, R. Y., & Chen, X. L. (2016). iPhone-Assisted Augmented Reality Localization of Basal Ganglia Hypertensive Hematoma. *World Neurosurgery, 94*, 480–492. https://doi.org/10.1016/j.wneu.2016.07.047

Khandelwal, P., Swarnalatha, P., Bisht, N., & Prabu, S. (2015). Detection of Features to Track Objects and Segmentation Using GrabCut for Application in Marker-less Augmented Reality. *Procedia Computer Science, 58*, 698–705. https://doi.org/10.1016/j.procs.2015.08.090

Pelargos, P. E., Nagasawa, D. T., Lagman, C., Tenn, S., Demos, J. V., Lee, S. J., … Yang, I. (2016). Utilizing virtual and augmented reality for educational and clinical enhancements in neurosurgery. *Journal of Clinical Neuroscience*. https://doi.org/10.1016/j.jocn.2016.09.002

Ribeiro, J., Alves, V., Silva, S., & Campos, J. (2015). *A 3D Computed Tomography Based Tool for Orthopedic Surgery Planning*. https://doi.org/10.1007/978-3-319-13407-9_8

Siltanen, S. (2012). Theory and applications of marker-based augmented reality. *Espoo 2012. VTT Science Series 3*. Retrieved from http://www.vtt.fi/publications/index.jsp

Thomas, D. J. (2016). Augmented reality in surgery: The Computer-Aided Medicine revolution. *International Journal of Surgery, 36*(October), 25. doi:10.1016/j.ijsu.2016.10.003 PMID:27741424

Chapter 8

Recommendation System:
A Potential Tool for Achieving Pervasive Health Care

Shashi Kant Srivastava
Indian Institute of Management Indore, India

Sudipendra Nath Roy
Indian Institute of Management Indore, India

ABSTRACT

Health is the most critical but very less celebrated application area of recommendation system. The purpose of this work is to put forward the present development and potential future applications of the recommendation system for the physical health of an individual and community. These recommendations are aimed to mitigate the probable future health risks. Present chapter ensembles the existing literature to illustrate the current applications of the subject. Furthermore, this put forward future scope and knowledge boundary for health recommendation system research. Because of present innovations i.e. wearable health technologies, the application of recommendation system for health has become possible. The present chapter evaluates the existing wearable health technologies and its suitability for the deployment of a responsive health recommendation system.

INTRODUCTION

Human illness is an unfortunate event seriously disrupting individual's life and his family. Mostly it brings grave emotional and economic losses. These losses are often of considerable magnitude, and many times, it is beyond the individual's ability to cope. Out of all illnesses, sudden illness is most critical since it gives very limited time to react. An alarm or a pre-signal in the event of sudden illness may result in saving of life. Timely alarm or pre-signal is feasible because nine out of ten cases reported as 'sudden illness' are in fact 'neglected' cases that deteriorated suddenly (Anogianakis et al., 1998). Presently, timely reporting of individual's health status area receives increasing attention from multiple disciplines of research. In the present chapter, we have elaborated one of the applications of information

DOI: 10.4018/978-1-5225-2851-7.ch008

hours. Also, when alarmed, patients might restrain himself or herself from doing some activities like becoming anxious, stressed or angry in a life situation for cardiac patients; and control eating habits for hyperlipidemia or obese patients. So, the incidence of attack will eventually be lesser in number under constant monitoring system which is a necessary criterion to control a lifestyle disease.

CONCEPT OF RECOMMENDATION SYSTEM

Recommendation system (RS) is one of the very common applications of IT in recent years (Huang et al., 2015). Most of the present applications of RS are business applications. These applications are, such as recommending products to the customers on Amazon.com (Linden, Smith, & York, 2003), suggesting movies to watch by Netflix (Koren, 2008) and MovieLens (Miller, Albert, Lam, Konstan, & Riedl, 2003), recommending music to listen to Last.fm and Pandora Radio, and recommendation news to read by VERSIFI Technologies (Billsus, Brunk, Evans, Gladish, & Pazzani, 2002). The efforts to use the technology of RS beyond business application are very rare. However, researchers have attempted to explore the application of RS for disaster mitigation (Srivastava & Ray, 2016).

Recommendation system is defined as the system which recommends an appropriate product or service after learning the customers' need (Choi, Kang, & Jeon, 2006). A health recommender systems (HRS) is a specialization of a Recommender Systems (RS) (Francesco Ricci, Lior Rokach, Bracha Shapira, & Paul B. Kantor, 2011; Wiesner & Pfeifer, 2014). Francesco Ricci et al. (2011) defined HRS as a piece of non-confidential and scientifically proven medical recommendation that is of interest not linked to the individual's medical history. However, this definition is not consistent with the accepted definition of RS, where RS is personalized based on individual interest and need. Therefore, based on the existing definition of the RS and HRS, we define HRS as the system that recommends most suitable health advice after learning from the available health related data of the patient/ customer in the event of a probable future health risk.

As HRS is a relatively new concept and previous commercial examples of recommender systems which we have discussed in the first paragraph of this section, were, by and large suggests only on the basis of specific requirement of a particular consumer, is missing in the definition of HRS suggested by Francesco Ricci et al. (2011). As per their definition health recommendation is independent of a patient's previous medical record and rather a contextual momentous suggestion. From the perspective of clinicians, this seems little bizarre because one must be aware of a patient's previous ailments, food habits, age, sex, any idiosyncratic feature like the allergy to certain medicines (sulfur containing medicines), etc. before giving a health suggestion to a healthy or ill individual for preventive or curative purpose. We have incorporated recommendation on the basis of previous information for a specific person just like movie recommender system or product recommendations system. In fact, without taking consideration of a patient's medical history, there is a high probability that a health suggestion may aggravate a disease or worsen his health condition. So we have incorporated this necessary medically relevant angle while defining HRS in our definition.

The technology of recommendation system is very recent. On the contrary, health recommendations are as old as the human civilization. Therefore, before recommender system, there are various existing models of HRS. Some of these are as follow:

- Health prescription by a qualified medical practitioner
- Exercise prescription by Gym trainer
- Diet prescription by nutritionist
- Vernacular health recommendation by elders

COMPARISON AND CONTRAST RS AND HRS

RS is defined as the system that recommends customer an appropriate product or service after learning from his needs (Choi, Kang, & Jeon, 2006). There are various other ways also by which RS is defined. It is advisable to understand these differences so that we may understand the various applications of RS and get and better insight into the potential applications of HRS. Another definition of the recommender system is that it is a system that predicts user preferences for consumables based on information about users (Masters, Madhyastha, & Shakouri, 2008). The first definition of recommendation is based on the needs of the individual whereas in second it is based on the user characteristics. Therefore, the concepts of user preference and user information are the two key components of RS. Mavridou, Kehagias, Tzovaras, and Hassapis (2013) define a recommender system as any system that produces individualized recommendations as output or has the effect of guiding the user in a personalized way to interesting or useful objects in a large space of possible options. Another definition also is in line with the previous definition of RS, as a system that selects a set of objects from a superset according to user's preference (Montes-Garcia, Alvarez-Rodriguez, Labra-Goyo, & Martinez-Merino, 2013). Furthermore, other researchers defined RS as a system that produces personalized suggestions to the user from a large space of possible options (Ferreira-Satler et al., 2012). All three definitions had emphasized on choosing the best option keeping user information from a larger option basket. Another definition suggested a recommender system as estimating ratings for unseen items by a user (Mei, Yang, Hua, & Li, 2011). A health recommender systems (HRS) is a specialization of Recommender Systems (RS) (Francesco Ricci et al., 2011; Wiesner & Pfeifer, 2014). Francesco Ricci et al. (2011) and Wiesner and Pfeifer (2014) define HRS as a piece of non-secretive and proven scientific medical information used to recommendable item of interest that is not linked to the individual's medical history. However, this definition is not consistent with the accepted definition of RS, where RS is personalized based on individual interest and need. Therefore, based on the existing definition of the RS and HRS, we define health recommendation system as the system that recommends most suitable health advice after learning from the available health related data of the patient/ customer as soon as the event of a probable future health risk occurs. There are multiple options available in case of RS, and it is in need of a user whether to go for it or not. But, in the case of HRS, the criteria of options may not be suitable and in most of the cases, recommendation will be of compulsory type. Because if a patient is not adhering to the recommended suggestion, it might harm him/her to a dangerous extent.

RELATIONSHIP BETWEEN RECOMMENDATION SYSTEM AND HEALTH

HRS is a technology phenomenon that is yet to become common among masses. Also, utility and impact of HRS is enormous if opted at a large scale and updated suitably for each ill patient cases. The signifi-

cance of the technology of RS a
of health is innumerable.

Instant medical advice at th
patients suffering from any acu
patient health, monitoring in a
Nevertheless, for some cases li
forgetful patients HRS can also
be resulted in a severe deterior
cannot be cured by medicines;
prescription which has been su
diminished ailment aggravation
this context.

Real-time Medication Mon
in Europe has already been pro
to the therapeutic protocols as
had been done for six months a
oral hypoglycemic agents. The
patients when combined with re
medicine therapy dyad (Vervlo
a dose, any missed dose in a d
time intervals. In extended stu
diabetic patients receiving oral
people. Patients were randomi
the similar pattern to the trial
the prescribed therapeutic regi
stick to the standardized medic
platform, it is limpid that we ca
gestions or medical advice that
receiving the guidance through
of literature concerning with cl
based HRS system has been st
can be convinced that it will or
ensure healthy living for the hu

Health recommender system
informs and update patients fr
analysis constitutes of real-time
status. Then the medical profess
ity to be pursued by the patient
Greatest difference of HRS wit
system and mainly developed d
health condition from past data
which were being monitored. A
ics personnel issues most prop

Wearable Health Gadgets

The real-time HRS has become a reality only because of the existence of wearable health gadgets. A wearable health gadget can capture real-time health information of an individual. Presently, the various form of this health data ais: energy burned, walking done, running performed, pulse rate, and measuring individual's blood pressure. With the help of present gadgets, one may plan his/her exercise schedule and can receive real-time suggestions based on his/her earlier prepared plan which can be provided as recommendation to him/her.

In recent times, where wearable health gadgets are becoming popular every day, it can take this concept to a socially implementable format. Synchronization of such health gadgets with a mobile phone (Android and iOS platform) has given a new dimension to mHealth initiatives. Wearable health gadgets are an important precondition for the real-time HRS. Wearable gadgets for the purpose of activity monitoring have become very common in the developed countries. The capability of these gadgets includes activity monitoring like walking, running, step climbing, etc. and then enumerate an overall result and inform the user about the total amount of calories burned on a particular day. This information helps an individual to plan his day accordingly, to meet his/her exercise target. Many of these gadgets also provide recommendations to perform activities based on preplanned exercise target. The present development and future scenario of these gadgets are shown as in Table 1. A thorough scrutiny of existing devices that are available via e-tailing companies like Amazon, Flipkart, Snapdeal, etc. is tabulated in the aforementioned table. The brief search finally results from six different existing devices which are compatible with iOS (Apple platform) and Android mobile operating systems. Also, some of the mentions were being extracted from different scientific publications and technological advertisements related to the futuristic wearable gadgets for the purpose of monitoring health metrics. The eminent journal 'Nature' published one such article by Gao et al. (2016) for monitoring blood glucose, lactate, and other necessary blood ions (sodium and potassium) from the sweat analysis. US-based wearable health device manufacturer company Gentag is also quite optimistic about their newly innovated product nfc-skin-patch. It is an

Table 1. Existing and futuristic health devices

S.N.	Existing Devices	Platform	Measure	Price in USD
1	Apple showcases watch	iOS	Fitness tracker	40
2	Polar H7 Blue Tooth	iOS and Android	Heartrate and Fitness tracker	50-150
3	Fii iFever Smart Thermometer	iOS and Android	Temperature	35
4	Misfit Shine Activity Tracker and Sleep Monitor	Android	Activity and Sleep Monitor	55
5	Sokos Bluetooth Smart Fitness Tracker Armband I Wristband I Bracelet	iOS and Android	Heartrate and Fitness tracker	40
6	Philips Health Watch	iOS and Android	Activity, Heartrate, and Sleep	200
S.N.	**Futuristic Devices**	**Source**	**Measure**	
1	The wearable sweat monitor	Published in Nature	Glucose, Lactate, Sodium, and Potassium	Not Available
2	Gentag smart skin patches	gentag.com/nfc-skin-patches/	Diabetes monitoring	Not Available

advanced device in the same product line of the organization which has a very diverse application arena from temperature monitoring and at the same time can serve as a painless diabetic patch (Gentag, 2016). We tabulated all the eight such major health gadgets of the market in Table 1.

Table 1 demonstrates the capability of these gadgets. Besides activity monitoring, there are gadgets that can monitor heartbeat, sleep pattern, and blood pressure. Also, monitoring of glucose, lactate, sodium, and potassium within the human body is not far. Real-time monitoring of all these health information provides innumerable data analytics and recommendation opportunities. The stakeholders involved in these opportunities are doctors, medical researchers, data scientists, and last but not the least patients. As a result, most of the lifestyle diseases can be monitored thoroughly, and appropriate recommendation can be provided to the patients based on the real-time data.

Mobile Apps

Mobile and computer technology had demonstrated a rapid growth in the past two decades. This growth has resulted in the new and innovative use of these technologies that were not imagined earlier. In the year 2003, the need for strengthening eHealth was realized (Almarri & Bhatti, 2015). Then, mHealth was conceptualized to further improve the healthcare network in the year 2009 by connecting wireless technologies in healthcare network (Almarri & Bhatti, 2015). As a result, in training, the healthcare professional's mobile apps have started playing a role. However, the role of mobile apps in the healthcare delivery to the patient is quite limited even today. To assess the role of mobile apps in the healthcare business, researchers conducted a research and reviewed the 500 medical mobile applications (Obiodu & Obiodu, 2012). These applications were in the market in the way back 2012 and were used for various purposes. Then, it was found that most of these apps were free of cost. As far as, the use of mobile apps at a patient end is concerned, according to Handel (2011), mobile applications are becoming very effective tools for a patients as well. They are sources of health information for patient and also serve as self-management tools. Although most of the mobile apps at present are used by individuals but mobile apps have a possibility to be used for public healthcare programs (Almarri & Bhatti, 2015). Researchers empirically found that there is a positive attitude towards apps and predicted that in future the use of mobile apps for healthcare will increase (Koehler, Vujovic, & McMenamin, 2013).

Medical Data Analytics

Because of the use of Internet, health gadgets, and mobile apps, there are unprecedented changes happening in healthcare services domain. Applications of these agents in healthcare has given an enormous amount of data, and improvements in the IT industry has given the capacity to store this data. Furthermore, development in IT human capability and capacity has made a complex analysis of this data possible.

We have explained earlier that sensors of wearable devices can measure physiological conditions of an individual. On the scale of time, these data are monitored for hours, minutes, and eventually for seconds. Therefore, these data are ready for data analytics. A correlation between the data observed from a sensor and medical diagnoses can be found with the help of machine learning algorithms. Data of multiple individuals will result in the big data example. Analysis of the big data may result in the further improvements of the medical diagnosis. Also, the data availability gives data analyst an opportunity of potential innovative insights. However, one must not forget that yet this data does not have an acceptable relational study to clinical conditions. And presently society does not have enough technical necessary information resulted from the analysis. We all know sweat is rich in chemical and hence rich in relevant information for disease. Along with that, it is quite prudent to monitor whether a person in dehydrated/fatigue by sweat analysis. Imagine the world when your biological indicators were being constantly known to the back-end clinicians in real-time, and they are suggesting you an apt therapeutic medication depending on the previous medical record and current test results. Health recommendation if hinged on diagnostic test results, will not only become much more accurate to provide a quality medical care, but also help a patient to act in timely manner for an illness (Cooper, 2016).

The future is not very far when our household items like chair, door or refrigerators were being connected to the internet and we will turn off the light of washroom via the internet which we forgot to switch off while leaving the house. This kind of technology is known as "Internet of Things" and are getting well nurtured to build smart homes in near future. However, our interest lies in providing you proper health guidance in a timely fashion and in order to do so, we must cling to existing technological landscape and the already invented products. One of such product is 'Smart Cushion' by Darma Inc. to monitor a person's sitting posture, stress level and sitting time to provide necessary recommendation via an Android mobile app. Depending on how much time a person is sitting or sitting posture, cushion provides information; utilizing which, recommendation had been appeared in the mobile app to rectify the sitting position or other suggestion for healthy leaving. Although a cushion is not a wearable device, it entirely relies on the principle of health recommendation system to work and the days are probably not far when the cushion will be replaced by a small device in your back pocket purse (Darma Cushion, 2016).

We often get irritated by our own devices like mobile, tablet, laptop or smart watch when it shows 'low charge' icon. It is really a herculean task to remember charge level of each of one's devices at proper time! Apart from it, we also must remember without the renewable energy, neither our ecosystem will be sustainable and nor any technological gadget. Keeping environment sustainability in mind, 'AMPY Mov Live Charged' had been manufactured. This wearable motion charger can convert kinetic energy of movements into battery power for smartphone or other wearable (AMPY, 2016). Imagine if your own wearable device that provides you healthy living, takes care of the environment as well. Nonetheless, you don't need to charge it too! Doesn't it sound good?

The possibility of new invention is enormous and with the upcoming trend of Internet of things, linking with multiple gadgets and synchronizing with wearable device can contribute to the HRS technology to determine healthy living of a person to a great extent. So, the future of this upcoming technology is both manifold and promising to a great level.

SUMMARY

Present society is altogether different to what it was used to be in the previous generations. Mechanization and computerization are an essential part of the present civilization. These have led to an increase in mental work by humans on the cost of physical work. The fine balance of physical and mental activity is distorted leading to the diseases commonly termed as lifestyle diseases. These diseases are numerous in numbers but mostly related to metabolic disorders. The unfortunate part of these diseases are that; they surface mostly at the critical stage of disease and the progress of these diseases remain unmonitored. These diseases are entirely dependent on individual's lifestyle and cannot be generalized to a larger population to deliver a permanent cure. Therefore, they need personalized attention. Recommendation system is one such technology that gives a personalized recommendation to the individuals based on his/her personal need. If personalized health status can be monitored on the real-time basis, this technology has the potential to give health recommendations for an individual. Broadly, personalized health recommendation based on recommender system principle is termed as Health Recommender System (HRS). Sensing and storing the individual's health metrics has become viable due to advances in the modern sensors and IT hardware's. Present wearable health gadget gives this health related data as energy burned/calories utilized, walking speed and duration, running performed, pulse rate, and measuring individual's blood pressure. Real-time glucose, potassium, sodium, and lactate monitoring is also in verse. These new innovations have made human capable to track the lifestyle diseases almost on real-time basis. Medical data analytics performed on the health-related sensors data which has been obtained through the gadgets; can provide the real-time health status of an individual. Based on which the HRS center can deliver the messages, obeying upon which he or she may prepare his/her health plans. Although, technically HRS is feasible in the present world; it is, however not without challenges. There are innumerable social challenges that are associated with this life changing technology. Privacy of data and its repercussion on the insurance business is one of such major challenge. HRS being an IT related subject has the vulnerability for its manipulation with mal-intention which is also a challenge that cannot be overlooked. However, it can be undoubtedly a major breakthrough in assisting twenty-first century's human health care if these challenges have been taken care of by the competent authorities.

REFERENCES

Al Ameen, M., Liu, J., & Kwak, K. (2012). Security and Privacy Issues in Wireless Sensor Networks for Healthcare Applications. *Journal of Medical Systems*, *36*(1), 93–101. doi:10.1007/s10916-010-9449-4 PMID:20703745

Almarri, A., & Bhatti, T. (2015). Consumers Attitude towards the Use of Mobile Health Apps: An Empirical Review. *Proceedings of Second International Conference on Electrical and Electronics Engineering, Clean Energy and Green Computing*, 56–61.

AMPY. (2016). *AMPY Mov Live charged*. Retrieved August 8, 2016, from http://www.getampy.com/

Angius, G., & Raffo, L. (2008). A Sleep Apnoea Keeper in a Wearable Device for Continuous Detection and Screening during Daily Life. *Computers in Cardiology*, *35*, 433–436.

Anogianakis, G., Maglavera, S., Pomportsis, A., Bountzioukas, S., Beltrame, F., & Orsi, G. (1998). Medical emergency aid through telematics: Design, implementation guidelines and analysis of user requirements for the MERMAID project. *International Journal of Medical Informatics*, *52*(1–3), 93–103. doi:10.1016/S1386-5056(98)00128-2 PMID:9848406

Billsus, D., Brunk, C., Evans, C., Gladish, B., & Pazzani, M. (2002). Adaptive Interfaces for Ubiquitous Web Access: Allowing mobile users to access any information at any time from any location. *Communications of the ACM*, *45*(5), 34–38. doi:10.1145/506218.506240

Chakraborty, B., & Yoshida, T. (2016). Design of a Framework for Wellness Determination and Subsequent Recommendation with Personal Informatics. *2016 AAAI Spring Symposium Series*, 332–336.

Mavridou, E., Kehagias, D. D., Tzovaras, D., & Hassapis, G. (2013). Mining affective needs of automotive industry customers for building a mass-customization recommender system. *Journal of Intelligent Manufacturing*, *24*(2), 251–265. doi:10.1007/s10845-011-0579-4

MedicineNet. (2016). *Dentition of Lifestyle disease*. Retrieved September 12, 2016, from http://www.medicinenet.com/script/main/art.asp?articlekey=38316

Mei, T., Yang, B., Hua, X.-S., & Li, S. (2011). Contextual Video Recommendation by Multimodal Relevance and User Feedback. *ACM Transactions on Information Systems*, *29*(2), 10. doi:10.1145/1961209.1961213

Miller, B. N., Albert, I., Lam, S. K., Konstan, J. a., & Riedl, J. T. (2003). MovieLens unplugged: experiences with an occasionally connected recommender. *Proceedings of the 8th international conference on Intelligent user interfaces - IUI '03*, 263–266. doi:10.1145/604045.604094

Montes-Garcia, A., Alvarez-Rodriguez, J. M., Labra-Goyo, J. E., & Martinez-Merino, M. (2013). Towards a journalist-based news recommendation system : The Wesomender approach. *Expert Systems with Applications*, *40*(17), 6735–6741. doi:10.1016/j.eswa.2013.06.032

Morrell, T. G., & Kerschberg, L. (2012). Personal Health Explorer : A Semantic Health Recommendation System. In *Data Engineering Workshops (ICDEW), 2012 IEEE 28th International Conference on.* IEEE. doi:10.1109/ICDEW.2012.64

Obiodu, V., & Obiodu, E. (2012). An Empirical Review of the Top 500 Medical Apps in a European Android Market. *Journal of Mobile Technology in Medicine*, *1*(4), 22–37. doi:10.7309/jmtm.74

Ricci, Rokach, Shapira, & Kantor. (2011). *Recommender systems handbook*. 10.1007/978-0-387-85820-3

Rivero-Rodríguez, A., Konstantinidis, S. T., Sanchez-Bocanegra, & Fernández-Luque, C. L. (2013). A Health Information Recommender System : enriching YouTube Health Videos with Medline Plus Information by the use of SnomedCT terms. *Proceedings of the 26th IEEE International Symposium on Computer-Based Medical Systems,* 257–261. doi:10.1109/CBMS.2013.6627798

Sardini, E., & Serpelloni, M. (2010). Instrumented Wearable Belt for Wireless Health Monitoring. *Procedia Engineering*, *5*, 580–583. doi:10.1016/j.proeng.2010.09.176

Schoonen, A. J. M., Schmidt, F. J., Hasper, H., Verbrugge, D. A., Tiessen, R. G., & Lerk, C. F. (1990). Development of a potentially wearable glucose sensor for patients with diabetes mellitus : Design and in- vitro evaluation. *Biosensors & Bioelectronics*, *5*(1), 37–46. doi:10.1016/0956-5663(90)80025-9 PMID:2310541

Sezgin, E., & Ozkan, S. (2013). A systematic literature review on Health Recommender Systems A Systematic Literature Review on Health Recommender Systems. *The 4th IEEE International Conference on E-Health and Bioengineering - EHB*. doi:<ALIGNMENT.qj></ALIGNMENT>10.1109/EHB.2013.6707249

Srivastava, S. K., & Ray, S. (2016). Disasters and Recommender System: Setting the Research Agenda for Developing Nations. *International Journal of Innovation, Management and Technology*, *7*, 52–56. doi:10.18178/ijimt.2016.7.2.644

Timmerer, C., Ebrahimi, T., & Pereira, F. (2015). Toward a new assessment of quality. *Computer*, *48*(3), 108–110. doi:10.1109/MC.2015.89

Vervloet, M., Van Dijk, L., Santen-reestman, J., Van Vlijmen, B., Bouvy, M. L., & De Bakker, D. H. (2011). Improving medication adherence in diabetes type 2 patients through Real-time Medication Monitoring : A Randomised Controlled Trial to evaluate the effect of monitoring patients ' medication use combined with short message service (SMS) reminders. *BMC Health Services Research*, *11*(1), 1. doi:10.1186/1472-6963-11-5 PMID:21199575

Vervloet, M., Van Dijk, L., Van Vlijmen, B., Van Wingerden, P., Bouvy, M. L., & De Bakker, D. H. (2012). SMS reminders improve adherence to oral medication in type 2 diabetes patients who are real-time electronically monitored. *International Journal of Medical Informatics*, *81*(9), 594–604. doi:10.1016/j.ijmedinf.2012.05.005 PMID:22652012

Wendel, S., Dellaert, B. G. C., Ronteltap, A., & Van Trijp, H. C. M. (2013). Consumers' intention to use health recommendation systems to receive personalized nutrition advice. *BMC Health Services Research*, *13*(1), 126. doi:10.1186/1472-6963-13-126 PMID:23557363

Wiesner, M., & Pfeifer, D. (2014). Health recommender systems: Concepts, requirements, technical basics and challenges. *International Journal of Environmental Research and Public Health*, *11*(3), 2580–2607. doi:10.3390/ijerph110302580 PMID:24595212

Zaverucha, G. M., & Cercone, N. (2007). Web Based Health Recommender System Using Rough Sets, Survival Analysis and Rule Based Expert Systems. In *Rough Sets* (pp. 491–499). Fuzzy Sets, Data Mining and Granular Computing.

Chapter 9
Real-Time Healthcare Intelligence in Organ Transplantation:
Real-Time Intelligence in Organ Transplantation

Bruno Fernandes
University of Minho, Portugal

Cecília Coimbra
University of Minho, Portugal

António Abelha
University of Minho, Portugal

ABSTRACT

Organ transplantation is the best and often the only treatment for patients with end-stage organ failure. However, the universal shortage of deceased donors results in a worrying situation that must be addressed. Brain dead donors constitute the largest share of organ donors, but identifying a patient that may progress to brain death can be a complex task. Therefore, the urgent need of intelligent solutions to support the decision-making process is crucial in critical areas as the organ transplantation is. This work aims at acquiring knowledge on the potential organ donor criteria for further detection and implementing a platform to assist the process of identification of potential organ donors at Centro Hospitalar do Porto – Hospital de Santo António. The developed system is currently implemented and displays a steady and competent behavior providing consequently a way to have more control of the information needed for the decision-making process

DOI: 10.4018/978-1-5225-2851-7.ch009

INTRODUCTION

In the field of organ donation, an early detection of potential donors is crucial. There are many factors that influence the number of potential donors but, regardless of that, it is known that the main source of all deceased donations come from Brain Dead (BD) donors, implying that most potential deceased donors must be localized in the Intensive Care Units (ICUs) and Emergency Departments (EDs) in patients who are victims of stroke or other severe brain events (Rudge, Matesanz, Delmonico, & Chapman, 2012; Fernandes, Gomes, Ermida, & Vardasca, 2015).

A comprehensive review of organ donation considers BD patients as the ideal multiorgan donors and, as a result, the major source of solid organs for transplantation are provided by BD patients (Rudge, Matesanz, Delmonico, & Chapman, 2012; Erwin, Kompanje, Jansen, & de Groot, 2013).

Particularly focusing on BD donation, the main objective is to monitor deceased organ donation potential, evaluate performance and identify key areas for improvement (Matesanz, 2001).

In this regard, clinical medical records can be valuable if used to full advantage since they hold a wealth of information about the patient's medical history, prescriptions, physician notes, etc. collected from the various Healthcare Information Systems (HIS) (Gong, et al., 2008; Raja, Mitchell, Day, & Hardin, 2008; Zhou, Han, Chankai, Prestrud, & Brooks, 2006).

To grant accurate and timely information, these HIS that provide access to electronic patient records play an expressive role in optimizing the support of adequate decision-making. Therefore, it is no surprise that in hospitals, the complexity of environments where people and information are distributed expects considerable coordination and communication among the professionals that work in such settings (Machado, Alves, Abelha, & Neves, 2007).

Indeed, the exchange and share of clinical knowledge among medical information systems is an important feature to improve healthcare systems, quality of diagnosis, but mainly, to improve quality in patient treatment (Peixoto, Santos, Abelha, & Machado, 2012).

Another important part of this process is actual people. Individuals who are responsible for making decisions in organizations are aware that timely and precise information is powerful enough to improve business performance (Santos & Ramos, 2006). That's where a Decision Support System (DSS) fits in as a system that intends to support business decision makers in semi-structured or unstructured decision situations working with decision makers as adjuncts, extending their capabilities but not replacing their judgment. As a matter of fact, this type of systems was aimed at decisions that required judgment or could not be completely supported by algorithms (Turban, Sharda, & Delen, 2011).

That said, and knowing that coding, storing and transmitting knowledge in organizations is not new, recently the organizational and managerial practice has become more knowledge-focused, and hospitals are not indifferent to that (Hahn & Subramani, 2000; Alavi & Leidner, 2005).

To best describe the decision support solution's architecture and practice, the concept of Business Intelligence (BI) is gaining ground (Cortes, 2005). BI characterizes a variety of activities to collect all the necessary data to make solid business decisions such as creating a data warehouse and/or data mart to store the data and handling front-end analytical tools. Altogether, this set of tools delivers end-users a high-level solution so they can make better, informed decisions counting on reports, predictions and/or analytical views (Turban, Rainer, & Potter, 2005).

Thus, BI is mainly referred to as a broad category of applications and technologies for gathering, storing, analyzing and providing access to data in order to deliver decision makers all the tools they need to obtain competitive advantages through quick business understanding and critical insights (Airinei & Homocianu, 2009; Ivan & Velicanu, 2015).

For purposes of increasing the availability of organs in CHP and trying to solve the problem of crippling delay in the potential donor referral, the main goal of this project is to acquire knowledge on how to design and develop new features resulting in a high-level solution applicable in clinical context. That must result in a useful and accurate tool so that the transplant team at CHP can improve their results.

As a result of a work previously done, a repository of potential organ donors and the mechanisms responsible for feeding it in real-time are already defined and will be used in this project.

Given the complexity of a project with this magnitude, it was decided that it would be better to divide it into several specific objectives:

- Regarding the potential organ donors identification model:
  - Perform a longitudinal study from the actual transplanted at CHP in the past years for feature extraction based on the frequency analysis in order to define a more accurate potential donor pattern;
  - Discuss the observed results with the transplant team at CHP in order to describe the structure of the model to apply.
- Regarding the repository of potential organ donors:
  - Analyze and study the existent HIS at CHP to ensure their interoperability, as well as the architecture of the previously defined repository;
  - Correct any possible situations that are not being captured correctly or that may be excluded by computer error;
  - Introduce new potential donor detection filters defined in the previous stage.
- Regarding the web platform:
  - Develop an intuitive user interface allowing a real-time graphical tracking of potential donors;
  - Define a notification system to alert responsible members whenever a new possible donor with a certain level of potential is identified;
  - Provide BI tools for statistical analysis and study of the data collected.

All things considered, it is possible to construct complex and rigorous Clinical Decision Support Systems (CDSSs) based on BI technologies with data from the various HIS that, when built upon a firm basis, can take the clinical decision-making to a whole new level.

BACKGROUND

Organ donation counts on many variables that must be taken into account when identifying potential organ donors. The use of IT solutions can provide an added value in facilitating the process of potential donors referral using the different existing HIS.

Healthcare organizations, as many others, are striving to make sense of the rapidly increasing volume and variety of data generated by both internal and external resources (Işık, Jones, & Sidorova, 2013). To face the challenge of how to make sense of the raw data inside relational databases and produce meaningful information for executive professionals to make effective decisions in the diverse clinical areas, the concept of CDSSs emerged (Kawamoto, Houlihan, Balas, & Lobach, 2005; Ali, Nassif, & Capretz, 2013).

By applying the right set of information technologies, it is possible to develop CDSSs that use the information provided by the various HIS for decision-making in more or less critical situations supporting the decision made by healthcare providers. Combined with BI, these systems can provide relevant information for the decision-making process improving the availability and overall quality of that information (Santos & Ramos, 2006).

The development of this type of systems is being encouraged to support new knowledge construction, processes improvement, pattern recognition and interpretation in large amounts of data, localization and development of organizational competencies and experience sharing (Santos & Ramos, 2006).

Within the scope of transplantation, some promising solutions and proposals are emerging to solve the inherent difficulty and complexity in order to improve the potential organ donors screening efficiency.

HEALTHCARE INTELLIGENCE IN ORGAN TRANSPLANTATION

Organ Donation and Transplantation Activities

Transplantation is the treatment of choice for severe organ failure. Despite this, the number of patients waiting for one or more organs is still increasing in Europe and as the shortage of organs has become more critical, new proposals have been developed to increase the organ donation potential (Jansen, et al., 2010; Irving, et al., 2012).

In Portugal, as in most countries, many systematic approaches and programs to increase organ donor rates and also to develop deceased donation to its maximum potential have been implemented, such as the initiation of the presumed consent legislation (Rudge, Matesanz, Delmonico, & Chapman, 2012). (Matesanz, 2001; Erwin, Kompanje, Jansen, & de Groot, 2013; Matesanz, 2001).

Even though there is no consensus on uniform criteria for defining a potential organ donor, a comprehensive review of organ donation considers BD patients the ideal multiorgan donors. As a result, the major source of solid organs for transplantation is provided by BD patients (Erwin, Kompanje, Jansen, & de Groot, 2013; Rudge, Matesanz, Delmonico, & Chapman, 2012). The work of the transplant team at CHP focuses on determining precursors of brain death that can provide significant results in creating a reliable pool of potential organ donors. As so, potential organ donors should be identified as soon as possible and should never be missed or delayed and it is desirable to identify a potential organ donor as early as possible to achieve a donor conversion rate as high as possible (Jansen, et al., 2010).

However, detection and management of potential organ donors is a complex process which takes several elements in consideration (Irving, et al., 2012).

Healthcare Information Systems

In medical science, where lives are at stake, a perfect scenario would be for all healthcare professionals to be perfectly skilled and informed, and for healthcare to be a field of order, knowledge and defined procedures even though uncertainty is a part of everyday life in surgical decision-making. However, one of the greatest concerns in nowadays' organizations is to introduce technology into their environments, and hospitals are not an exception. Consequently, HIS have been introduced in order to improve the quality of healthcare delivery (Jalote-Parmar, 2009; Palazzo, et al., 2013; Cardoso, et al., 2014; Khodambashi, 2013).

The Data Sources level represents all the operational environment of the application. These Data Sources are represented as databases including the data from different operational systems, responsible for feeding the Data Warehouse. They represent the origin of information intended to collect and make available through the Data Warehouse and they also represent the diverse operational activity's support systems used in an organization, in the form of HIS (Cortes, 2005).

The Data Warehouse (DW) level represents the storage environment that include the data validation and transformation before storing it in the DW. There always exist some kind of treatment to perform over the data before integrating it into the analytic repository. The area where this happens is called the Data Staging Area. Here, sequential search algorithms and text transformation procedures predominate, called the Extract, Transform and Load (ETL) procedures.

Above the Data Staging Area is the DW which is the analytical repository where data is stored after correctly transformed and integrated. It is over the DW that a set of services with the objective to provide information to end-users is implemented. This set of services includes a variety of utilities such as multidimensional analysis servers that can be later accessed by Online Analytical Processing (OLAP) tools, BI servers, Data Mining engines, amongst others (Cortes, 2005; Gardner, 1998).

The Business Analytics level is characterized as the set of technologies that support real-time analytics, enabling end-users to interact and explore the data from the repository previously created. Here the user is provided with a set of dynamic analysis tools that can be used to query data, generate reports or identify trends and patterns in data. That's where the interaction with the users takes place and where they can communicate with the system and analyze the presented results. This is one of the reasons why the user interface must be specially designed for an intuitive interaction.

KNOWLEDGE DISCOVERY IN DATABASES

Knowledge Discovery in Databases (KDD) is a fast-evolving research field which development is targeted to the benefit of practical, social and economic fields, amongst others. The motivation for this growth is linked primarily to the existence of a powerful technology for collecting, storing and managing large amounts of data, also known as big data. Most of this data hold valuable information like patterns and trends that can be utilized to improve business decisions. However, considering that the data is collected into databases, it became necessary to develop automatic processes for data analysis, like Data Mining (DM) (Rezende, 2003).

To best analyze and comprehend large volumes of data, several studies have been conducted in order to develop knowledge extraction techniques, also known as Data Mining. This process of KDD aims at finding knowledge from a set of data so it can be used in decision-making processes. Therefore, an important requirement is that this knowledge is human-understandable, as well as useful and interesting for end-users, generally the decision-makers, in a way this knowledge can support their decision-making process (Rezende, 2003; Fayyad, Piatetsky-Shapiro, & Smyth, 1996).

TEXT MINING

As the Data Mining techniques have been developed to deal with structured data, specific Text Mining techniques to deal with unstructured data were conceived (Rezende, 2003).

By applying the right set of information technologies, it is possible to develop CDSSs that use the information provided by the various HIS for decision-making in more or less critical situations supporting the decision made by healthcare providers. Combined with BI, these systems can provide relevant information for the decision-making process improving the availability and overall quality of that information (Santos & Ramos, 2006).

The development of this type of systems is being encouraged to support new knowledge construction, processes improvement, pattern recognition and interpretation in large amounts of data, localization and development of organizational competencies and experience sharing (Santos & Ramos, 2006).

Within the scope of transplantation, some promising solutions and proposals are emerging to solve the inherent difficulty and complexity in order to improve the potential organ donors screening efficiency.

HEALTHCARE INTELLIGENCE IN ORGAN TRANSPLANTATION

Organ Donation and Transplantation Activities

Transplantation is the treatment of choice for severe organ failure. Despite this, the number of patients waiting for one or more organs is still increasing in Europe and as the shortage of organs has become more critical, new proposals have been developed to increase the organ donation potential (Jansen, et al., 2010; Irving, et al., 2012).

In Portugal, as in most countries, many systematic approaches and programs to increase organ donor rates and also to develop deceased donation to its maximum potential have been implemented, such as the initiation of the presumed consent legislation (Rudge, Matesanz, Delmonico, & Chapman, 2012). (Matesanz, 2001; Erwin, Kompanje, Jansen, & de Groot, 2013; Matesanz, 2001).

Even though there is no consensus on uniform criteria for defining a potential organ donor, a comprehensive review of organ donation considers BD patients the ideal multiorgan donors. As a result, the major source of solid organs for transplantation is provided by BD patients (Erwin, Kompanje, Jansen, & de Groot, 2013; Rudge, Matesanz, Delmonico, & Chapman, 2012). The work of the transplant team at CHP focuses on determining precursors of brain death that can provide significant results in creating a reliable pool of potential organ donors. As so, potential organ donors should be identified as soon as possible and should never be missed or delayed and it is desirable to identify a potential organ donor as early as possible to achieve a donor conversion rate as high as possible (Jansen, et al., 2010).

However, detection and management of potential organ donors is a complex process which takes several elements in consideration (Irving, et al., 2012).

Healthcare Information Systems

In medical science, where lives are at stake, a perfect scenario would be for all healthcare professionals to be perfectly skilled and informed, and for healthcare to be a field of order, knowledge and defined procedures even though uncertainty is a part of everyday life in surgical decision-making. However, one of the greatest concerns in nowadays' organizations is to introduce technology into their environments, and hospitals are not an exception. Consequently, HIS have been introduced in order to improve the quality of healthcare delivery (Jalote-Parmar, 2009; Palazzo, et al., 2013; Cardoso, et al., 2014; Khodambashi, 2013).

HIS can be defined as the socio-technical subsystems that comprise all management and organization information processing, as well as the healthcare professionals roles (Haux, Winter, Ammenwerth, & Brigl, 2013; Duarte, Portela, Abelha, Machado, & Santos, 2011). The design and implementation of HIS must focus on ensuring the efficient production of information in order to provide clinical decision-making capabilities (Duarte, Portela, Abelha, Machado, & Santos, 2011; Costa, Novais, Machado, Alberto, & Neves, 2007). As to provide complete and useful features, HIS must also allow the extraction of clinical and management indicators as a way to improve the decision-making, planning and logistics processes (Cardoso, Marins, Portela, Abelha, & Machado, 2014; Chaudhry, et al., 2006).

Clinical Decision Support Systems

Making decisions is characterized as the process of developing and analyzing alternatives to make a decision which is nothing more than a choice from the available alternatives. The majority of the decisions are made in response to a problem and involve judgement, which are the cognitive aspects of the decision-making process (Škrobáčková & Kopáčková, 2006).

CDSSs fit in as "any electronic system designed to aid directly in clinical decision making in which characteristics of individual patients are used to generate patient-specific assessments or recommendations that are then presented to clinicians for consideration" (Kawamoto, Houlihan, Balas, & Lobach, 2005).

In their classic form, CDSSs include alerts, reminders, order sets that automatically remind the clinical of a determined action, or care summary dashboards that provide feedback on quality and performance indicators for further improvement (Bright, et al., 2012).

Such systems have been shown to improve overall healthcare quality and efficiency by enhancing the delivery of preventive care services, and improve adherence to recommended care standards (Shea, DuMouchel, & Bahamonde, 1996; Balas, et al., 2000; Hunt, Haynes, Hanna, & Smith, 1998).

Reviews on the deployment of CDSSs showed that (Berner, 2009):

- Computer-based decision support is more effective than manual processes for decision support;
- CDSSs interventions that are presented automatically and fit into the workflow of the clinicians are more likely to be used;
- CDSSs that recommend actions for users are more effective than the ones that simply provide assessments;
- CDSSs' interventions that provide information at the time and place of decision-making are more likely to have an impact.

Nevertheless, it is important to understand that a CDSS 's target is not to replace clinicians but to support their daily work by reconstructing the way clinical episodes are seen.

Business Intelligence

Some sources describe BI as systems that combine data from different sources with analytic tools in order to provide relevant information for the decision-making process. The aim of such systems is to improve the availability and overall quality of that information (Santos & Ramos, 2006; Cody, Kreulen, Krishna, & Spangler, 2002).

When compared to DSS, BI is defined as a broad category of applications, practices, and technologies for gathering, storing, analyzing and providing access to data to support the business users in making better decisions. This includes all the ways an enterprise can explore, access and analyze information in the data warehouse to develop insights that will utterly lead to improved, informed decisions (Škrobáčková & Kopáčková, 2006; Olszak & Batko, 2012).

In fact, nowadays, BI is considered a top priority for many organizations and although healthcare still lags behind other industries in adopting BI, leading practitioners agree that taking a more enterprise-wide, platform-based approach to BI provides large gains to the institution (Olszak & Batko, 2012).

Depending on the requirements of every project, technologies can be merged and combined, creating a reliable DSS architecture. This DSS 's architecture must back up all the technological requirements BI might need. After a literature analysis, the framework that best suited this work is composed of three levels, from a development point of view, from bottom to top: The Data Sources level, the Data Warehouse level, and the Business Analytics level as represented in Figure 1 (Bâra & Lungu, 2012).

This approach was proposed by Han and Kamber (Jiawei & Kamber, 2001) and Eckerson (2003).

Figure 1. Adopted BI's support infrastructure architecture
Adapted from Cortes (2005)

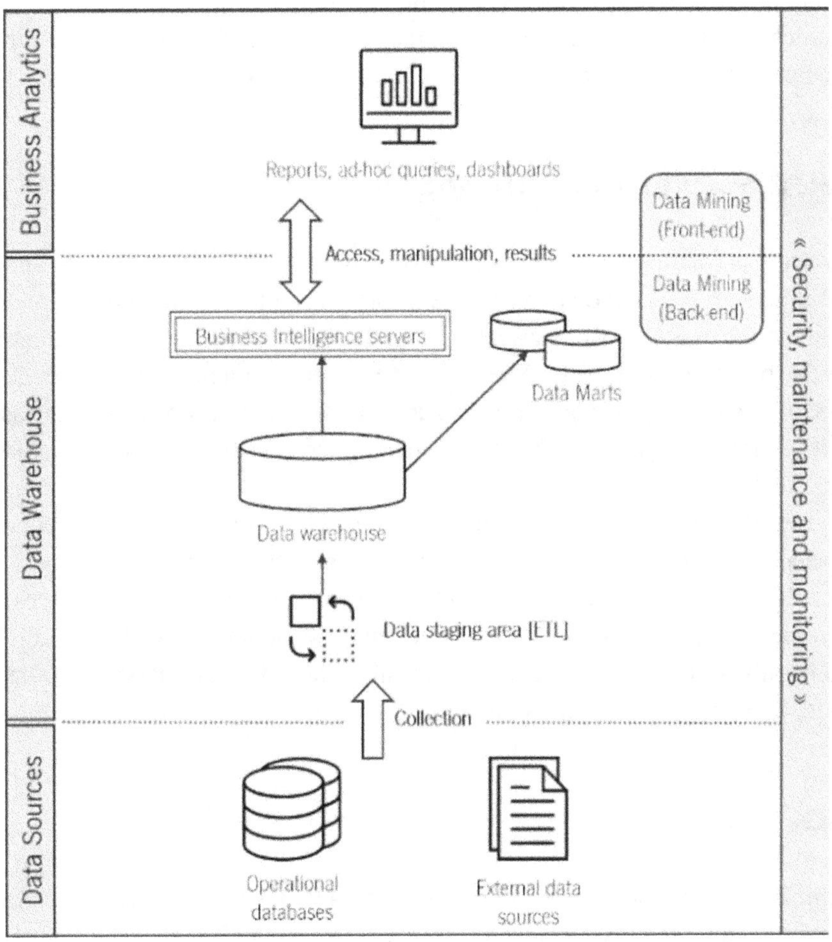

The Data Sources level represents all the operational environment of the application. These Data Sources are represented as databases including the data from different operational systems, responsible for feeding the Data Warehouse. They represent the origin of information intended to collect and make available through the Data Warehouse and they also represent the diverse operational activity's support systems used in an organization, in the form of HIS (Cortes, 2005).

The Data Warehouse (DW) level represents the storage environment that include the data validation and transformation before storing it in the DW. There always exist some kind of treatment to perform over the data before integrating it into the analytic repository. The area where this happens is called the Data Staging Area. Here, sequential search algorithms and text transformation procedures predominate, called the Extract, Transform and Load (ETL) procedures.

Above the Data Staging Area is the DW which is the analytical repository where data is stored after correctly transformed and integrated. It is over the DW that a set of services with the objective to provide information to end-users is implemented. This set of services includes a variety of utilities such as multidimensional analysis servers that can be later accessed by Online Analytical Processing (OLAP) tools, BI servers, Data Mining engines, amongst others (Cortes, 2005; Gardner, 1998).

The Business Analytics level is characterized as the set of technologies that support real-time analytics, enabling end-users to interact and explore the data from the repository previously created. Here the user is provided with a set of dynamic analysis tools that can be used to query data, generate reports or identify trends and patterns in data. That's where the interaction with the users takes place and where they can communicate with the system and analyze the presented results. This is one of the reasons why the user interface must be specially designed for an intuitive interaction.

KNOWLEDGE DISCOVERY IN DATABASES

Knowledge Discovery in Databases (KDD) is a fast-evolving research field which development is targeted to the benefit of practical, social and economic fields, amongst others. The motivation for this growth is linked primarily to the existence of a powerful technology for collecting, storing and managing large amounts of data, also known as big data. Most of this data hold valuable information like patterns and trends that can be utilized to improve business decisions. However, considering that the data is collected into databases, it became necessary to develop automatic processes for data analysis, like Data Mining (DM) (Rezende, 2003).

To best analyze and comprehend large volumes of data, several studies have been conducted in order to develop knowledge extraction techniques, also known as Data Mining. This process of KDD aims at finding knowledge from a set of data so it can be used in decision-making processes. Therefore, an important requirement is that this knowledge is human-understandable, as well as useful and interesting for end-users, generally the decision-makers, in a way this knowledge can support their decision-making process (Rezende, 2003; Fayyad, Piatetsky-Shapiro, & Smyth, 1996).

TEXT MINING

As the Data Mining techniques have been developed to deal with structured data, specific Text Mining techniques to deal with unstructured data were conceived (Rezende, 2003).

Text Mining is described as a process of knowledge discovery based on technologies such as Natural Language Processing (NLP) information extraction and Data Mining that makes it possible to discover patterns and trends semi-automatically from huge collections of unstructured text (Uramoto, et al., 2004; Hearst, 1999; Brusic & Zeleznikow, 1999; Swanson & Smalheiser, 1997; Agrawal & Srikant, 1994; Chen, Fuller, Friedman, & Hersh, 2006; Turban, Aronson, & Liang, 2005).

Text Mining system's preprocessing operations focus on the identification and extraction of representative features from natural language documents. These preprocessing operations are responsible for modeling unstructured text stored in document collections (implicit knowledge) into structured content (explicit knowledge) (Chen, Fuller, Friedman, & Hersh, 2006; Feldman & Sanger, 2007).

In healthcare, physicians often express opinions in terms of words that contain useful information that can be further used to develop intelligent models to improve the healthcare process. Hence, Text Mining proves to be an effective tool in healthcare datasets if correctly applied within clinical record archives leading to an accurate prediction of future outcomes in various healthcare settings (Raja, Mitchell, Day, & Hardin, 2008). Hirschman notes in his review of milestones in biomedical Text Mining research that the field began by focusing on three approaches to process text: linguistic context of text, pattern matching, and word co-occurrence. This last one, word co-occurrence, proves to be very effective on occurrence statistics-based predictions (Hirschman, Park, Tsujii, Wong, & Wu, 2002).

As the output of a NLP system is intended to be employed by a healthcare application, it must hold adequate recall, precision and specificity for the intended clinical application, but it should also be possible to adjust its performance according to the needs of the application. Any application involving NLP must undergo a performance evaluation before being deployed to ensure it is appropriate to address such clinical settings (Chen, Fuller, Friedman, & Hersh, 2006).

One evident challenge in the Text Mining field lies on the pertinent declaration of negatives in text which makes it harder to determine whether a finding within narrative medical records is present or absent. Indeed, the most frequently described findings are the ones that deny these findings on the patient (Chapman, Bridewell, Hanbury, Cooper, & Buchanan, 2001). Thus, the development of methods to automatically discriminate between terms that are mentioned as being present and terms that are negated provide a crucial improvement for this type of systems where negation in predicate logic is well defined and syntactically present.

SOLUTIONS AND RECOMMENDATIONS

Defining the Potential Organ Donor Criteria

At a preliminary stage, a crucial criterion for identifying a death that may yield a potential organ donor consists on filtering medical record reviews indicating primary brain death.

This definition of potential organ donor returns patients' records clinically consistent with organ donor potential based on ICD-9-CM codes.

In that sense, a list of ICD-9-CM codes was developed by the transplant team at CHP based on retrospective data analysis from recent years and includes a set of diagnostics that may yield a potential BD donor. For example, the list contains ICD-9-CM codes for subarachnoid hemorrhage (SAH), traumatic brain injury (TBI) and intracerebral hemorrhage (ICH) which are known to precede brain death in over 80% of the cases, according to the literature (Lovelock, Rinkel, & Rothwell, 2010).

The complete list of ICD-9-CM codes used for this purpose is represented in Table 1.

A set of automatic procedures was then conceived to search, retrieve and store patients' records on the diverse hospital databases that are consistent with the any of the codes listed in Table 1, using Java.

Another expressive way of detecting patients that may lead to BD donors rests on the evaluation of the patient's Cranio-Encephalic Computerized Tomography (CE CT) scan reports looking for medical evidence of devastating neurological events (Fernandes, 2013).

To best classify and identify potential donors, a systematic approach for detection was adopted. This approach was designed to retrieve a set of most common keywords and expressions in potential organ donors' CE CT scan reports so it can be applied to the software-based screening system.

In order to get clinically relevant and accurate results, the context of this approach was narrowed to the CE CT scan reports from those patients who became actual organ donors from 2010 to 2015 at CHP.

Table 1. ICD-9-CM codes for inclusion of potential organ donors

ICD-9-CM Code	Description
191	Malignant neoplasm of brain
192	Malignant neoplasm of other and unspecified parts of nervous system
225	Benign neoplasm of brain and other parts of nervous system
320	Bacterial meningitis
324	Intracranial and intraspinal abscess
348.1	Anoxic brain damage
348.4	Compression of brain
348.5	Cerebral edema
348.8	Other conditions of brain
348.9	Unspecified condition of brain
430	Subarachnoid hemorrhage
431	Intracerebral hemorrhage
432	Other and unspecified intracranial hemorrhage
433	Occlusion and stenosis of precerebral arteries
434	Occlusion of cerebral arteries
435	Transient cerebral ischemia
436	Acute, but ill-defined, cerebrovascular disease
800	Fracture of vault of skull
801	Fracture of base of skull
803	Other and unqualified skull fractures
804	Multiple fractures involving skull or face with other bones
850	Concussion
851	Cerebral laceration and contusion
852	Subarachnoid, subdural, and extradural hemorrhage, following injury
853	Other and unspecified intracranial hemorrhage following injury
854	Intracranial injury of other and unspecified nature

As to meet its specifications, this system aims to (a) extract critical medical findings and related information in the free text scan reports and (b) deploy that structured knowledge for future events detection.

Keywords/Expressions Extraction Module

The process began with a collection of documents to be analyzed, that is, the collection of CE CT scan reports from actual organ donors from the past 5 years. Data extraction and cleaning procedures are the first step and required meticulous and precise attention to ensure that the data was valid and the information was complete. A stop list of words to be ignored in the document while performing the analysis was adopted. It contained commonly occurring terms that do not carry much value to the analysis process, providing more reliable results. Domain knowledge played a fundamental role at this stage.

Thereafter, an algorithm run for n-gram frequency extraction was performed resulting in a table of all the n-grams set along with their corresponding frequency in the collection of documents. This stage required general understanding of algorithms capable of converting raw textual data into useful numeric information that users can comprehend and was performed using R Studio and the tm package, specific for text mining.

A total of 134 CE CT scan reports performed by 62 actual donors from 2010 to 2015 were analyzed.

Due to the essential participation of the transplant teams in this type of solutions, the final set of keywords and expressions was discussed with responsible medical professional at CHP. This way it was possible to integrate their field expertise in deciding the criticality of a word occurrence, according to the defaults of medical findings related to devastating neurological events. This permitted the removal of some expressions that wouldn't produce any added value to the system since they represent common terms in any CE CT scan report, often names of brain structures such as "parenchyma" and "cerebellar tonsils", just to name a few.

Also, some synonyms were specified in order to increase the potential of this tool, and additional keywords were introduced.

The final set of clinical conditions represented in the form of keywords and expressions is displayed in Table 2.

This concludes a two-step process for keywords and expressions extraction: preprocessing the large volume of textual data and developing useful predictions based on that data.

To draw up a schematic view on this, Figure 2 represents the extraction module architecture.

CE CT Scan Reports Classification Module

At this point, a set of keywords and expressions was already decided and ready to implement into the next step. Next, a retrieval module was constructed which is responsible for building a connection between the set of keywords previously defined and the scan reports database.

Anytime this module finds a CE CT scan report, it applies a natural language algorithm in order to identify the affirmation of any of the expressions defined previously in Table 2, using a simple negation module to disregard negated findings due to the underlying characteristics of medical reporting.

Table 2. Final set of keywords and expressions

Keywords or Expressions	
aneurism	injury
contusion	ischemic (or ischemia)
craniectomy	mass effect
edema	midline shift
effacement of the sulci	space conflict
heart attack	space occupying lesion
hematoma	stroke
hemorrhage (or hemorrhagic)	subarachnoid hemorrhage
hernia	trauma
hypodensity	thrombosis
hydrocephalus	ventricular dilatation

Figure 2. Keywords/expressions extraction module architecture

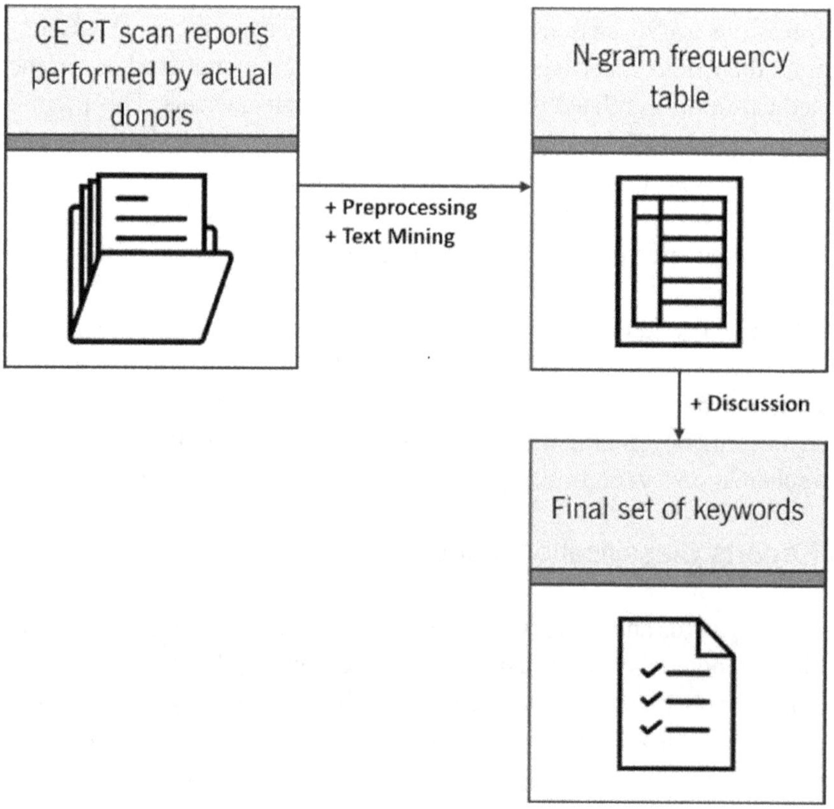

This approach is based on the ConText algorithm, which is, respectively, based on a negation algorithm called NegEx (Chapman, Bridewell, Hanbury, Cooper, & Buchanan, 2001; Chapman, Chu, & Downling, 2007). This is a regular-expression-based algorithm for determining the status of the contextual features in medical reports and has proven to perform very well at identifying negated conditions (Chapman, Chu, & Downling, 2007).

This adapted version of the algorithm takes as input CE CT scan reports and a set of clinical conditions in the form of keywords and/or expressions as previously defined and outputs, for each condition, the value for contextual features or modifiers. This adaptation of ConText only determines values for the Negation modifier - affirmed or negated (Chapman, Chu, & Downling, 2007).

By identifying the existence of trigger terms such as "no sign of" and "without", the algorithm searches for the keywords/expressions that fall within the scope of that trigger term and determines if those clinical conditions should be negated (Chapman, Chu, & Downling, 2007).

If the algorithm classifies the match as an affirmation of any of the keywords, it adds the patient's sequential number and the exam ID to a special table referencing all the detected cases.

Figure 3 represents the classification module architecture.

This module is particularly notable for its application within the DSS described next. By signaling patients with highest potential of becoming BD donors, an SMS and email alert notification is then forwarded to the transplant team providing an added value to the system, improving their awareness on patients evolution.

All things considered, it is now possible to portray an algorithm to best describe the potential organ donor profile regarding both the list of ICD-9-CM codes and the set of keywords present in CE CT scan reports. Figure 4 portrays the critical pathway for deceased organ donation suggested using the information from the previous steps.

In an initial phase of identification, any patient with a clinical diagnosis consistent with any of the defined in Table 1 representing severe brain damage is immediately added to the pool of potential organ donors.

In a subsequent monitoring phase, if any of these patients in the actual pool of potential organ donors perform a CE CT scan whose results indicate the affirmation of at least one of the keywords defined in Table 2 a notification alert is forwarded to the transplant team.

Figure 3. Classification module architecture

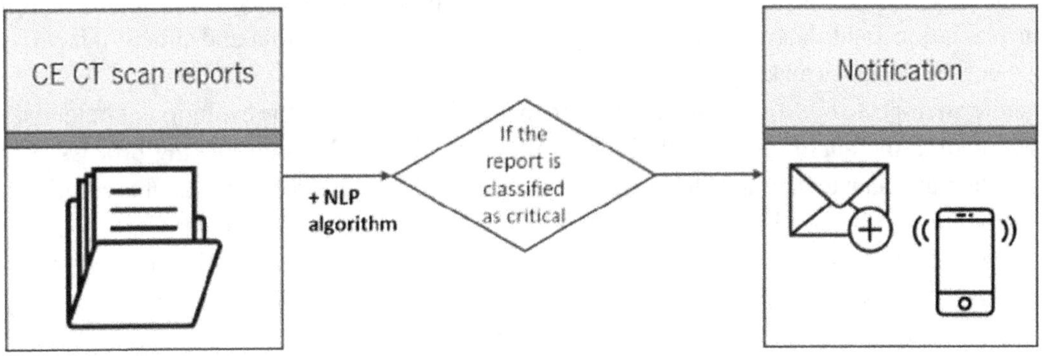

Figure 4. The critical pathway for deceased organ donation

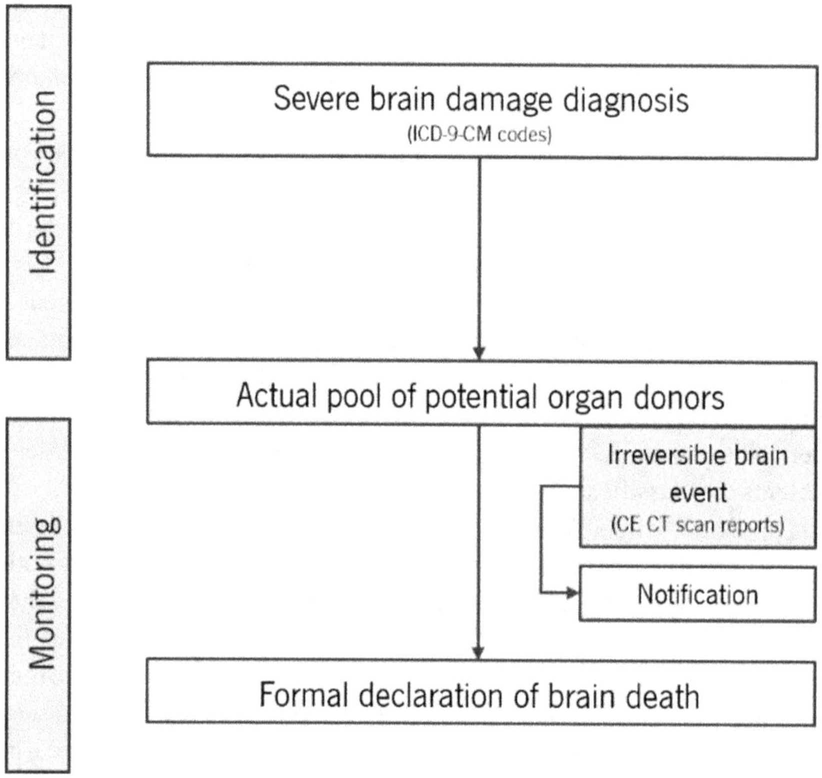

Using these criteria, the responsible team has the ability to monitor the identified potential organ donors more accurately and timely until a formal declaration of brain death occurs. Once a patient is declared BD, the transplant team must take fast actions to achieve the best results.

A REAL-TIME PLATFORM FOR DECISION SUPPORT IN ORGAN TRANSPLANTATION: ORGANITE

One of the major purposes of this work was to develop a prototype of a decision support platform in the transplantation field, later called Organite, in order to provide reliable and timely information to complement the decision-making process.

Organite attempts to build a high-level solution to identify and follow the evolution of potential organ donors providing the qualified staff all the tools they need in the decision-making process. Through Organite, the transplant team is able to access and interact with data from diverse databases and services in the form of a web-based platform using a standard web browser, locally at CHP.

Such a system proves to be very efficient since the manual process of identification and monitoring of a potential donor is very complex and time-consuming. As data comes from various HIS, it may happen that some cases might go unnoticed in the large amount of data.

Organite follows a REpresentational State Transfer (REST) architecture which is a client-server web architecture for network applications that partitions tasks offered by the providers of a resource or service - servers - and content or service requesters - clients. These two communicate over a computer network on separate machines using simple Hypertext Transfer Protocol (HTTP) requests initiated by the client and waiting for a response from the server. The client component was constructed using AngularJS and the server component uses Flask for the construction of REST APIs.

Organite counts with several technologies to support real-time analytics, enabling end-users to interact and explore the data from the repository previously created. Its objective lies on providing results to end-users through a set of visualization tools from reporting to decision support web applications. (Cortes, 2005) Due to how this type of data must be analyzed, a set of tables and graphical elements for statistical means was developed, as listed below:

- History of potential donors;
- Current potential donors;
- Statistical Graphics;
- Statistical Data.

The history of potential donors presents all the potential donors identified by the platform since its implementation in the form of a table with relevant data to accurately identify and access the patients' details.

The set of attributes available in this first table includes the patients' Sequential Number (Número Sequencial), his/her most recent diagnosis' Clinical Episode ID (ID Episódio), Notes (Anotações), Specialty (Especialidade) and Date (Data do Diagnóstico). A column showing the patients' Medical Condition (Estado) is also available and can be:

- **Deceased (Faleceu):** If the patient is dead;
- **Admitted (Internado):** If the patient is currently admitted in the hospital;
- **Admitted in the ER (Urgências):** If the patient is currently admitted in the ER;
- **Medical Discharge (Alta):** If the patient has already had medical discharge;
- **Unknown (Desconhecido):** If the patient's condition is none of the above and can't be correctly determined;
- **Entry (Entrada):** Before the automatic procedure determine the patient's medical condition from any of the above, this parameter is identified as an entry.

On the table, each medical condition has a color to ease the identification process.

To provide this section with some input options from the user, it is also possible to order the results based on the Clinical Episode ID, Specialty, Date of Diagnosis or Medical Condition's column and filter the results shown based on the Clinical Episode ID, Date of Diagnosis and patients' Sequential Number input data from users.

This page is purposed to provide the medical team all the means on the background of the system for statistical and learning purposes.

A fully detailed view of each patient can also be accessed from this page by clicking over the patient's Sequential Number.

Figure 5 shows an overview of this page.

The current potential donors section presents all the applicable identified potential donors, also in the form of a table with the same set of attributes and features as the previous section.

This page concatenates the actual cases that the transplant team must considerate, that is, it excludes the patients that had deceased or have had medical discharge, and plays an essential role in the whole platform since it includes the most probable cases of becoming an actual organ donor.

The detailed view of each patient can also be accessed from this page by clicking over the patient's Sequential Number.

This detailed view reveals detailed aspects on the patient's condition. Some necessary parameters like the patient's medical and clinical tests are very relevant to determine the patient's potential of becoming an actual donor.

The list of fields about the patient that this view offers includes:

- Sequential Number (Número Sequencial);
- Process Number (Número de Processo);
- Gender (Género);
- Date of Birth (Data de Nascimento);
- Medical Condition (Estado);
- Most Recent Diagnosis (Diagnóstico mais recente);
- Electronic Health Record (PCE).

Figure 5. History of potential donors' page

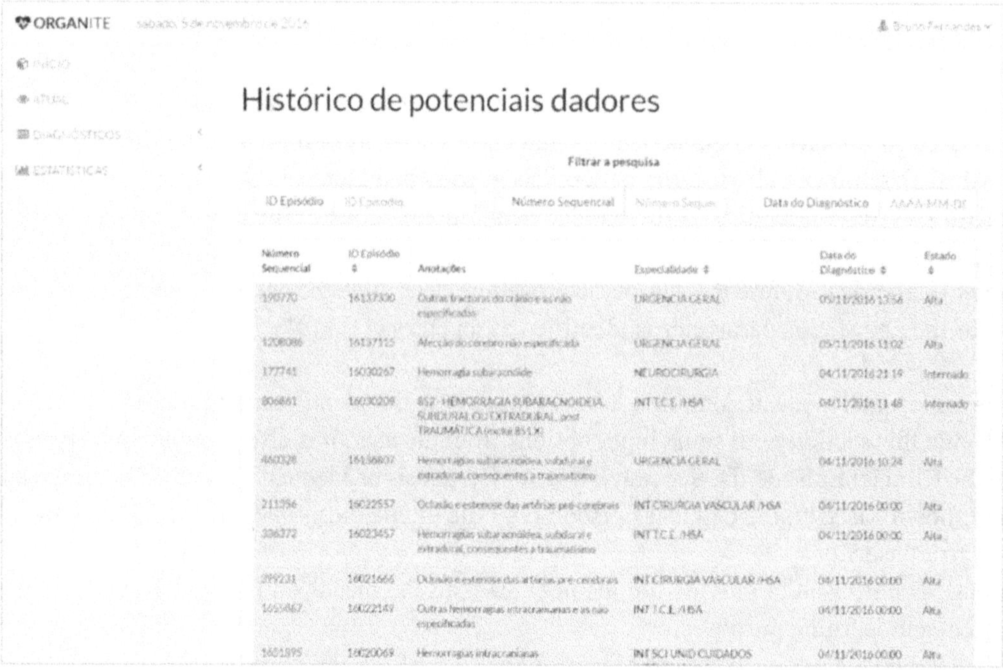

The Medical Condition field holds some additional information for each situation and the Electronic Health Record field provides full access to the patient's details along with his/her course in the hospital.

Three tabs displaying all the identified diagnosis, medical tests and clinical tests of the referred patient are also available allowing the transplant team to access this type of information without needing to resort to other systems. A link to the medical and clinical test reports is also available.

Figure 6 shows an overview of this page.

To provide an overview of the data collected by the system, a set of graphical elements was developed in order to facilitate data analysis by the transplant team.

Assuming the form of dashboards, these elements contain data aggregated into different perspectives revealing the most important aspects to be analyzed. At the same time, this section offers the possibility to generate simple, downloadable reports in the form of text files that the transplant team members can utilize for further offline analysis.

The Statistical Graphics section offers the following set of dashboards:

- Counter of all the identified cases in the last 24 hours;
- Bar chart representing the total number of entries per clinical module within the last week;
- Interactive radial chart representing the total number of entries per clinical module, specialty and ICD-9-CM code;
- Donut chart representing the total relative distribution of entries per medical specialty;
- Stacked area chart representing the total number of entries per clinical module, within the last year, grouped by month. This graphic offers the possibility to alternate between the stacked, stream and expanded views.

Figure 6. Detailed view on a patient

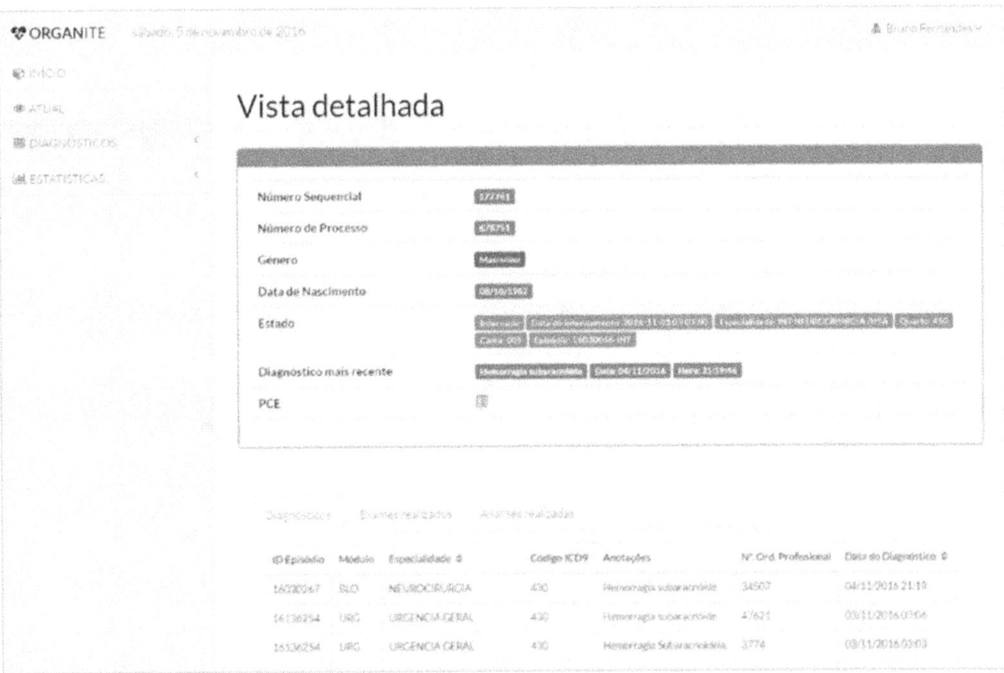

Figure 7 represents a view of this page.

If correctly analyzed, the data provided by these elements can help develop new methodologies and techniques on how to detect and monitor potential organ donors, since it is possible to identify, for example, the clinical areas with most identified cases. This feature can be essential in developing an ever-improving potential organ donor identification criteria.

Another feature also available in Organite provides the transplant team with specific data organized into yearly patient-centered categories. This component also complements the system with the ability to generate downloadable, text-based reports, since there is an option to download a text file with the required data.

The data represented in this section is organized on a table with drop-down buttons to ease data visualization and understanding. Considering that the data relates to the year the user must preselect, the complete set of parameters represented is:

- Total number of entries;
- Average number of entries per day;
- Total number of entries per month;
- Total number of entries per gender;
- Total number of entries per age group. This parameter is divided into four age groups: 0-18; 19-35; 36-50 and 50+.

Figure 8 represents an overview of this page.

Figure 7. Overview of the statistical graphics page

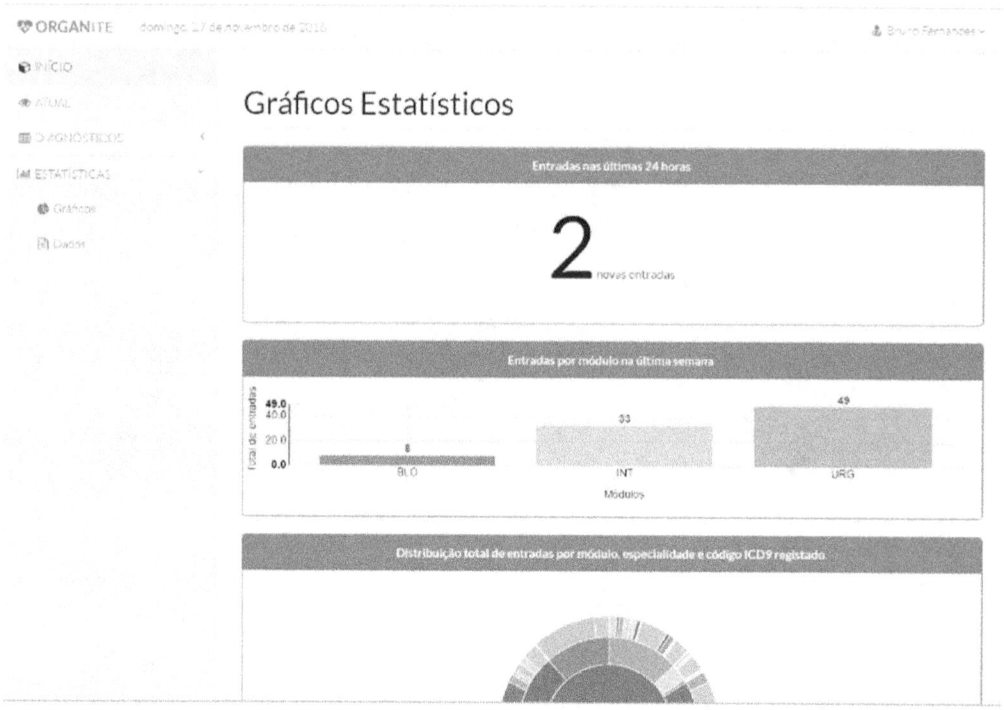

Figure 8. Statistical data on identified cases per year

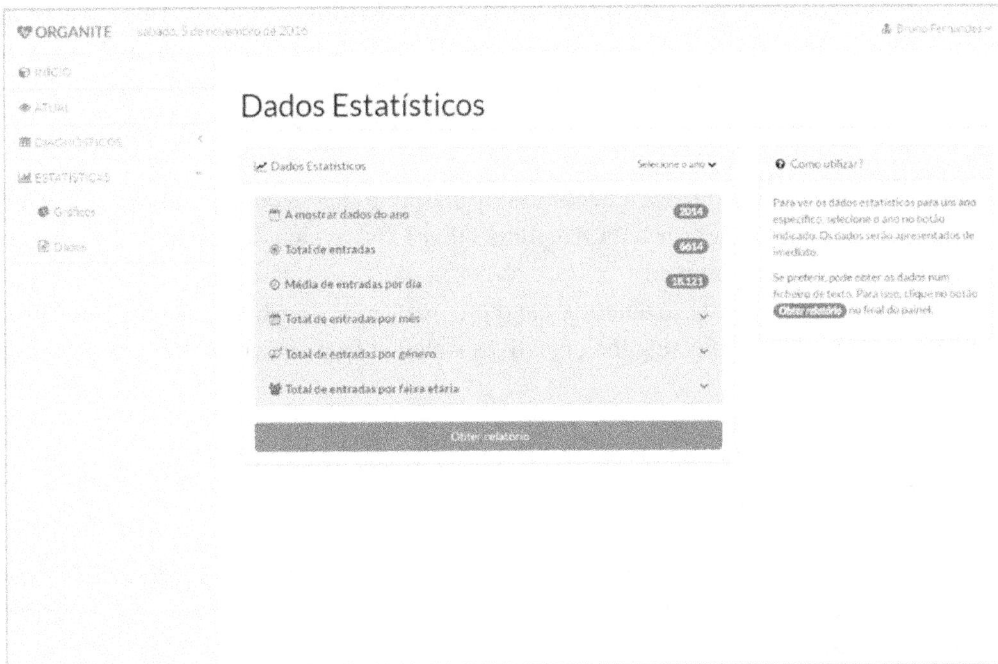

This set of parameters complements the information provided in the Statistical Graphics section. Users can now get information on the total number of entries verified and compare the values among the different years and months within years to understand the evolution in the number of identified cases.

It is now also possible to recognize which age group has a greater contribute as well as which gender dominates the number of identified cases.

In general, users can now make sense of a large amount of data and, through this indicators, get useful insights and define better strategies to attain the best results.

To provide an overall discussion on the main topics that arose during the system's design and implementation, the next paragraphs will point out some key thoughts and impressions on the system's outcomes and future directions.

This work enabled the exploration of concepts like BI and Knowledge Discovery to introduce a valuable solution that may contribute to the continuous optimization of such a crucial and sensitive field as the organ transplantation is. As so, it is a solution in constant development and innovation that should meet the field demands.

After stating the main problem and inherent questions, an artifact was designed and implemented, in this particular case, the functional prototype of the system, and further evaluated according to criteria implicit in the proposal. This includes both the definition of effective potential organ donor criteria and the web-based platform.

The definition of effective potential organ donor criteria demonstrates the power of analyzing real data from actual organ donors by applying Text Mining to quickly identify keywords from a large quantity of textual data. This helps to answer the question of the eligibility criteria of a potential organ donor.

In what concerns the repository of potential organ donors, the implementation of correction measures and new filters proved to meet the objectives of continuous improvement and refinement of the results obtained.

The web-based platform was a natural evolution by adopting new, simpler and more efficient technologies to make it lighter and cleaner with AngularJS and Flask which demonstrated to respond very well in the context which it was applied.

The resulting strategy utilizes these outcomes and provides an actionable plan to increase productivity and provide a greater service meeting the objectives stated at first and answering the raised research problem.

FUTURE RESEARCH DIRECTIONS

The innovative feature of this project reflects its ability to evolve in virtually every direction as there will always be space for improvements besides the required continuous maintenance and the manifestation of new clinical circumstances.

Further knowledge on predictive indicators that evidence a patient's potential for organ donation must be assessed in order to upgrade the potential organ donor criteria. Also, DM models concerning new pathways must be addressed in order to explore other targets.

It would be interesting to explore more clinical records to assess the patient's probability of evolving into an actual organ donor such as the Glasgow Coma Scale (GCS), pupil reactivity, amongst others. The collection of such data would be of great help if combined with intelligence algorithms to identify patterns and trends in the patient's records.

It would also be relevant to implement a logistics module responsible for implementing either an exclusion criteria model and the donor/recipient pair selection as stated by the Portuguese law and the hospital's principles. This would include contraindications for donation such as risk behaviors and the presence of a potentially transmissible infectious disease. Also, if the potential donor has registered in life in Registo Nacional de não Dadores (RENDA), the Portuguese framework for non-donors, his/her contribution must be rejected.

Furthermore, it may also have considerable impact in donation if the platform offered any kind of donor/recipient pair selection tools that would allow the input of some data concerning the recipient's clinical tests (blood type, HLA typing and crossmatching) and it would output the best matched potential organ donors organized in some way. Additionally, a number of relevant trials should be addressed together with the transplant team at CHP in order to adapt the platform to their needs and correct any eventual limitations concerning the quality of information, time in getting information, time in decision-making, multi-query ability, graphical aspect of the platform and system usability. This type of trials could easily fit in the form of questionnaires.

CONCLUSION

The system developed represents an innovative way of supporting decision making in the transplants environment. Following this systematic approach, it is now possible to automatically acquire, process and present useful data to end-users reducing drastically the time between the period of possible brain death recognition and a formal brain death diagnosis, contributing to a valuable method to increase the number of actual donors.

The KDD component proved to be a very reasonable method for defining the potential organ donor criteria based on CE CT scan reports. Taking real clinical information from actual donations from the past five years as input and applying more or less complex text mining procedures, the output is likely to produce more realistic predictive models.

Unlike other similar tools, this type of screening system complements itself with the two-step mechanism. It takes all patients diagnosed with any of the ICD-9-CM codes defined, centralizes that information and displays it in a graphical interface specially designed to allow a fast, interactive understanding by end-users.

At the same time, end-users can now follow-up potential organ donors along with their course in the hospital having all the data they need in a single site, accessible anytime and anywhere inside the hospital's intranet.

The notification system improves the transplant team members' awareness of patients' evolution, signaling patients with the highest potential of becoming BD donors, that is, those who need more attention and may, therefore, result in actual organ donors.

The clinical indicators in the form of graphics constitute an effective method that can contribute, through evidence, for an improved clinical decision-making.

The main contributions of this dissertation can, then, be summarized as:

- The definition of more accurate potential organ donor selection criteria;
- The construction, using the selection criteria model, of a potential donors pool;
- The follow-up of potential donors through a structured interface anytime and anywhere inside the hospital's intranet;
- The notification of the occurrence of devastating neurological events on potential donors CE CT scan reports.

Finally, through the presentation of Organite together with the transplant team at CHP it has been proved that the adoption of a technological tool to complement the medical team's traditional methods may be more satisfactorily accepted if end-users acknowledge the project's objectives and the gains it may bring for their daily work. The fact that some members might not be inclined to change their professional routines may constitute a limitation for the implementation of such solutions. If these issues are not resolved the systems run the risk of being rejected and fall into disuse.

REFERENCES

Agrawal, R., & Srikant, R. (1994). Fast algorithms for mining association rules. *Proc. 20th int. conf. very large data bases, VLDB*, 487-499.

Airinei, D., & Homocianu, D. (2009). DSS vs. business intelligence. *Revista Economica.*

Alavi, M., & Leidner, D. E. (2005). Review: Knowledge management and knowledge management systems: conceptual foundations and research issues. *Knowledge Management: Critical Perspectives on Business and Management*, 163.

Ali, O. T., Nassif, A. B., & Capretz, L. F. (2013). Business intelligence solutions in healthcare a case study: Transforming OLTP system to BI solution. *Communications and Information Technology (IC-CIT), 2013 Third International Conference* (pp. 209-214). IEEE.

Balas, E. A., Weingarten, S., Garb, C. T., Blumenthal, D., Boren, S. A., & Brown, G. B. (2000). Improving preventive care by prompting physicians. *Archives of Internal Medicine*, *160*(3), 301–308. doi:10.1001/archinte.160.3.301 PMID:10668831

Bâra, A., & Lungu, I. (2012). *Improving Decision Support Systems with Data Mining Techniques*. IN-TECH Open Access Publisher. doi:10.5772/47788

Berner, E. S. (2009). *Clinical decision support systems: state of the art.* AHRQ Publication.

Bright, T. J., Wong, A., Dhurjati, R., Bristow, E., Bastian, L., Coeytaux, R. R., & Musty, M. D. et al. (2012). Effect of clinical decision-support systems: A systematic review. *Annals of Internal Medicine*, *157*(1), 29–43. doi:10.7326/0003-4819-157-1-201207030-00450 PMID:22751758

Brusic, V., & Zeleznikow, J. (1999). Knowledge discovery and data mining in biological databases. *The Knowledge Engineering Review*, *14*(3), 257–277. doi:10.1017/S0269888999003069

Cardoso, L., Marins, F., Portela, F., Abelha, A., & Machado, J. (2014). Healthcare interoperability through intelligent agent technology. *Procedia Technology*, 1334-1341.

Cardoso, L., Marins, F., Portela, F., Santos, M., Abelha, A., & Machado, J. (2014). The next generation of interoperability agents in healthcare. *International Journal of Environmental Research and Public Health*, *11*(5), 5349–5371. doi:10.3390/ijerph110505349 PMID:24840351

Chapman, W. W., Bridewell, W., Hanbury, P., Cooper, G. F., & Buchanan, B. G. (2001). A simple algorithm for identifying negated findings and diseases in discharge summaries. *Journal of Biomedical Informatics*, *34*(5), 301–310. doi:10.1006/jbin.2001.1029 PMID:12123149

Chapman, W. W., Chu, D., & Downling, J. N. (2007). Context: An algorithm for identifying contextual features from clinical text. *Proceedings of the Workshop on BioNLP 2007: Biological, Translational, and Clinical Language Processing*, 81-88. doi:10.3115/1572392.1572408

Chaudhry, B., Wang, J., Wu, S., Maglione, M., Mojica, W., Roth, E., & Shekelle, P. G. et al. (2006). Systematic review: Impact of health information technology on quality, efficiency, and costs of medical care. *Annals of Internal Medicine*, *144*(10), 742–752. doi:10.7326/0003-4819-144-10-200605160-00125 PMID:16702590

Chen, H., Fuller, S. S., Friedman, C., & Hersh, W. (2006). *Medical informatics: knowledge management and data mining in biomedicine* (Vol. 8). Springer Science & Business Media.

Cody, W. F., Kreulen, J. T., Krishna, V., & Spangler, W. S. (2002). The integration of business intelligence and knowledge management. *IBM Systems Journal*, *41*(4), 697–713. doi:10.1147/sj.414.0697

Cortes, B. (2005). *Sistemas de suporte à decisão*. FCA-Editora Informática.

Costa, R., Novais, P., Machado, J., Alberto, C., & Neves, J. (2007). Inter-organization cooperation for care of the elderly. *Integration and Innovation Orient to E-Society*, *2*, 200–208.

Duarte, J., Portela, C. F., Abelha, A., Machado, J., & Santos, M. F. (2011). Electronic health record in dermatology service. *International Conference on ENTERprise Information Systems*, 156-164.

Eckerson, W. (2003). *Smart companies in the 21st century: The secrets of creating successful business intelligence solutions*. Academic Press.

Erwin, J., Kompanje, O., Jansen, N. E., & de Groot, Y. J. (2013). 'in plain language': Uniform criteria for organ donor recognition. *Intensive Care Medicine*.

Fayyad, U., Piatetsky-Shapiro, G., & Smyth, P. (1996). From data mining to knowledge discovery in databases. *AI Magazine*, 37.

Feldman, R., & Sanger, J. (2007). *The text mining handbook: advanced approaches in analyzing unstructured data*. Cambridge University Press.

Fernandes, A. (2013). *Early imagiology criteria for the screening of possible brain-death donors at the emergency room*. University of Barcelona.

Fernandes, A., Gomes, A., Ermida, D., & Vardasca, T. (2015). Imaging screening of catastrophic neurological events using a software tool: Preliminary results. *Transplantation Proceedings*, *47*(4), 1001–1004. doi:10.1016/j.transproceed.2015.03.021 PMID:26036504

Gardner, S. R. (1998). Building the data warehouse. *Communications of the ACM*, 53.

Gong, T., Tan, C. L., Leong, T. Y., Pang, B. C., Lim, C. T., Tian, Q., & Zhang, Z. et al. (2008). Text mining in radiology reports. *2008 Eighth IEEE International Conference on Data Mining* (pp. 815-820). IEEE. doi:10.1109/ICDM.2008.150

Hahn, J., & Subramani, M. R. (2000). A framework of knowledge management systems: issues and challenges for theory and practice. *Proceedings of the twenty first international conference on Information systems*, 302-312.

Haux, R., Winter, A., Ammenwerth, E., & Brigl, B. (2013). *Strategic information management in hospitals: an introduction to hospital information systems*. Springer Science & Business Media.

Hearst, M. A. (1999). Untangling text data mining. *Proceedings of the 37th annual meeting of the Association for Computational Linguistics on Computational Linguistics*, 3-10. doi:10.3115/1034678.1034679

Hirschman, L., Park, J. C., Tsujii, J., Wong, L., & Wu, C. H. (2002). Accomplishments and challenges in literature data mining for biology. *Bioinformatics (Oxford, England)*, *18*(12), 1553–1561. doi:10.1093/bioinformatics/18.12.1553 PMID:12490438

Hunt, D. L., Haynes, R. B., Hanna, S. E., & Smith, K. (1998). Effects of computer-based clinical decision support systems on physician performance and patient outcomes: A systematic review. *Journal of the American Medical Association*, *280*(15), 1339–1346. doi:10.1001/jama.280.15.1339 PMID:9794315

Irving, M. J., Tong, A., Jan, S., Cass, A., Rose, J., Chadban, S., & Howard, K. et al. (2012). Factors that influence the decision to be an organ donor: A systematic review of the qualitative literature. *Nephrology, Dialysis, Transplantation*, *27*(6), 2526–2533. doi:10.1093/ndt/gfr683 PMID:22193049

Işık, Ö., Jones, M. C., & Sidorova, A. (2013). Business intelligence success: The roles of BI capabilities and decision environments. *Information & Management*, *50*(1), 13–23. doi:10.1016/j.im.2012.12.001

Ivan, M., & Velicanu, M. (2015). Healthcare industry improvement with business intelligence. *Informatica Economica*, 81.

Jalote-Parmar, A. (2009). Workflow Driven Decision Support Systems: A case of an intra-operative visualization system for surgeons. TU Delft, Delft University of Technology.

Jansen, N. E., de Groot, Y. J., Bakker, J., Kuiper, M. A., Aerdts, S., & Maas, A. I. (2010). Imminent brain death: point of departure for potential heart-beating organ donor recognition. *Intensive Care*, 1488-1494.

Jiawei, H., & Kamber, M. (2001). Data mining: Concepts and techniques. San Francisco, CA: Morgan Kaufmann.

Kawamoto, K., Houlihan, C. A., Balas, E. A., & Lobach, D. F. (2005). Improving clinical practice using clinical decision support systems: A systematic review of trials to identify features critical to success. *BMJ (Clinical Research Ed.)*, 465. PMID:15767266

Khodambashi, S. (2013). Business process re-engineering application in healthcare in a relation to health information systems. *Procedia Technology*, 949-957.

Lovelock, C., Rinkel, G., & Rothwell, P. (2010). Time trends in outcome of subarachnoid hemorrhage population-based study and systematic review. *Neurology*, *74*(19), 1494–1501. doi:10.1212/WNL.0b013e3181dd42b3 PMID:20375310

Machado, J., Alves, V., Abelha, A., & Neves, J. (2007). Ambient intelligence via multiagent systems in the medical arena. *Engineering Intelligent Systems for Electrical Engineering and Communications*, 151–157.

Matesanz, R. (2001). A decade of continuous improvement in cadaveric organ donation: The spanish model. *Nefrologia*, 59–67. PMID:11881417

Matesanz, R., Dominguez-Gil, B., Coll, E., de la Rosa, G., & Marazuela, R. (2011). Spanish experience as a leading country: What kind of measures were taken?. *Transplant International*, *24*(4), 333–343. doi:10.1111/j.1432-2277.2010.01204.x PMID:21210863

Olszak, C., & Batko, K. (2012). Business intelligence systems. new chances and possibilities for healthcare organizations. *Informatyka Ekonomiczna*, 123-138.

Palazzo, L., Sernani, P., Claudi, A., Dolcini, G., Biancucci, G., & Franco, A. F. (2013). A multi-agent architecture for health information systems. *International Workshop on Artificial Intelligence and Net-Medicine*, 41.

Peixoto, H., Santos, M., Abelha, A., & Machado, J. (2012). Intelligence in interoperability with AIDA. *International Symposium on Methodologies for Intelligent Systems*, 264-273.

Raja, U., Mitchell, T., Day, T., & Hardin, J. M. (2008). Text mining in healthcare. applications and opportunities. *Journal of Healthcare Information Management*, 52–56. PMID:19267032

Rezende, S. O. (2003). *Sistemas inteligentes: fundamentos e aplicações*. Editora Manole Ltda.

Rudge, C., Matesanz, R., Delmonico, F., & Chapman, J. (2012). International practices of organ donation. *British Journal of Anaesthesia*, *108*(suppl 1), 48–55. doi:10.1093/bja/aer399 PMID:22194431

Santos, M. Y., & Ramos, I. (2006). *Business Intelligence: Tecnologias da informação na gestão do conhecimento*. FCA-Editora de Informática.

Shea, S., DuMouchel, W., & Bahamonde, L. (1996). A meta-analysis of 16 randomized controlled trials to evaluate computer-based clinical reminder systems for preventive care in the ambulatory setting. *Journal of the American Medical Informatics Association*, *3*(6), 399–409. doi:10.1136/jamia.1996.97084513 PMID:8930856

Škrobáčková, M., & Kopáčková, H. (2006). *Decision support systems or business intelligence: what can help in decision making?. Scientific papers of the University of Pardubice. Series D*. Faculty of Economics and Administration.

Swanson, D. R., & Smalheiser, N. R. (1997). An interactive system for finding complementary literatures: A stimulus to scientific discovery. *Artificial Intelligence*, *91*(2), 183–203. doi:10.1016/S0004-3702(97)00008-8

Turban, E., Aronson, J., & Liang, T.-P. (2005). *Decision Support Systems and Intelligent Systems* (7th ed.). Pearson Prentice Hall.

Turban, E., Rainer, R., & Potter, R. (2005). *Introduction to information technology*. Academic Press.

Turban, E., Sharda, R., & Delen, D. (2011). *Decision support and business intelligence systems*. Pearson Education India.

Uramoto, N., Matsuzawa, H., Nagano, T., Murakami, A., Takeuchi, H., & Takeda, K. (2004). A text-mining system for knowledge discovery from biomedical documents. *IBM Systems Journal*, *43*(3), 516–533. doi:10.1147/sj.433.0516

Zhou, X., Han, H., Chankai, I., Prestrud, A., & Brooks, A. (2006). Approaches to text mining for clinical medical records. *Proceedings of the 2006 ACM symposium on Applied computing*, 235-239. doi:10.1145/1141277.1141330

KEY TERMS AND DEFINITIONS

Brain Dead (BD): Patient whose brain function is complete and irreversibly lost (including involuntary activity necessary to sustain life) and need machines in order to stay alive.

Client-Server Architecture: Distributed application structure that partitions tasks or workloads between the providers of a resource or service, called servers, and service requesters, called clients.

Clinical Indicator: A measure, process, or outcome used to judge a particular clinical situation and indicate whether the care delivered was appropriate.

Cranio-Encephalic Computerized Tomography (CE CT): Noninvasive diagnostic imaging procedure that uses a combination of X-Rays and computer technology to produce horizontal, or axial, images (often called slices) of the brain. A CE CT scan may be performed to assess the brain for tumors and other lesions, injuries, intracranial bleeding, structural anomalies such as hydrocephalus, infections, brain function or other conditions.

Text Mining: The analysis of data contained in natural language text documents.

Chapter 10
Advanced Issues of Health Informatics and Clinical Decision Support System in Global Health Care

Kijpokin Kasemsap
Suan Sunandha Rajabhat University, Thailand

ABSTRACT

This chapter indicates the advanced issues of health informatics; the advanced issues of Clinical Decision Support System (CDSS); CDSS and Computerized Physician Order Entry (CPOE); the false positive alerts in CDSS; and CDSS and biomedical engineering. Health informatics and CDSS are the advanced health care technologies with the support of many technological fields. Health informatics and CDSS apply various computerized devices to provide enhanced health-related outcomes in terms of problem solving, analytical thinking, and decision making. Health informatics and CDSS help clinicians and health care providers to make complex information useful in supporting clinical decisions, thus delivering the best standard of care for each patient. The chapter argues that utilizing health informatics and CDSS has the potential to increase health outcomes and reach strategic goals in global health care.

INTRODUCTION

Nowadays, medicine and health fields are getting more and more involved with computer science (El-Fakdi, Gamero, Melendez, Auffret, & Haigron, 2014). Health informatics is an emerging field that is important to the effective delivery of modern health care (Lui, 2013) and applies the information science methods to analyze the health care information, to execute from raw data to knowledge, for the effective problem solving, decision making, and care delivery (Dalrymple, 2011). Medical and health activities can greatly benefit from the effective utilization of health informatics (Michell, Rosenorn-Lanng, Gulliver, & Currie, 2014). The increasing application of information and communication technology (ICT) in health care has created the needs to secure the health professionals' knowledge and skills in health and nursing informatics (Saranto, Jylhä, & Kinnunen, 2011).

DOI: 10.4018/978-1-5225-2851-7.ch010

The field of health informatics is at the intersection of information, computer science, behavioral science, and health care (Knott & Weller, 2014). Health informatics is a relatively new area which deals with mining large amounts of data to gain the useful insights (Narasimhamurthy, 2017). There is a need for health informatics to be fully integrated with each other and provide interoperability across various organizational domains for ubiquitous access and sharing (Naseer & Stergioulas, 2010). The interoperability framework, identifying citizens, providers, policymakers, and researchers is related to the improvement of understanding, access, trust, discourse, and practice toward the effective health care system (Juzwishin, 2010).

Clinical reasoning of healthcare professionals is rarely considered in the development of paper-based guidelines (Kilsdonk, Peute, Riezebos, Kremer, & Jaspers, 2016). Clinical guidelines are the important methods to improve the quality of health care while reducing the health care-related cost and supporting the medical staff (Douali & Jaulent, 2013). Poor design of CDSS interface can readily slow down health care practitioners as they may spend more time in searching for relevant information than in reviewing recommendations (Kilsdonk et al., 2016).

CDSS is the software designed to help clinicians make decisions about patient diagnosis using technical devices (Moon & Galea, 2017) toward bringing more confidence in health care for the physicians (Ruiz-Fernandez & Soriano-Paya, 2011). CDSS can improve guideline adherence by health care practitioners and support health care practitioners in the effective medical decision making (Jaspers, Smeulers, Vermeulen, & Peute, 2011). CDSS tends to be integrated into many systems, such as sensor technology, hardware, software, and communications (Pombo, Garcia, Bousson, & Felizardo, 2015), enough to help diagnose the patient's disease and prescribe the proper medication (Kareem & Bajwa, 2013).

This chapter is based on a literature review of health informatics and CDSS. The extensive literature of health informatics and CDSS provides a contribution to practitioners and researchers in order to maximize their impact in global health care.

BACKGROUND

The market of tools, devices, and processes for both medical treatments and medical diagnosis has been growing at a very fast pace, driven by the multidisciplinary development of innovative technologies (Catapano & Verkerke, 2011). Health care providers require the timely and accurate information about their patients (El Morr, 2014). Health informatics is the use of devices and resources to collect, store, move, and retrieve data to support health care (Mahmood, 2008). Health care systems are complex and often approach a deterministic chaos in the number and types of interactions that occur among health care providers and patients (Johnson & Tashiro, 2011).

Health informatics is the science of health information (Perry et al., 2008). Regarding health informatics, ICT helps improve the communication along processes in health care settings (Saboor, Hörbst, & Ammenwerth, 2013). From a technical perspective, the rapid transformation of the health care sector through health informatics is achievable (Brear, 2010). A fundamental premise of continuity in patient care and safety suggests the timely sharing of health information through health informatics among different health care providers at the point of care and after the visit (Gundlapalli, Reid, Root, & Xu, 2011). The practice of health informatics is faced with the complexities of multijurisdictional, multidisciplinary, and multicultural partner-based approaches to the problem-solving perspectives (LeRouge, Tolentino, Fuller, & Tuma, 2013).

Over decades, the importance of decision support system has increasingly identified as an enabler to the achievement of medical industry's strategic and operational objectives (Miah, 2014). Decision making is an integral aspect in the health-care routine that the ability to make the right decisions at crucial moments can lead to the patient's health improvements (Osop & Sahama, 2016). CDSS utilizes the passive or active decision support to modify the clinician behavior through the recommendations of specific actions (Rothman, Leonard, & Vigoda, 2012). The adoption of CDSS leads to the increased clinical performance through improved clinician decision making, adherence to evidence-based guidelines, medical error reduction, and more efficient information transfer (Carney, Weaver, McDaniel, Jones, & Haggstrom, 2016).

Clinical decisions need to be segmented in terms of whether they apply to individual cases, groups of patients or whole populations (Parry, 2012). CDSS interacts with practitioners and electronic health record (EHR) systems to receive the patient data as the input and provide the recommendations for patient diagnosis, treatment, and long-term care planning (Kazemzadeh, Sartipi, & Jayaratna, 2012).

IMPORTANT ASPECTS OF HEALTH INFORMATICS AND CLINICAL DECISION SUPPORT SYSTEM

This section provides the advanced issues of health informatics; the advanced issues of CDSS; CDSS and CPOE; the false positive alerts in CDSS; and CDSS and biomedical engineering.

Advanced Issues of Health Informatics

Informatics, the maximization of data utilization and acquisition through the intersection of information and computer science, becomes universal across a wide range of applications (Mackert, Whitten, & Holtz, 2010) toward enabling the collection, storage, retrieval, and analysis of data (Pasupathy, 2011). Clinical decisions based on the wrong sources of information can lead to medical errors, high treatment costs, and poor patient outcomes (Zaheer, 2014). Reducing medical errors, increasing patient safety, and improving the quality of health care are the major goals in the health care industry (Kasemsap, 2017a). Concerning health informatics, both Internet usage and accessibility have grown at a staggering rate, thus affecting technology utilization for health care purposes (Hung et al., 2013).

Standards in health informatics enable access to the patient health records to read and add the new data relevant to other health care providers taking care of the patient (Kern, 2009). Health informatics is capable of storing the valuable data concerning telemedicine (Treurnicht & van Dyk, 2012). The health informatics-related skills are essential for the health care-related profession to play a leadership role in design, implementation, and operation of next-generation health care (Hussey & Kennedy, 2016). Health informaticians have staked the health care-related claim to the evidence-based practice with their work on decision-support tools (Murphy, 2010).

There is a need to better understand where models from human computer interaction (HCI) can assist in the adoption of health informatics in health care (Price, 2011). Improved health care technologies and their accessibility, and societal improvements including higher income, better housing, improved food availability, and stronger welfare support mean that people are living longer (Rigby, 2014). Investments in the clinical information technology (IT) systems can be beneficial only when the systems are used by the physicians for the accurate diagnosis and prescriptions (Chang, Hwang, Hung, & Li, 2007).

Using health informatics can improve the quality of health care through the effective utilization of information systems (Abuidhail, 2009). Nursing informatics is the subcategory of health informatics and covers all areas of health care where nurses work, such as clinical task, administrative duty, research, and education (Strachan, Murray, & Erdley, 2011). Nursing informatics is the retrieval of data and information to enhance the nursing clinical practices concerning information management systems (Sneed, 2011). If the usage rate is low, the technology can no longer be effective for health care organizations (Chang, Chen, & Chang, 2009).

Advanced Issues of Clinical Decision Support System

Information is used as a critical tool for health care activities (Luukkonen, Toivanen, Mursu, Saranto, & Korpela, 2013). There is the growing health-care information that overloads physicians while facing the urgent cases (Akaichi & Mhadhbi, 2016). In making clinical decisions, clinicians often review medical literature to ensure the reliability of diagnosis, test, and treatment because the medical literature can answer clinical questions and assist clinicians making clinical decisions (Jiang et al., 2016). The quality of medical decision making relies on access to the available information, the quality of the information, and the quantity of relevant information (Bircher, 2010).

The application of CDSS in health care contributes to service quality enhancement, but it should not be forgotten that the final decision in health care is always made by a medical expert (Parshutin & Kirshners, 2013). CDSS provides physicians, patients, and health professionals with knowledge and person-specific information, that is intelligently filtered and retrieved at appropriate times, to enhance patient health and health care (Osheroff et al., 2007). Many hospitals rely on CDSS to assist in the prescription reviewing process (Beaudoin, Kabanza, Nault, & Valiquette, 2016). Examples of CDSS tools include the order sets created for the specific conditions or types of patients; databases that can provide information relevant to the particular patients; reminders for preventive care; and alerts about the potentially dangerous situations (Liu et al., 2015).

CDSS running within EHR can activate alerts when deviation from recommended care is detected through an electronic reminder system (Ali, Giordano, Lakhani, & Walker, 2016). Clinical trial (CT) inclusion and exclusion criteria can be readily used to implement the CDSS for patient eligibility determination (Marcos, Maldonado, Martinez-Salvador, Bosca, & Robles, 2013). Extracting medical knowledge by structured data mining of many medical records and from unstructured data mining of natural language source text on the Internet will become increasingly important for CDSS (Robson & Boray, 2016). Data mining is the process of applying the computational methods in showing the unknown data formats in large data sets (Kasemsap, 2015). Data mining plays a key role in organizing huge amount of data and condensing it into valuable information (Kasemsap, 2016).

The medical decision is mostly based upon the physicians' knowledge and experience rather than on the intensive knowledge of the patient's medical history (Al-Hyari, Al-Taee, & Al-Taee, 2014). The insufficient knowledge coverage for the detailed clinical pathways makes it difficult to provide the accurate information to improve the patient safety (Li, 2015). Lack of consideration for the interaction between decision makers and CDSS is a major reason for poor system adoption (Miller et al., 2015). In a chronic disease (e.g., diabetes), documentation is a critical component of disease management (Ali et al., 2016). When deploying the new CDSS, it is essential to monitor it to ensure that it normally operates, that the operational rules are correctly used (Lee et al., 2014). While CDSS can improve the health care-related documentation, it may not in itself improve patient compliance, which depends on the coordination between patient and health care provider (Morrow et al., 2012). Inconsistency and incompleteness in documentation are related to a lack of coordination among the activities involved in the processes of care (Schnipper et al., 2010).

CDSS, an important part of clinical practice, is comprised of three important perspectives: knowledge base; program for integrating the patient-specific information with the knowledge base; and user interface that allows clinicians to interact with the system and get the right information needed to make the right decision for the right patient at the right time (Eberhardt, Bilchik, & Stojadinovic, 2012). CDSS has focused on the formal clinical reasoning (Raghupathi, 2010). Clinical reasoning requires the holistic approach, incorporating the characteristics of softness, openness, complexity, flexibility, and generality of CDSS, while traditional rule-based approaches are sufficient for the clinical function applications (Raghupathi, 2010). Karra et al. (2014) indicated that the types and frequency of clinical decisions made by the intensive care nurses are related to the features of intensive care unit (ICU) work environment, their professional autonomy and accountability, as well as their perceptions of their clinical role.

Many health care institutions are deploying the distributed data warehouse (DWH) applications as the effective CDSS for the strategic decision making (Stolba, Nguyen, & Tjoa, 2010). Health-related data will be generated and accumulated, resulting in an enormous volume of data (Akerkar, 2016). CDSS provides the guidance related to the patient, thus importing the patient data into the CDSS application and providing the relevant information (Shrestha, 2013). Artificial intelligence (AI) is the area of computer science that emphasizes the creation of intelligent machines that work and react like humans (Kasemsap, 2017b). AI is used in CDSS applications, and plays significant role in the applied medical techniques (Al-Khasawneh & Hijazi,2014). Currently, evolution of health services is strongly influenced by the development of information and communication technology (Fernández, 2010).

Clinical Decision Support System and Computerized Physician Order Entry

Computerized physician order entry (CPOE) is the good example that describes how health informatics can be utilized as an effective solution to the health-care policy concerns (Al-Khudairy, 2014). CDSS is usually integrated with the existing CPOE systems to optimize the quality of clinical practices by providing physicians with alerts at the point-of-care (Tsai, Wang, Hsu, & Li, 2016). CPOE systems in hospital settings has been shown to reduce both prescription errors and adverse drug events (Ammenwerth, Schnell-Inderst, Machan, & Siebert, 2008).

medication safety for end-users, however many deficiencies have been reported, such as the lack of allergy alerts and the integration with other hospital systems (Khajouei, Wierenga, Hasman, & Jaspers, 2011). Alert fatigue occurs when there is a high number of non-clinically alerts, thus resulting alerts both relevant and not-relevant being ignored (de Wit et al., 2015).

False Positive Alerts in Clinical Decision Support System

False positive alerts in the patient-safety-related CDSS systems are recognized as the alerts which incorrectly prompt when no-risk patients are encountered (Tsai et al., 2016). The alert-based CDSS has shown to improve the physicians' practice in reducing medical errors and improving adherence to clinical guidelines in various clinical settings (Holstiege, Mathes, & Pieper, 2015). When alert system performance or physician responses to alert systems are measured, most studies reported on physicians' adherence rate, or other commonly used terms, such as acceptance rate, compliance rate, and adoption rate of the alert systems (Ranji, Rennke, & Wachter, 2014).

Excessive false positive alerts lead to the alert fatigue, which means if physicians were exposed to a large number of false positive alerts, they may be desensitized to most alerts (Tsai et al., 2016). Desensitization is an approach to overriding the true positive alerts (Seidling et al., 2014) and can lead to the adverse events on patient outcomes (Carspecken, Sharek, Longhurst, & Pageler, 2013). The alert fatigue phenomenon in CDSS has been mostly proposed in observational studies and before–after studies (Heringa, Floor-Schreudering, Tromp, Smet, & Bouvy, 2015), but rarely in the randomized controlled trials (RCTs). In the design of RCTs, the baseline characteristics of population studied are important in determining the effectiveness and reliability of outcomes (Chaudhry et al., 2006).

Clinical Decision Support System and Biomedical Engineering

The ability of computers to utilize the clinical and biomedical knowledge represents an important transition in human history (Robson & Baek, 2009). Computer aided medical diagnosis is one of the most important research fields in biomedical engineering (Goletsis, Exarchos, Giannakeas, Tsipouras, & Fotiadis, 2011). The multidisciplinary field of biomedical engineering is critical to the continuous evolution of medical technologies (Shukla & Tiwari, 2011) and engineering perspectives (Devedzic, Ristic, Stefanovic, Cukovic, & Lukovic, 2012). New developments in medical technology have paved the way for the ongoing studies of cognitive neuroscience and biomedical engineering for health care (Wu, 2013). Biomedical engineering unites the engineering methods with biological and medical sciences in order to enhance the quality of individuals' lives (Azar, 2013).

Biomedical engineers utilize engineering and biology knowledge to design, fabricate, and analyze of biomedical systems, devices, diagnostics, and therapeutics that address problems and opportunities associated with human health and performance. Regarding CDSS, medical data is the observation regarding a patient, including demographic details (e.g., age), medical history (e.g., diabetes and obesity), laboratory examinations (e.g., triglyceride), biomedical signals, and medical images (Goletsis et al., 2011). A typical nanotechnology application example in biomedical engineering is its usage as drug eluting interfaces for implantable devices, such as orthopedic implants and dental implants (Akujuobi, 2017). The factors contributing to biomedical engineering include the reasonable knowledge of the health care professional and the situations requiring the accurate decision making (Mishra, 2011).

FUTURE RESEARCH DIRECTIONS

The classification of the extensive literature in the domains of health informatics and CDSS will provide the potential opportunities for future research. The information concerning health informatics and CDSS must be filtered, organized, and presented in an effective way that supports the current workflow, allowing the users to effectively make the informed decision and take action in modern health care. Recent developments in the robotic age have made robots and robotics more intelligent, affordable, and user-friendly in modern operations, ranging from manufacturing to health care (Kasemsap, 2017c). An examination of linkages among health informatics, CDSS, and robotics in health care settings should be further studied.

CONCLUSION

This chapter indicated the advanced issues of health informatics; the advanced issues of CDSS; CDSS and CPOE; the false positive alerts in CDSS; and CDSS and biomedical engineering. Health informatics and CDSS are the advanced health care technologies with the support of many technological fields. Health informatics and CDSS apply various computerized devices to provide enhanced health-related outcomes in terms of problem solving, analytical thinking, and decision making. Health informatics and CDSS help clinicians and health care providers to make complex information useful in supporting clinical decisions, thus delivering the best standard of care for each patient. Utilizing health informatics and CDSS has the potential to increase health outcomes and reach strategic goals in global health care.

REFERENCES

Abuidhail, J. (2009). Women's health and health informatics: Perinatal care health education. In D. Parry & E. Parry (Eds.), *Medical informatics in obstetrics and gynecology* (pp. 263–277). Hershey, PA: IGI Global. doi:10.4018/978-1-60566-078-3.ch013

Akaichi, J., & Mhadhbi, L. (2016). A clinical decision support system: Ontology-driven approach for effective emergency management. In J. Moon & M. Galea (Eds.), *Improving health management through clinical decision support systems* (pp. 270–294). Hershey, PA: IGI Global. doi:10.4018/978-1-4666-9432-3.ch013

Akerkar, R. (2016). Towards an intelligent integrated approach for clinical decision support. In A. Aggarwal (Ed.), *Managing big data integration in the public sector* (pp. 187–205). Hershey, PA: IGI Global. doi:10.4018/978-1-4666-9649-5.ch011

Akujuobi, C. M. (2017). Nanotechnology applications in biomedical engineering. In Oncology: Breakthroughs in research and practice (pp. 352–365). Hershey, PA: IGI Global. doi:10.4018/978-1-5225-0549-5.ch012

Al-Hyari, A. Y., Al-Taee, A. M., & Al-Taee, M. A. (2014). Diagnosis and classification of chronic renal failure utilising intelligent data mining classifiers. *International Journal of Information Technology and Web Engineering*, *9*(4), 1–12. doi:10.4018/ijitwe.2014100101

Al-Khasawneh, A., & Hijazi, H. (2014). A predictive e-health information system: Diagnosing diabetes mellitus using neural network based decision support system. *International Journal of Decision Support System Technology*, *6*(4), 31–48. doi:10.4018/ijdsst.2014100103

Al-Khudairy, S. (2014). Caring for our aging population: Using CPOE and telehomecare systems as a response to health policy concerns. In C. El Morr (Ed.), *Research perspectives on the role of informatics in health policy and management* (pp. 153–166). Hershey, PA: IGI Global. doi:10.4018/978-1-4666-4321-5.ch010

Ali, S. M., Giordano, R., Lakhani, S., & Walker, D. M. (2016). A review of randomized controlled trials of medical record powered clinical decision support system to improve quality of diabetes care. *International Journal of Medical Informatics*, *87*, 91–100. doi:10.1016/j.ijmedinf.2015.12.017 PMID:26806716

Ammenwerth, E., Schnell-Inderst, P., Machan, C., & Siebert, U. (2008). The effect of electronic prescribing on medication errors and adverse drug events: A systematic review. *Journal of the American Medical Informatics Association*, *15*(5), 585–600. doi:10.1197/jamia.M2667 PMID:18579832

Azar, A. T. (2013). Overview of biomedical engineering. In *Bioinformatics: Concepts, methodologies, tools, and applications* (pp. 1–28). Hershey, PA: IGI Global. doi:10.4018/978-1-4666-3604-0.ch001

Beaudoin, M., Kabanza, F., Nault, V., & Valiquette, L. (2016). Evaluation of a machine learning capability for a clinical decision support system to enhance antimicrobial stewardship programs. *Artificial Intelligence in Medicine*, *68*, 29–36. doi:10.1016/j.artmed.2016.02.001 PMID:26947174

Bircher, N. G. (2010). The electronic patient record: A practicing physician's perspective. In S. Kabene (Ed.), *Healthcare and the effect of technology: Developments, challenges and advancements* (pp. 84–100). Hershey, PA: IGI Global. doi:10.4018/978-1-61520-733-6.ch006

Brear, M. (2010). Organizational factors: Their role in health informatics implementation. In J. Rodrigues (Ed.), *Health information systems: Concepts, methodologies, tools, and applications* (pp. 1295–1303). Hershey, PA: IGI Global. doi:10.4018/978-1-60566-988-5.ch081

Carney, T. J., Weaver, M., McDaniel, A. M., Jones, J., & Haggstrom, D. A. (2016). Organizational factors influencing the use of clinical decision support for improving cancer screening within community health centers. In *E-health and telemedicine: Concepts, methodologies, tools, and applications* (pp. 118–148). Hershey, PA: IGI Global. doi:10.4018/978-1-4666-8756-1.ch007

Carspecken, C. W., Sharek, P. J., Longhurst, C., & Pageler, N. M. (2013). A clinical case of electronic health record drug alert fatigue: Consequences for patient outcome. *Pediatrics*, *131*(6), e1970–e1973.

Catapano, G., & Verkerke, G. J. (2011). Artificial organs. *International Journal of Biomaterials Research and Engineering*, *1*(2), 41–76. doi:10.4018/ijbre.2013070104

Chang, I. C., Hwang, H. G., Hung, W. F., & Li, Y. C. (2007). Physicians' acceptance of pharmacokinetics-based clinical decision support systems. *Expert Systems with Applications*, *33*(2), 296–303. doi:10.1016/j.eswa.2006.05.001

Chang, J. Y., Chen, L. K., & Chang, C. C. (2009). Perspectives and expectations for telemedicine opportunities from families of nursing home residents and caregivers in nursing homes. *International Journal of Medical Informatics*, *78*(7), 494–502. doi:10.1016/j.ijmedinf.2009.02.009 PMID:19345640

Chaudhry, B., Wang, J., Wu, S., Maglione, M., Mojica, W., Roth, E., & Shekelle, P. G. et al. (2006). Systematic review: Impact of health information technology on quality, efficiency, and costs of medical care. *Annals of Internal Medicine*, *144*(10), 742–752. doi:10.7326/0003-4819-144-10-200605160-00125 PMID:16702590

Dalrymple, P. W. (2011). Data, information, knowledge: The emerging field of health informatics. *Bulletin of the Association for Information Science and Technology*, *37*(5), 41–44. doi:10.1002/bult.2011.1720370512

de Wit, H. A. J. M., Gonzalvo, C. M., Cardenas, J., Derijks, H. J., Janknegt, R., & van der Kuy, P. H. M. (2015). Evaluation of clinical rules in a standalone pharmacy based clinical decision support system for hospitalized and nursing home patients. *International Journal of Medical Informatics*, *84*(6), 396–405. doi:10.1016/j.ijmedinf.2015.02.004 PMID:25746461

Devedzic, G., Ristic, B., Stefanovic, M., Cukovic, S., & Lukovic, T. (2012). Development of 3D parametric model of human spine and simulator for biomedical engineering education and scoliosis screening. *Computer Applications in Engineering Education*, *20*(3), 434–444. doi:10.1002/cae.20411

Douali, N., & Jaulent, M. (2013). Clinical practice guidelines formalization for personalized medicine. *International Journal of Applied Evolutionary Computation*, *4*(3), 26–33. doi:10.4018/jaec.2013070103

Eberhardt, J., Bilchik, A., & Stojadinovic, A. (2012). Clinical decision support systems: Potential with pitfalls. *Journal of Surgical Oncology*, *105*(5), 502–510. doi:10.1002/jso.23053 PMID:22441903

El-Fakdi, A., Gamero, F., Melendez, J., Auffret, V., & Haigron, P. (2014). eXiTCDSS: A framework for a workflow-based CBR for interventional clinical decision support systems and its application to TAVI. *Expert Systems with Applications*, *41*(2), 284–294. doi:10.1016/j.eswa.2013.05.067

El Morr, C. (2014). *Research perspectives on the role of informatics in health policy and management.* Hershey, PA: IGI Global. doi:10.4018/978-1-4666-4321-5

Fernández, D. R. (2010). An agent-based architecture to ubiquitous health. In S. Mohammed & J. Fiaidhi (Eds.), *Ubiquitous health and medical informatics: The ubiquity 2.0 trend and beyond* (pp. 213–232). Hershey, PA: IGI Global. doi:10.4018/978-1-61520-777-0.ch011

Goletsis, Y., Exarchos, T. P., Giannakeas, N., Tsipouras, M. G., & Fotiadis, D. I. (2011). Integration of clinical and genomic data for decision support in cancer. In *Clinical technologies: Concepts, methodologies, tools and applications* (pp. 412–421). Hershey, PA: IGI Global. doi:10.4018/978-1-60960-561-2.ch212

Gundlapalli, A. V., Reid, J. H., Root, J., & Xu, W. (2011). Regional and community health information exchange in the United States. In A. Shukla & R. Tiwari (Eds.), *Biomedical engineering and information systems: Technologies, tools and applications* (pp. 198–218). Hershey, PA: IGI Global. doi:10.4018/978-1-61692-004-3.ch011

Heringa, M., Floor-Schreudering, A., Tromp, P. C., Smet, P. A., & Bouvy, M. L. (2015). Nature and frequency of drug therapy alerts generated by clinical decision support in community pharmacy. *Pharmacoepidemiology and Drug Safety*, *25*(1), 82–89. doi:10.1002/pds.3915 PMID:26602064

Holstiege, J., Mathes, T., & Pieper, D. (2015). Effects of computer-aided clinical decision support systems in improving antibiotic prescribing by primary care providers: A systematic review. *Journal of the American Medical Informatics Association*, *22*(1), 236–242. doi:10.1136/amiajnl-2014-002886 PMID:25125688

Hung, M., Conrad, J., Hon, S. D., Cheng, C., Franklin, J. D., & Tang, P. (2013). Uncovering patterns of technology use in consumer health informatics. *Wiley Interdisciplinary Reviews: Computational Statistics*, *5*(6), 432–447. doi:10.1002/wics.1276 PMID:24904713

Hussey, P. A., & Kennedy, M. A. (2016). Instantiating informatics in nursing practice for integrated patient centred holistic models of care: A discussion paper. *Journal of Advanced Nursing*, *72*(5), 1030–1041. doi:10.1111/jan.12927 PMID:26890201

Jaspers, M. W., Smeulers, M., Vermeulen, H., & Peute, L. W. (2011). Effects of clinical decision-support systems on practitioner performance and patient outcomes: A synthesis of high-quality systematic review findings. *Journal of the American Medical Informatics Association*, *18*(3), 327–334. doi:10.1136/amiajnl-2011-000094 PMID:21422100

Jiang, J., Zheng, J., Zhao, C., Su, J., Guan, Y., & Yu, Q. (2016). Clinical-decision support based on medical literature: A complex network approach. *Physica A: Statistical Mechanics and Its Applications*, *459*, 42–54.

Johnson, K., & Tashiro, J. (2011). Interprofessional care and health care complexity: Factors shaping human resources effectiveness in health information management. In S. Kabene (Ed.), *Human resources in healthcare, health informatics and healthcare systems* (pp. 250–280). Hershey, PA: IGI Global. doi:10.4018/978-1-61520-885-2.ch015

Juzwishin, D. W. (2010). Enabling technologies and challenges for the future of ubiquitous health: The interoperability framework. In S. Mohammed & J. Fiaidhi (Eds.), *Ubiquitous health and medical informatics: The ubiquity 2.0 trend and beyond* (pp. 596–622). Hershey, PA: IGI Global. doi:10.4018/978-1-61520-777-0.ch028

Kareem, S., & Bajwa, I. S. (2013). Virtual telemedicine and virtual telehealth: A natural language based implementation to address time constraint problem. In *Data mining: Concepts, methodologies, tools, and applications* (pp. 881–892). Hershey, PA: IGI Global. doi:10.4018/978-1-4666-2455-9.ch045

Karra, V., Papathanassoglou, E. D., Lemonidou, C., Sourtzi, P., & Giannakopoulou, M. (2014). Exploration and classification of intensive care nurses' clinical decisions: A Greek perspective. *Nursing in Critical Care*, *19*(2), 87–97. doi:10.1111/nicc.12018 PMID:24400657

Kasemsap, K. (2015). The role of data mining for business intelligence in knowledge management. In A. Azevedo & M. Santos (Eds.), *Integration of data mining in business intelligence systems* (pp. 12–33). Hershey, PA: IGI Global. doi:10.4018/978-1-4666-6477-7.ch002

Kasemsap, K. (2016). Multifaceted applications of data mining, business intelligence, and knowledge management. *International Journal of Social and Organizational Dynamics in IT*, *5*(1), 57–69. doi:10.4018/IJSODIT.2016010104

Kasemsap, K. (2017a). The perspectives of medical errors in the health care industry. In M. Riga (Ed.), *Impact of medical errors and malpractice on health economics, quality, and patient safety* (pp. 113–143). Hershey, PA: IGI Global. doi:10.4018/978-1-5225-2337-6.ch005

Kasemsap, K. (2017b). Artificial intelligence: Current issues and applications. In R. Das & M. Pradhan (Eds.), *Handbook of research on manufacturing process modeling and optimization strategies* (pp. 454–474). Hershey, PA: IGI Global. doi:10.4018/978-1-5225-2440-3.ch022

Kasemsap, K. (2017c). Robotics: Theory and applications. In M. Moore (Ed.), *Cybersecurity breaches and issues surrounding online threat protection* (pp. 311–345). Hershey, PA: IGI Global. doi:10.4018/978-1-5225-1941-6.ch013

Kazemzadeh, R. S., Sartipi, K., & Jayaratna, P. (2012). A framework for data and mined knowledge interoperability in clinical decision support systems. In J. Tan (Ed.), *Advancing technologies and intelligence in healthcare and clinical environments breakthroughs* (pp. 84–110). Hershey, PA: IGI Global. doi:10.4018/978-1-4666-1755-1.ch006

Kern, J. (2009). Standardization in health and medical informatics. In J. Tan (Ed.), *Medical informatics: Concepts, methodologies, tools, and applications* (pp. 2059–2065). Hershey, PA: IGI Global. doi:10.4018/978-1-60566-050-9.ch156

Khajouei, R., Wierenga, P. C., Hasman, A., & Jaspers, M. W. (2011). Clinicians satisfaction with CPOE ease of use and effect on clinicians' workflow, efficiency and medication safety. *International Journal of Medical Informatics*, *80*(5), 297–309. doi:10.1016/j.ijmedinf.2011.02.009 PMID:21419695

Kilsdonk, E., Peute, L. W., Riezebos, R. J., Kremer, L. C., & Jaspers, M. W. M. (2016). Uncovering healthcare practitioners' information processing using the think-aloud method: From paper-based guideline to clinical decision support system. *International Journal of Medical Informatics*, *86*, 10–19. doi:10.1016/j.ijmedinf.2015.11.011 PMID:26725690

Knott, V. E., & Weller, D. (2014). Informatics and e-health: Advancing knowledge and improving cancer care. *European Journal of Cancer Care*, *23*(6), 713–715. doi:10.1111/ecc.12268 PMID:25352463

Lee, J., Han, H., Ock, M., Lee, S. I., Lee, S., & Jo, M. W. (2014). Impact of a clinical decision support system for high-alert medications on the prevention of prescription errors. *International Journal of Medical Informatics*, *83*(12), 929–940. doi:10.1016/j.ijmedinf.2014.08.006 PMID:25256067

LeRouge, C., Tolentino, H., Fuller, S., & Tuma, A. (2013). Doing and understanding: Use of case studies for health informatics education and training. In S. Sarnikar, D. Bennett, & M. Gaynor (Eds.), *Cases on healthcare information technology for patient care management* (pp. 1–34). Hershey, PA: IGI Global. doi:10.4018/978-1-4666-2671-3.ch001

Li, W. (2015). Clinical pathway enhanced by knowledge management technology: A critical step towards medical quality improvement. In *Healthcare administration: Concepts, methodologies, tools, and applications* (pp. 978–996). Hershey, PA: IGI Global. doi:10.4018/978-1-4666-6339-8.ch051

Liu, G. C., Odell, J. D., Whipple, E. C., Ralston, R., Carroll, A. E., & Downs, S. M. (2015). Data visualization for truth maintenance in clinical decision support systems. *International Journal of Pediatrics and Adolescent Medicine*, *2*(2), 64–69. doi:10.1016/j.ijpam.2015.06.001

Lui, K. (2013). The health informatics professional. In *User-driven healthcare: Concepts, methodologies, tools, and applications* (pp. 120–141). Hershey, PA: IGI Global. doi:10.4018/978-1-4666-2770-3.ch007

Luukkonen, I., Toivanen, M., Mursu, A., Saranto, K., & Korpela, M. (2013). Researching an activity-driven approach to information systems development. In M. Cruz-Cunha, I. Miranda, & P. Gonçalves (Eds.), *Handbook of research on ICTs and management systems for improving efficiency in healthcare and social care* (pp. 431–450). Hershey, PA: IGI Global. doi:10.4018/978-1-4666-3990-4.ch022

Mackert, M., Whitten, P., & Holtz, B. (2010). Health infonomics: Intelligent applications of information technology. In M. Pankowska (Ed.), *Infonomics for distributed business and decision-making environments: Creating information system ecology* (pp. 217–232). Hershey, PA: IGI Global. doi:10.4018/978-1-60566-890-1.ch012

Mahmood, O. (2008). Application of wireless data grids for health informatics. In N. Wickramasinghe & E. Geisler (Eds.), *Encyclopedia of healthcare information systems* (pp. 61–67). Hershey, PA: IGI Global. doi:10.4018/978-1-59904-889-5.ch009

Marcos, M., Maldonado, J. A., Martinez-Salvador, B., Bosca, D., & Robles, M. (2013). Interoperability of clinical decision-support systems and electronic health records using archetypes: A case study in clinical trial eligibility. *Journal of Biomedical Informatics*, *46*(4), 676–689. doi:10.1016/j.jbi.2013.05.004 PMID:23707417

Miah, S. J. (2014). A demand-driven cloud-based business intelligence for healthcare decision making. In Z. Sun & J. Yearwood (Eds.), *Handbook of research on demand-driven web services: Theory, technologies, and applications* (pp. 324–339). Hershey, PA: IGI Global. doi:10.4018/978-1-4666-5884-4.ch015

Michell, V., Rosenorn-Lanng, D. J., Gulliver, S. R., & Currie, W. (Eds.). (2014). *Handbook of research on patient safety and quality care through health informatics*. Hershey, PA: IGI Global. doi:10.4018/978-1-4666-4546-2

Miller, A., Moon, B., Anders, S., Walden, R., Brown, S., & Montella, D. (2015). Integrating computerized clinical decision support systems into clinical work: A meta-synthesis of qualitative research. *International Journal of Medical Informatics*, *84*(12), 1009–1018. doi:10.1016/j.ijmedinf.2015.09.005 PMID:26391601

Mishra, S. (2011). Social and ethical concerns of biomedical engineering research and practice. In A. Shukla & R. Tiwari (Eds.), *Biomedical engineering and information systems: Technologies, tools and applications* (pp. 54–80). Hershey, PA: IGI Global. doi:10.4018/978-1-61692-004-3.ch003

Moon, J. D., & Galea, M. P. (2017). Overview of clinical decision support systems in healthcare. In *Medical imaging: Concepts, methodologies, tools, and applications* (pp. 1501–1527). Hershey, PA: IGI Global. doi:10.4018/978-1-5225-0571-6.ch064

Morrow, D. G., Conner-Garcia, T., Graumlich, J. F., Wolf, M. S., McKeever, S., Madison, A., & Kaiser, D. et al. (2012). An EMR-based tool to support collaborative planning for medication use among adults with diabetes: Design of a multi-site randomized control trial. *Contemporary Clinical Trials*, *33*(5), 1023–1032. doi:10.1016/j.cct.2012.05.010 PMID:22664648

Murphy, J. (2010). Health science librarianship's legacy to health informatics. *Health Information and Libraries Journal*, *27*(1), 75–79. doi:10.1111/j.1471-1842.2010.00882.x PMID:20402807

Narasimhamurthy, A. (2017). An overview of machine learning in medical image analysis: Trends in health informatics. In *Medical imaging: Concepts, methodologies, tools, and applications* (pp. 36–58). Hershey, PA: IGI Global. doi:10.4018/978-1-5225-0571-6.ch002

Naseer, A., & Stergioulas, L. K. (2010). HealthGrids in health informatics: A taxonomy. In K. Khoumbati, Y. Dwivedi, A. Srivastava, & B. Lal (Eds.), *Handbook of research on advances in health informatics and electronic healthcare applications: Global adoption and impact of information communication technologies* (pp. 124–143). Hershey, PA: IGI Global. doi:10.4018/978-1-60566-030-1.ch008

Osheroff, J. A., Teich, J. M., Middleton, B., Steen, E. B., Wright, A., & Detmer, D. E. (2007). A roadmap for national action on clinical decision support. *Journal of the American Medical Informatics Association, 14*(2), 141–145. doi:10.1197/jamia.M2334 PMID:17213487

Osop, H., & Sahama, T. (2016). Data-driven and practice-based evidence: Design and development of efficient and effective clinical decision support system. In J. Moon & M. Galea (Eds.), *Improving health management through clinical decision support systems* (pp. 295–328). Hershey, PA: IGI Global. doi:10.4018/978-1-4666-9432-3.ch014

Parry, D. (2012). Computerised decision support for women's health informatics. In *Machine learning: Concepts, methodologies, tools and applications* (pp. 1404–1416). Hershey, PA: IGI Global. doi:10.4018/978-1-60960-818-7.ch513

Parshutin, S., & Kirshners, A. (2013). Research on clinical decision support systems development for atrophic gastritis screening. *Expert Systems with Applications, 40*(15), 6041–6046. doi:10.1016/j.eswa.2013.05.011

Pasupathy, K. S. (2011). Systems engineering and health informatics. In *Clinical technologies: Concepts, methodologies, tools and applications* (pp. 1684–1705). Hershey, PA: IGI Global. doi:10.4018/978-1-60960-561-2.ch606

Perry, T. L., Tucker, T., Hudson, L. R., Gandy, W., Neftzger, A. L., & Hamar, G. B. (2008). The application of data mining techniques in health plan population management: A disease management approach. In J. Wang (Ed.), *Data warehousing and mining: Concepts, methodologies, tools, and applications* (pp. 1799–1809). Hershey, PA: IGI Global. doi:10.4018/978-1-59904-951-9.ch106

Pombo, N., Garcia, N., Bousson, K., & Felizardo, V. (2015). Machine learning approaches to automated medical decision support systems. In P. Vasant (Ed.), *Handbook of research on artificial intelligence techniques and algorithms* (pp. 183–203). Hershey, PA: IGI Global. doi:10.4018/978-1-4666-7258-1.ch006

Price, M. (2011). A bio-psycho-social review of usability methods and their applications in healthcare. In *Clinical technologies: Concepts, methodologies, tools and applications* (pp. 1874–1899). Hershey, PA: IGI Global. doi:10.4018/978-1-60960-561-2.ch704

Raghupathi, W. (2010). Designing clinical decision support systems in health care: A systemic view. In M. Hunter (Ed.), *Strategic information systems: Concepts, methodologies, tools, and applications* (pp. 652–661). Hershey, PA: IGI Global. doi:10.4018/978-1-60566-677-8.ch043

Ranji, S. R., Rennke, S., & Wachter, R. M. (2014). Computerised provider order entry combined with clinical decision support systems to improve medication safety: A narrative review. *BMJ Quality & Safety, 23*(9), 773–780. doi:10.1136/bmjqs-2013-002165 PMID:24728888

Rigby, M. (2014). The core vision of person-centred care in a modern information-based society. In I. Meyer, S. Müller, & L. Kubitschke (Eds.), *Achieving effective integrated e-care beyond the silos* (pp. 1–21). Hershey, PA: IGI Global. doi:10.4018/978-1-4666-6138-7.ch001

Robson, B., & Baek, O. K. (2009). *The engines of Hippocrates: From the dawn of medicine to medical and pharmaceutical informatics*. Hoboken, NJ: John Wiley & Sons. doi:10.1002/9780470461808

Robson, B., & Boray, S. (2016). Data-mining to build a knowledge representation store for clinical decision support. Studies on curation and validation based on machine performance in multiple choice medical licensing examinations. *Computers in Biology and Medicine*, *73*, 71–93. doi:10.1016/j.compbiomed.2016.02.010 PMID:27089305

Rothman, B., Leonard, J. C., & Vigoda, M. M. (2012). Future of electronic health records: Implications for decision support. *Mount Sinai Journal of Medicine: A Journal of Translational and Personalized Medicine, 79*(6), 757–768. doi:10.1002/msj.21351

Ruiz-Fernandez, D., & Soriano-Paya, A. (2011). A distributed approach of a clinical decision support system based on cooperation. In *Clinical technologies: Concepts, methodologies, tools and applications* (pp. 1782–1799). Hershey, PA: IGI Global. doi:10.4018/978-1-60960-561-2.ch612

Saboor, S., Hörbst, A., & Ammenwerth, E. (2013). Modeling and automated examination of communication processes in integrated health information systems: A systematic approach. *International Journal of Knowledge-Based Organizations*, *3*(1), 19–36. doi:10.4018/ijkbo.2013010102

Saranto, K., Jylhä, V., & Kinnunen, U. (2011). Are nurses prepared for engagement to evidence-based practice with new technologies? In A. Cashin & R. Cook (Eds.), *Evidence-based practice in nursing informatics: Concepts and applications* (pp. 98–112). Hershey, PA: IGI Global. doi:10.4018/978-1-60960-034-1.ch008

Schnipper, J. L., Linder, J. A., Palchuk, M. B., Yu, D. T., McColgan, K. E., & Volk, L. A. et al.. (2010). Effects of documentation-based decision support on chronic disease management. *The American Journal of Managed Care*, *16*(12), SP72–SP81. PMID:21314226

Seidling, H. M., Klein, U., Schaier, M., Czock, D., Theile, D., Pruszydlo, M. G., & Haefeli, W. E. et al. (2014). What, if all alerts were specific – estimating the potential impact on drug interaction alert burden. *International Journal of Medical Informatics*, *83*(4), 285–291. doi:10.1016/j.ijmedinf.2013.12.006 PMID:24484781

Shrestha, S. (2013). Clinical decision support system for diabetes prevention: An illustrative case. In S. Sarnikar, D. Bennett, & M. Gaynor (Eds.), *Cases on healthcare information technology for patient care management* (pp. 308–329). Hershey, PA: IGI Global. doi:10.4018/978-1-4666-2671-3.ch017

Shukla, A., & Tiwari, R. (2011). *Biomedical engineering and information systems: Technologies, tools and applications* (pp. 1–384). Hershey, PA: IGI Global. doi:10.4018/978-1-61692-004-3

Sneed, W. (2011). A treatise on rural public health nursing. In *Clinical technologies: Concepts, methodologies, tools and applications* (pp. 2013–2028). Hershey, PA: IGI Global. doi:10.4018/978-1-60960-561-2.ch711

Stolba, N., Nguyen, T. M., & Tjoa, A. M. (2010). Data warehouse facilitating evidence-based medicine. In T. Nguyen (Ed.), *Complex data warehousing and knowledge discovery for advanced retrieval development: Innovative methods and applications* (pp. 174–207). Hershey, PA: IGI Global. doi:10.4018/978-1-60566-748-5.ch008

Strachan, H., Murray, P., & Erdley, W. S. (2011). Nursing informatics history and its contributions to nursing knowledge. In A. Cashin & R. Cook (Eds.), *Evidence-based practice in nursing informatics: Concepts and applications* (pp. 78–97). Hershey, PA: IGI Global. doi:10.4018/978-1-60960-034-1.ch007

Treurnicht, M. J., & van Dyk, L. (2012). Clinical-pull approach to telemedicine implementation policies using health informatics in the developing world. In J. Rodrigues, I. de la Torre Díez, & B. Sainz de Abajo (Eds.), *Telemedicine and e-health services, policies, and applications: Advancements and developments* (pp. 424–450). Hershey, PA: IGI Global. doi:10.4018/978-1-4666-0888-7.ch016

Tsai, C. Y., Wang, S. H., Hsu, M. H., & Li, Y. C. (2016). Do false positive alerts in naïve clinical decision support system lead to false adoption by physicians? A randomized controlled trial. *Computer Methods and Programs in Biomedicine, 132*, 82–91. doi:10.1016/j.cmpb.2016.04.011 PMID:27282230

Wu, J. (2013). *Biomedical engineering and cognitive neuroscience for healthcare: Interdisciplinary applications* (pp. 1–472). Hershey, PA: IGI Global. doi:10.4018/978-1-4666-2113-8

Zaheer, S. (2014). Implementation of evidence-based practice and the PARIHS framework. In C. El Morr (Ed.), *Research perspectives on the role of informatics in health policy and management* (pp. 19–36). Hershey, PA: IGI Global. doi:10.4018/978-1-4666-4321-5.ch002

ADDITIONAL READING

Abugabah, A., Afarraj, O., & Sansogni, L. (2016). Information systems in healthcare with a special focus on developing countries. In *E-health and telemedicine: Concepts, methodologies, tools, and applications* (pp. 1688–1706). Hershey, PA: IGI Global. doi:10.4018/978-1-4666-8756-1.ch085

Barrett, J. S. (2015). Paediatric models in motion: Requirements for model-based decision support at the bedside. *British Journal of Clinical Pharmacology, 79*(1), 85–96. doi:10.1111/bcp.12287 PMID:24251868

Blum, D., Raj, S. X., Oberholzer, R., Riphagen, I. I., Strasser, F., & Kaasa, S. (2015). Computer-based clinical decision support systems and patient-reported outcomes: A systematic review. *Patient, 8*(5), 397–409. doi:10.1007/s40271-014-0100-1 PMID:25432150

Dalrymple, P. (2013). Health informatics: Introduction. *Bulletin of the Association for Information Science and Technology, 39*(5), 18–19. doi:10.1002/bult.2013.1720390504

Esmaeilzadeh, P., Sambasivan, M., Kumar, N., & Nezakati, H. (2015). Adoption of clinical decision support systems in a developing country: Antecedents and outcomes of physicians' threat to perceived professional autonomy. *International Journal of Medical Informatics, 84*(8), 548–560. doi:10.1016/j.ijmedinf.2015.03.007 PMID:25920928

Facelli, J. C., Hurdle, J. F., & Mitchell, J. A. (2013). Medical informatics and bioinformatics. In *Bioinformatics: Concepts, methodologies, tools, and applications* (pp. 195–221). Hershey, PA: IGI Global. doi:10.4018/978-1-4666-3604-0.ch010

Fossum, M., Alexander, G. L., Ehnfors, M., & Ehrenberg, A. (2011). Effects of a computerized decision support system on pressure ulcers and malnutrition in nursing homes for the elderly. *International Journal of Medical Informatics*, *80*(9), 607–617. doi:10.1016/j.ijmedinf.2011.06.009 PMID:21783409

Horsky, J., Schiff, G. D., Johnston, D., Mercincavage, L., Bell, D., & Middleton, B. (2012). Interface design principles for usable decision support: A targeted review of best practices for clinical prescribing interventions. *Journal of Biomedical Informatics*, *45*(6), 1202–1216. doi:10.1016/j.jbi.2012.09.002 PMID:22995208

Kabene, S. M. (2011). *Human resources in healthcare, health informatics and healthcare systems* (pp. 1–378). Hershey, PA: IGI Global. doi:10.4018/978-1-61520-885-2

Kane-Gill, S. L., Visweswaran, S., Saul, M. I., Wong, A. K., Penrod, L. E., & Handler, S. M. (2011). Computerized detection of adverse drug reactions in the medical intensive care unit. *International Journal of Medical Informatics*, *80*(8), 570–578. doi:10.1016/j.ijmedinf.2011.04.005 PMID:21621453

Kilsdonk, E., Peute, L. W., Riezebos, R. J., Kremer, L. C., & Jaspers, M. W. (2013). From an expert-driven paper guideline to a user-centred decision support system: A usability comparison study. *Artificial Intelligence in Medicine*, *59*(1), 5–13. doi:10.1016/j.artmed.2013.04.004 PMID:23684240

Knight, E. P., & Shea, K. (2014). A patient-focused framework integrating self-management and informatics. *Journal of Nursing Scholarship*, *46*(2), 91–97. doi:10.1111/jnu.12059 PMID:24354997

Lui, K. (2015). Ethics in health informatics and information technology. In M. Khosrow-Pour (Ed.), *Encyclopedia of information science and technology* (3rd ed.; pp. 3000–3010). Hershey, PA: IGI Global. doi:10.4018/978-1-4666-5888-2.ch293

Marcum, J. A. (2012). An integrated model of clinical reasoning: Dual-process theory of cognition and metacognition. *Journal of Evaluation in Clinical Practice*, *18*(5), 954–961. doi:10.1111/j.1365-2753.2012.01900.x PMID:22994991

Mendes, D. J., Rodrigues, I. P., Baeta, C. F., & Solano-Rodriguez, C. (2015). Extended clinical discourse representation structure for controlled natural language clinical decision support systems. *International Journal of Reliable and Quality E-Healthcare*, *4*(2), 1–11. doi:10.4018/IJRQEH.2015040101

Mokeddem, S., & Atmani, B. (2016). Assessment of clinical decision support systems for predicting coronary heart disease. *International Journal of Operations Research and Information Systems*, *7*(3), 57–73. doi:10.4018/IJORIS.2016070104

Najaftorkaman, M., Ghapanchi, A. H., Talaei-Khoei, A., & Ray, P. (2015). A taxonomy of antecedents to user adoption of health information systems: A synthesis of thirty years of research. *Journal of the Association for Information Science and Technology*, *66*(3), 576–598. doi:10.1002/asi.23181

Nallas, R., & Moon, J. (2016). Integration of automation and clinical decision support systems. In J. Moon & M. Galea (Eds.), *Improving health management through clinical decision support systems* (pp. 165–185). Hershey, PA: IGI Global. doi:10.4018/978-1-4666-9432-3.ch008

Paolucci, F., Ergas, H., Hannan, T., & Aarts, J. (2011). The effectiveness of health informatics. In *Clinical technologies: Concepts, methodologies, tools and applications* (pp. 25–49). Hershey, PA: IGI Global. doi:10.4018/978-1-60960-561-2.ch103

Raghupathi, W., & Nerur, S. (2012). The intellectual structure of health and medical informatics. In J. Tan (Ed.), *Advancing technologies and intelligence in healthcare and clinical environments breakthroughs* (pp. 1–16). Hershey, PA: IGI Global. doi:10.4018/978-1-4666-1755-1.ch001

Rommers, M. K., Teepe-Twiss, I. M., & Guchelaar, H. J. (2011). A computerized adverse drug event alerting system using clinical rules: A retrospective and prospective comparison with conventional medication surveillance in the Netherlands. *Drug Safety*, *34*(3), 233–242. doi:10.2165/11536500-000000000-00000 PMID:21332247

Tawadrous, D., Shariff, S. Z., Haynes, R. B., Iansavichus, A. V., Jain, A. K., & Garg, A. X. (2011). Use of clinical decision support systems for kidney-related drug prescribing: A systematic review. *American Journal of Kidney Diseases*, *58*(6), 903–914. doi:10.1053/j.ajkd.2011.07.022 PMID:21944664

White, M. (2013). Public health informatics: An invitation to the field. *Bulletin of the Association for Information Science and Technology*, *39*(5), 25–29. doi:10.1002/bult.2013.1720390506

Wilson, E. V. (2011). Applying personal health informatics to create effective patient-centered e-health. In *Clinical technologies: Concepts, methodologies, tools and applications* (pp. 1800–1811). Hershey, PA: IGI Global. doi:10.4018/978-1-60960-561-2.ch613

Wright, A., Sittig, D. F., Ash, J. S., Erickson, J. L., Hickman, T. T., Paterno, M., & Middleton, B. et al. (2015). Lessons learned from implementing service-oriented clinical decision support at four sites: A qualitative study. *International Journal of Medical Informatics*, *84*(11), 901–911. doi:10.1016/j.ijmedinf.2015.08.008 PMID:26343972

Zarikas, V., Papageorgiou, E., & Regner, P. (2015). Bayesian network construction using a fuzzy rule based approach for medical decision support. *Expert Systems: International Journal of Knowledge Engineering and Neural Networks*, *32*(3), 344–369. doi:10.1111/exsy.12089

KEY TERMS AND DEFINITIONS

Biomedical Engineering: The advanced engineering perspective concerning biology.

Clinical Decision Support System: The method toward effectively making health care-related decision.

Computerized Physician Order Entry: The way to electronically enter the medical orders in health care settings through applying various technologies.

Electronic Health Record: The digital health record for the health care providers that is shared among multiple facilities and agencies.

Health Care: The execution of illness that is used by health care providers in health care settings.
Health Informatics: The sophisticated procedure to organize the health information.
Information: The data that is used for many important tasks.
Intensive Care Unit: The section in hospital that takes care of seriously ill patients.
Knowledge: The understanding of complex methods and systems.

Chapter 11
Applied Business Intelligence in Surgery Waiting Lists Management

Cristiana Neto
University of Minho, Portugal

Inês Dias
University of Minho, Portugal

Maria Santos
University of Minho, Portugal

Hugo Peixoto
University of Minho, Portugal

José Machado
University of Minho, Portugal

ABSTRACT

With the advent of computer science in hospitals, Electronic Health Record comes up, with the aim of bringing the new information technologies to the hospital environment with the promise not only to replace the paper process, but also to improve and provide better patient care. The operationalization of the EHR in supporting evidence-based practice, complex and conscientious decision-making, and improving the quality of healthcare delivery has been supported by the Business Intelligence (BI) technology. Since the beginning of the 1990s, the Portuguese health system has been confronted with a chronic problem, waiting time for surgery, due to inability to respond to demand for surgical therapy. Therefore, using business intelligence and information, obtained with the construction of dashboards, can help, for example, allocating hospital resources and reducing waiting times.

DOI: 10.4018/978-1-5225-2851-7.ch011

INTRODUCTION

Because of the infinite amount of information, the sources of information in health units are complex, varied, immense and distributed. These days, it becomes more and more valuable to ensure a significant homogeneity between medical, administrative and clinical systems, leading to the integration of the different hospital systems.

It is a reality that the waiting times in hospitals for surgical treatment are high and, in Portugal, most of the health complaints result from high waiting times (Portela et al., 2011).

Access to health care is highly influenced by the existence of waiting lists and the existence of waiting lists lead to conclude that there is an inability of the health system to satisfy the elementary human health needs and raise concerns both at efficiency and equity levels (Barros, 2008). Despite being possible to reduce waiting lists' average duration to minimum values, it's considered to be impossible the absence of waiting lists (Hurst & Siciliani, 2003).

In Portugal, a patient is submitted to a primary care consultation and, if needed, proceeds to a specialist consultation at the hospital. A document designated P1, currently electronically registered is issued by the physician allowing the patient to be placed on the waiting list for a specialty consultation. After that, in need for surgical intervention, it proceeds to the waiting list for surgery (Fernandes et al., 2010).

For hospital values, waiting time is focused on the waiting time since there is a need for a specialty consultation until it is performed, and from the moment it is decided to proceed to a surgical intervention until the agenda of it (Portela et al., 2011). It's important to emphasize that waiting lists for surgery tend to be more pronounced in countries that combine health insurance (Barros, 2008).

For the last decades, Portugal has suffered an increase in waiting lists, which may be due to aging of the population, the introduction of new technologies, leading to an increased demand for surgical interventions. Also the malfunctions in resources' distribution and the number of operating rooms available, for example, interfere directly with those waiting times (OPSS, 2003).

Over the last few years, information systems (IS) have been implemented with the aim of combating waiting lists for surgery and they intend to help in patients' management. SIGIC – Integrated System for the Management of Enrolled Patients for Surgery was implemented within Portuguese health care institutions in 2004 and led to a better planning and programming of the institution's activity, reducing waiting times through management. In addition, the acknowledgment of different situations through information systems and a more efficient management of resources, tend to create a greater response capacity of health institutions (Oliveira, 2012).

Electronic Health Record (EHR) has recently become one of the most crucial sources of clinical information, due to the expansion of Health Information Systems (HIS) (Oliveira, 2012; Peixoto et al., 2010). It is a computerized health record that contains all the clinical information concerning a patient, such as biometric information, old prescriptions, lab and imaging results, clinical diagnosis, etc. It aims to help systems to bring together all the information provided to a certain patient, providing a cross-sectional analysis of the patient's medical history in different services and different institutions and, new advanced mechanisms that integrate EHR with decision support systems begin to appear (Oliveira, 2012).

The quantity and quality of the information available in an EHR for health professionals can have a strong impact on their performance, since it guides their decision-making path. It is therefore fundamental that multiple information axes intersect in a related and coherent way (Martins, 2011).

In order to analyze the potential use of a BI tool to access the waiting lists for surgery in Portugal, data were analyzed for several patients, which were later processed through ETL process, part of the Business Intelligence Process, with the consequent creation of dashboards with Indicators. In this article it is presented a theoretical contextualization about the processes previously mentioned and several indicators achieved using the selected BI tool.

HEALTH INFORMATION SYSTEMS

By creating new systems or using the ones that already exist, it's difficult sometimes to guarantee interoperability between different systems, to ensure the usability of the used platforms. It is difficult to access data and to know for sure whether the data is correct or not.

With that being said, and with the emergence of EHR, it becomes both necessary and feasible to define four main quality indicators, which are: Interoperability, Usability, Information Quality and Difficulty to Access Data (Marins, 2014; Miranda et al., 2010).

In their daily work, all people in a health facility use a set of independent technologies involving tons of different information. And, nowadays, this independence may be the cause of the difficulty in interoperability between information systems (Cardoso et al., 2014).

Interoperability describes the extent to which systems and devices can exchange data, and interpret that shared data. For two systems to be interoperable, they must be able to exchange data and subsequently present that data in a way that it can be understood by the user (Blumenthal & Glaser, 2007).

Concerning the second quality indicator, usability, it's important to know that it is crucial in promoting the widespread adoption and the "meaningful use" of EHR, and it describes how easily a task can be accomplished by the user when using a system in an efficient and accurate way. Missing critical functionalities, poor reliability of the software, or inadequate match between interface features and user tasks in general will have a strong impact on users' ability to conduct their work, independently from the usability of the available system features (Zhang & Walji, 2011).

In the BI context there is a clear difference between data and information (quality), since the main goal of BI is to provide high quality information for administrative decision making. There is a hierarchical relationship between data and information, since data quality is not guaranteed antecedent of information quality, implying that data quality is positively related to information quality (Wieder & Ossimitz, 2015). In health information systems, it's absolutely needed to guarantee that the information is completely trustworthy.

It is sometimes extremely difficult to access or obtain data for the EHR, especially due to the fact that, in several hospitals, the patient information is still in a paper chart and not in a digital version. In addition, much of the data, even in digital format, is in multiple places. Healthcare data also occurs in different formats (e.g., text, numeric, paper, digital, pictures, videos, etc.). Radiology uses images, old medical records exist in paper format, and today's EMRs can hold hundreds of rows of textual and numerical data (Mendes & Rodrigues, 2010).

In a society with so much worries about information, there is a constant need to build usable infrastructures in order to collect, storage, process, represent and distribute.

Defined as a set of data organized and presented in a specific context, the information is an essential element to the decision-making process. But, to complete its function, the information must fulfil the present characteristics: the information is useful only if it is recent; the information has to be exact to generate trust in the system; it is crucial that the system affects the decisions made; the users must be able to connect to the information in time; the information has to be published in a way it is easily read and understood (Luís et al., 2013).

These days, increased importance has been given to the management of information and knowledge in institutions in order to implement successful strategies, to continuously improve processes and to measure institutional performance. Clinical knowledge bases must be continuously updated in order to adequately address health care needs. Advanced medical computing applications require a wide variety of knowledge assets. Thus, clinical systems with a built-in decision support system have the tendency to reduce the incidence of medical errors and improve the quality of health services, leading to a significant reduction in costs (Fayyad et al., 1996).

Information on Surgery Waiting List

The waiting time (ET) for surgery due to inability to respond to demand for surgical therapy, has been a problem to the Portuguese health system since the beginning of the 1990s.

However, this situation has improved considerably since the creation of SIGIC in 2004, as already mentioned.

The amount of data collected in integrated systems has naturally increased over the years. In this context, the need for interoperability in health is mandatory, since the different information systems can differ about its main objective (care, unit management or research), its scope and the technologies they use and support (stand-alone, client-server, web-based).

Interoperability is a very important point when it comes to managing waiting lists for surgery. Considering that when a patient is enrolled in the list, there is a lot of information needed to complete the process, such as the history of the patient's illnesses, the history of previous surgeries, information about chronic diseases, personal information, given information by doctors regarding the patient's condition, among others. This information may be stored in several different systems, which may be a problem itself, and of course, in case of transfer of a patient who was waiting for surgery in a hospital to another hospital, the data must be compatible with the target hospital system, otherwise there may be serious loss of information.

The data we received have been extracted from several sources, which makes us reflect on the interoperability of the systems in question. The data we received contained various information, both on administrative records and records of the operating room. These records referred to the patient, the physician, the surgery itself, etc. There was also a lot of information that contained only a code, without any connection to other information, which could be in another system, which would therefore compromise the interoperability between systems.

A wrong diagnosis may occur due to the existence of inconsistent information that was included in the EHR and subsequently disseminated. In order to avoid this and some moral and ethical issues, a complete validation of the exchanged and integrated information must be carried out. The development of top-level interoperability frameworks is indispensable for the quality of the healthcare environment (Cardoso et al., 2014).

Problems with the quality of information are also routinely felt by all institutions, especially hospitals, with different levels of severity and injury. The negative impact translates into unnecessary costs, affected decision processes or loss of user's confidence. Problems with the quality of information on a waiting list for surgery can have serious consequences such as performing surgery at the wrong location, a relatively common mistake in Portuguese hospitals (for example, operating the left leg when the problem is in the right leg).

BUSINESS INTELLIGENCE

Data arises from several information sources, and it becomes necessary that the process effectively resorts to the integration of systems. Here enters the ETL Process that is based, as the name indicates in the information Extraction from a Database, Transformation, and Loading (Figure 1).

- **Extraction:** This phase consists of an initial extraction and later extraction of the altered data. Initially, the extraction is based on the first set of extracted data and its consequent loading into the Data Warehouse (DW). The extraction of altered data is parallel to the continuous updating of the DW.
- **Transformation:** In this phase, the cleaning, integration and optimization of the input data are done to obtain accurate data, which are correct, complete, consistent and unambiguous.
- **Load:** The *Load* step is based on the extracted and transformed data written for a multidimensional structure.

Briefly, the data from different data sources are extracted and processed. Subsequently they are propagated to an instance called the Data Staging Area where they go through a transformation that ends in the upload to a second DB, the DW (El-Sappagh et al. 2011; Ferreira et al., 2010).

Since large amounts of data are processed, the ETL process is considered the most critical step in the construction of a DW. Therefore, an ETL tool must improve communications efficiency between the various DBs and should always contain mechanisms capable of reading different formats.

Figure 1. ETL process schema
El Sappagh et al. (2011)

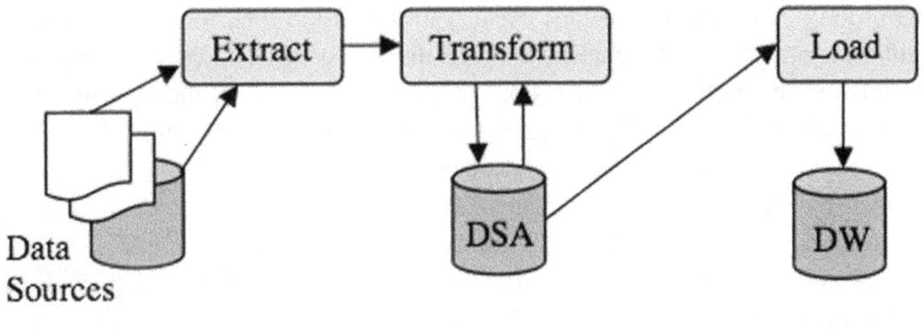

A Data Warehouse system is an intelligent data repository that allows adding and organizing data from one or multiple sources in order to make it easier to access. In other words, by extracting data from different applications we are able to construct a central repository that structures the information from which the Business Intelligence (BI) process can be acquired (Caldeira, 2012).

Since 80% of the data analysis time is spent in the transformation process (Khan et al., 2012), it is crucial to use a suitable Data Warehouse architecture to decrease it. This data storage architecture is based on a multidimensional data model, which allows the analysis of the data from several perspectives and provides the managers with a high power of decision making.

Having an architectural database model that facilitates the analysis of large volumes of data, allows a DW to aid in decision making. Thus, it should have several characteristics like easy access information, information presented consistently, adaptable and change-resistant system, help decision making and a single source of data (Kimball & Ross, 2002).

For multidimensional models, a DW can have different architectures, from the star schema, to the snowflake or to the constellation, allowing information to be viewed from different points of view depending on the subject in question (Sezões et al., 2006).

The most commonly used is the star model which comprises creating dimension tables linked by foreign keys to a fact table. The last one, as the name implies, stores facts as well as the foreign keys relative to the characteristics of the dimensional tables. In the other hand, the dimension tables contain all the detailed information regarding the attributes that describe the data contained in the central table.

A fundamental advantage of the described model is the single table of facts that contain all the data as well as the definition of only one primary key per dimension and the low maintenance need due to the low number of connections between tables (Sezões et al., 2006).

An example of an institution that would benefit from the implementation of a DW would be health institutions, which could result in very promising outcomes. In spite of the potential difficulties experienced in the implementation of the same, as well as the need to strengthen the personnel training to specialize in the subject, the high degree of automation of these institutions makes them excellent candidates in the development of these repositories (Mul et al., 2012).

The technology of analysis Online Analytical Process (OLAP) was born with the purpose of assisting the process of making decisions by obtaining information from databases. Basically, transitional data is transformed in interpretable data, that is, large quantities of information are analyzed in real time, being this information always open to be dynamically explored.

As already said in this analysis, the users have permission to obtain the organized information, being able to form data subgroups in a multidimensional structure in order to respond to specific questions. So, OLAP uses the Multidimensional Analysis or the Hypercube Analysis, like it is known, as shown in Figure 2.

There is a group of numerical measures, existent in the multidimensional data models, associated to a set of dimensions that give the context to a certain measure. Then, each dimension is united by some type of relations hierarchy. The dimension's aggregate, hierarchies and measures are designated as cube (Thalhammer et al., 2001). The bigger the number of analysis measures, the more the number of perspectives to understand and analyze the available information.

As advantages, the OLAP tool has an enormous flexibility to be used in reports, mainly because the information doesn't have to be normalized. As disadvantages, there is a lot of information organized in large numbers of tables, as the principal operation is 'insert', and not delete and update which are only used when errors occur (Romero & Abelló, 2010). Business Intelligence is not a new concept but it has

Figure 2. Multidimensional cube representation
Oliveira (2012)

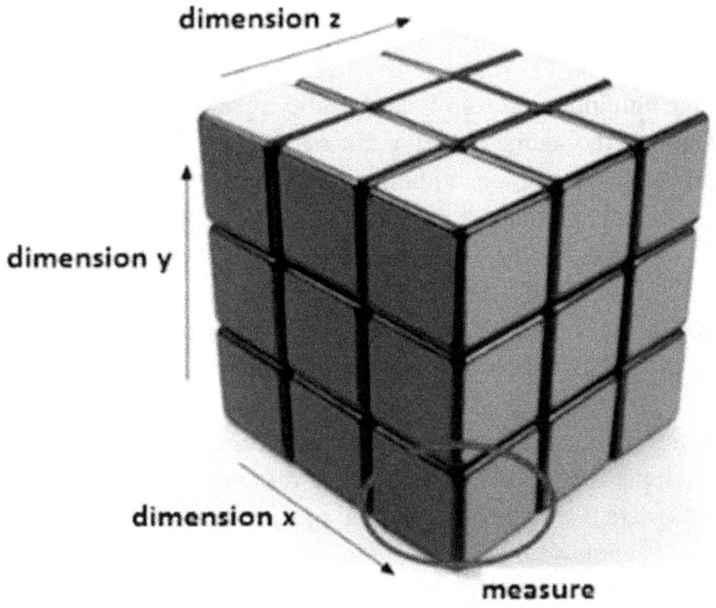

become increasingly important as an area of research and development with great impact since the new generation is more interactive and includes data warehouse technology (Barrento et al., 2010).

BI arose in the 70's and was characterized by the exhaustive programming, implying high costs in its' development. It was initially used in organizations only with the purpose of strategic support for decision making. However, BI systems are currently widely used as a system of data transformation into knowledge. In response to this increase of complexity, BI is now based on the Knowledge Extracting process and consists of three main steps: the accumulation of raw data through Data Warehousing, the ETL process and the analysis and reporting of Information to create knowledge for decision support.

As main goals, a Business Intelligence system has the access to reliable data, an increase in transparency and understanding of the business as well as being a support for analytical and decision making as it was already mentioned. In the other hand, besides being seen as an actual key to enhancing business value and performance, it is still important to reduce the latency between the moment the operational data is acquired and when the analysis of the data is processed, as it is the vital objective of this system (Sezões et al., 2006).

BI systems are known for their high applicability. In the health field, the information systems of health care institutions should support both clinical and administrative processes. However, some of these systems need to be rethought as there is still a major shortage of interoperability (Peixoto, H, 2010).

In conclusion, BI systems are defined as highly specialized tools for data analysis, data query, reporting, OLAP analysis and dashboards that support organizational decision making. Its' main tasks are the preparation of forecasts based on historical data and past events, the detailed analysis of the institution as well as the creation of scenarios that show the impact of changing certain variables (Majchrzak et al., 2011; Reed et al., 2002).

METHODOLOGY

At an early stage of the practical development of this project, it was necessary to establish some objectives in order to guide the work. These were:

- Construction of the multidimensional model (identifying dimensions and facts);
- Extraction of data from the source (Excel or other BD);
- Data transformation (Normalization, withdrawing unnecessary values, among others);
- Loading the data into MySQL database structure;
- Construction of the indicators (Power BI or Excel).

Initially, an exploration and analysis of the waiting list data for surgical intervention was performed. The data used in this project are a subset of some clinical data extracted from a hospital in the north of Portugal.

As we received the information in SQL format, all the DB manipulation was done with the support of the Oracle SQL Developer tool, an open integrated development environment. At this early stage, it was crucial to realize the data that had been provided to us in order to understand how they related to each other and what information would be relevant to the performance of our study.

During this first analysis, we realized that among so much information, the pertinent information for our work would be the one on the waiting list registers, as well as several information about the surgeries to perform (service, type of surgery…) and the patients that were in that same list (date of birth, sex, address…).

Obviously, it is necessary to take into account that the data we were manipulating were sometimes incomplete since, although they are real data, they are only a part of those used in the hospital reality. With this in mind, there were several decisions we had to make while handling the data. Thus, we made the decision that the data that were actually relevant would be those referring to waiting list records that were not canceled (i.e., no date or cancellation code), thus accounting for such records as being active. We also decided to keep records that had no date of operation, as the data provided were relatively recent, it would be likely that these cases would remain on the waiting list at the time of data manipulation. All this data transformation was performed in Excel since it is a tool that facilitates this process, although the data has been provided in SQL format. It allowed us for example to calculate ages given the patient's date of birth. Also with regard to the dates, it was also necessary to keep in mind its format, since Excel and MySQL accept different date formats.

For this project, it was also decided to use a star schema as multidimensional model to organize the data, which, as already mentioned, besides being the most common model, has as main advantages the existence of a single table of facts containing all the information without redundancies, the definition of only one primary key per dimension, the reduction of the number of interconnections and of course little need for maintenance. The fields and tables have been selected according to the choice of indicators we made, however the model is prepared to receive more fields if other indicators need to be calculated. That is, our dimensions and our table of facts were defined according to the data that we found interesting for the construction of indicators. So the main dimensions we created were specialty, sex, priority, subsystem, among others and the main measure was obviously the waiting time (and also the age).

Initially, we defined several dimensions that became unnecessary since they were not useful in the construction of indicators, as well as some were added already in the indicator construction phase. For example, we felt that it was interesting to do some indicators using age intervals, which led us to add a dimension to the model that describes the existing age intervals and which ages belong to it, as well as its column in the fact table.

This last task was complicated by the need to cross the data, for example, to obtain the date of birth and place it in the fact table next to respective patient's ID, it was necessary to cross the fact table (which has all the waiting list records) with the table that provided the personal information of all patients.

All these steps have always taken into account the improvement of the quality of the information, since this interferes directly with all the extraction of knowledge, as already mentioned. Now that the data is "clean" and organized, the quality of information is increased and obviously, the results of the analysis will be more reliable.

At the end of this process, that we may call ETL (Extract, Load, Transform), we got a waiting list with a total of 21932 records, registered between the years 2011 and 2016, loaded definitively in MySQL.

The next step taken was to load the project into Power BI establishing connection with MySQL through localhost, in order to initiate the construction of the indicators. In case we need to change something in the data, like adding a new dimension as we said before, it should be made in MySQL and then refreshed in Power BI. In Figure 3 is a schematic representation of the steps we take during this project.

Power BI

There are numerous BI tools in the market however for this project we used the Power BI tool.

Power BI is a suite of business analytics tools to analyze data and share insights provided by Microsoft. It is a system able to unify all the organization's data, publishing reports securely to an organization and setting up automatic data so everyone has the latest information.

Figure 3. Through extraction, transformation, and loading (ETL) processes, data from various sources are validated, cleaned, transformed, aggregated, and loaded into data warehouse, special sort of database system, optimized for reporting. And through use of special software tools, in our case Power BI, we can produce various dynamic analyses of data, known as BI results.
Vatovec (2011)

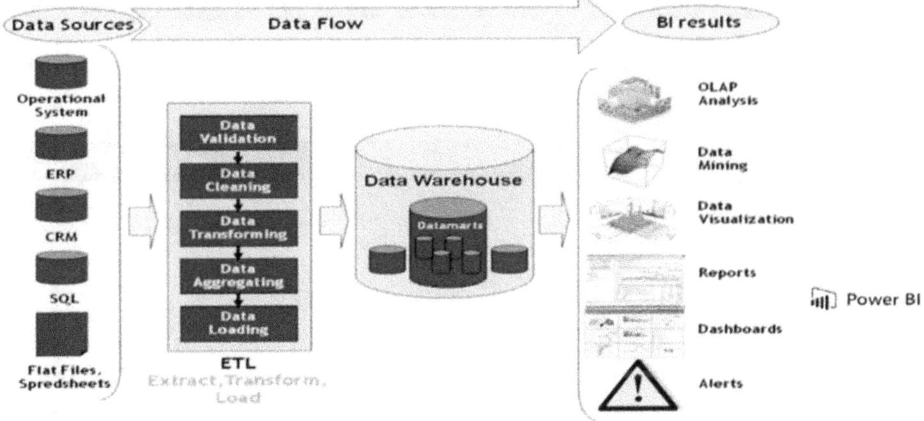

Power BI Dashboards provide all the perspectives for business users with their most important information in only one place, updated in real time and available on all of their devices. It can connect SQL Server databases, Analysis Services models, and many other data sources to the same dashboards in Power BI. This way, users can easily explore the data presented in the dashboard ending in the search for easy answers. The data and the reports update automatically and can be accessed from anywhere using Power BI apps (Microsoft, 2017).

RESULTS AND DISCUSSION

Indicators constitute an important element of business modelling as they offer criteria for determining whether an organization is fulfilling its objectives, be they strategic goals, quality requirements and analyze its performance. In the health area, especially hospitals, they are important to give an overview of the problems that need to be solved and the points that are having a good performance.

Taking the resulting data we have after the ETL process, several indicators were developed, mostly relating the different dimensions (specialty, gender, priority, etc.) with the waiting time in the waiting list for surgery. With the development of the indicators it was possible to compare the results with some statistical data that we found.

Firstly, we decided to make some general indicators, such as the number of participants on the waiting list for surgery and the average waiting time between dates (Figure 4), so that it was possible to see the evolution and compare with the Portuguese reality.

Analyzing the indicators of the Figure 5, we can see the total number of patients on the surgery waiting list and the average time, that varies with the selected dates in the slicer. In the bottom graphic, we can see that the registries on the surgery waiting list on this hospital has been almost the same over the years, although it been increasing in Portugal (ACSS, 2016).

Next, we decided to analyze the indicators about the specialties, such as the waiting time and the number of registrations by specialty.

Figure 4. General indicators

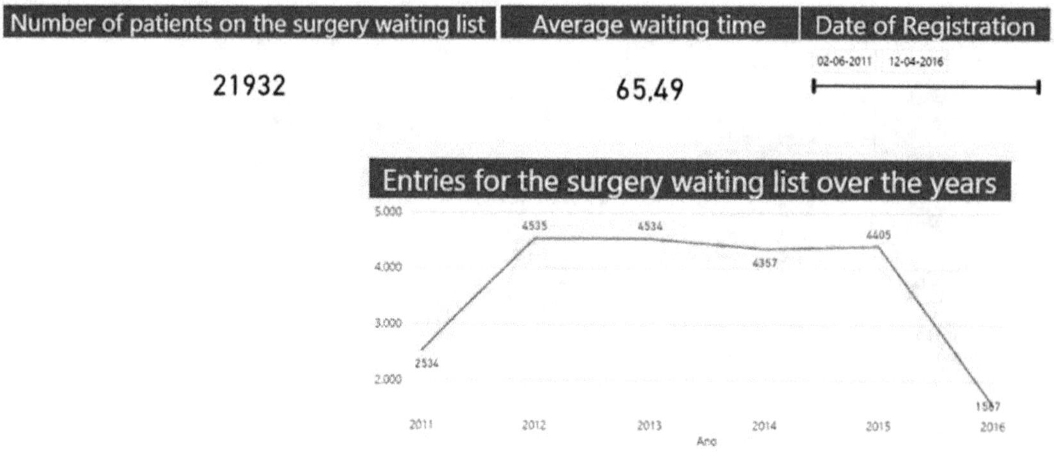

Figure 5. Indicators about specialties

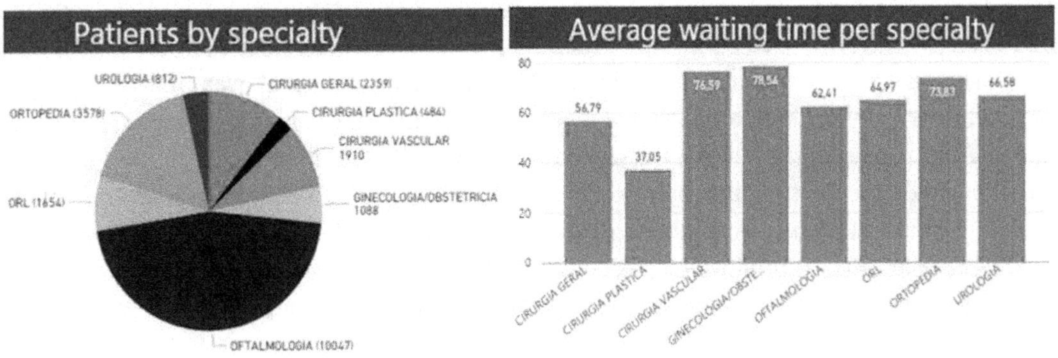

As we can see in the Figure 6 the most common specialty is ophthalmology and orthopedics. Regarding the waiting times, it is observed that the specialties with longer waiting times are orthopedics, vascular surgery and gynecology/obstetrics. It would be expected that the orthopedic and vascular surgery specialties occupied the first places with regard to the longer waiting time, since in the report (ACSS, 2016) these two specialties also occupied the places with the longest waiting time. What is surprising is the fact that gynecology/obstetrics leads the longest waiting period, considering that the national level has the shortest waiting time (ACSS, 2016), as it can be seen in the Figure 6, the waiting time for a gynecology/obstetrics surgery is much longer than the national time (being the only specialty having this issue).

These results suggest that the hospital from which these data were extracted presents problems in responding to surgeries registered in the gynecology/obstetrics area. This observation shows the usefulness of performing indicators, e.g. in this case it allowed the hospital in question to perceive that something was wrong in the gynecology/obstetrics service and can subsequently apply some measures to try to solve the problem.

Figure 6. Indicator about gynecology/obstetrics specialty

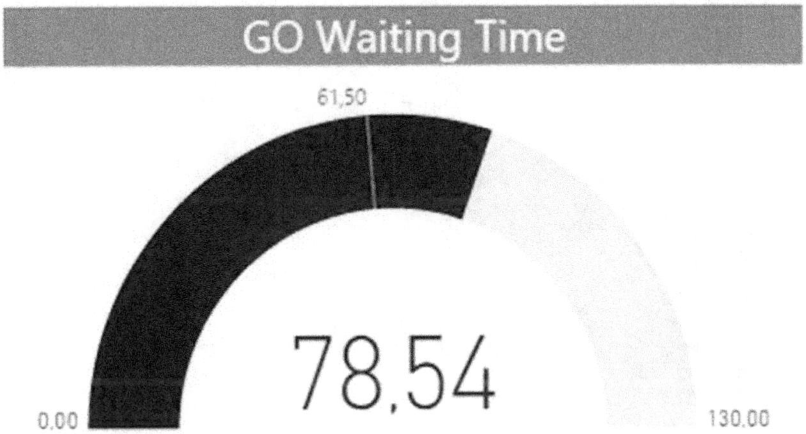

Another point that we found interesting to analyze was the waiting time by priority, and so, the indicator of Figure 7 was constructed. The three priorities types considered in this study were: normal, priority and without priority. Analyzing Figure 7, we can conclude that the vast majority of patients have a normal priority to be operated on and that there is a great discrepancy between the waiting time of normal priority and the priority one (which is much higher). This abnormal event may be explained by the fact that the priority patients were immediately operated on without being registered in the system, since the priority is to treat the patient, the record was eventually "forgotten".

With the data on the waiting time by priority, it was still possible to compare the average time with the TMGR ("Tempo Máximo Garantido de Resposta"), which means "maximum guaranteed response time" and represents the time until which it is considered clinically acceptable to treat the patient (ACSS, 2016). In general, the average value of waiting time for normal priority patients is below the TMGR (in days), as shown in Figure 8.

Figure 7. Indicators about priority

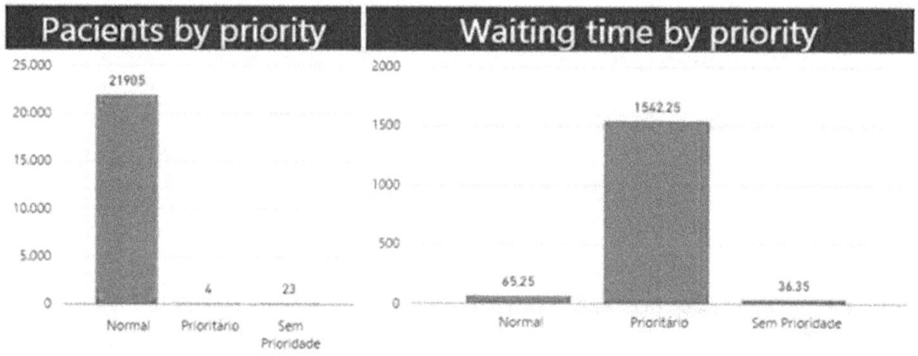

Figure 8. Indicator comparing the average waiting time of normal priority with the TMGR

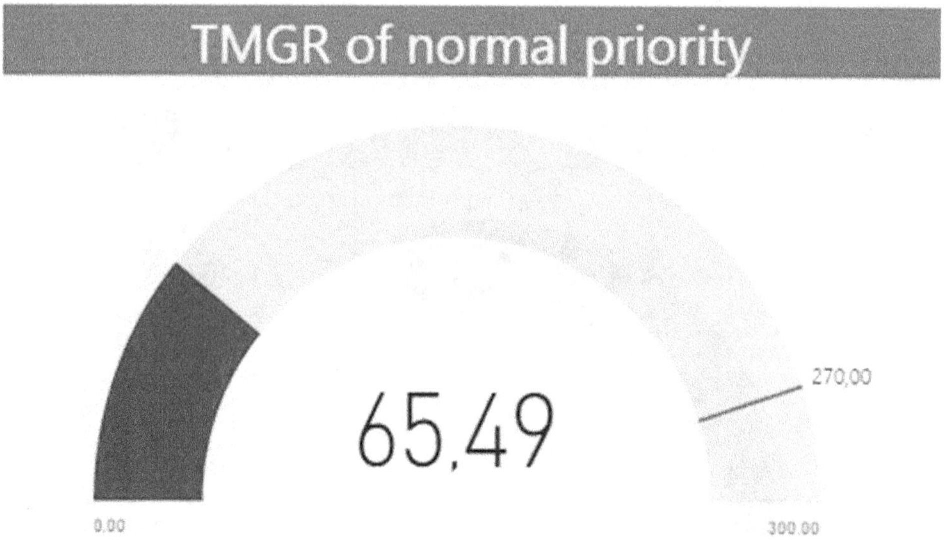

However, in our data, there was 747 patients that waited more than the TMGR, which represents 3,4% of the total patients. This percentage is way below the national statistic which was 12,2% in 2015, as described in the report.

Further conclusions were drawn: there are more women on the waiting list for surgery and they have longer waiting times, the main diagnoses observed are cataracts, varicose veins and myopia, which makes sense considering that the specialty with more demand is ophthalmology (45.81%), also, the main surgical intervention refers to ophthalmology and is phacoemulsification and aspiration of cataracts, the range of ages with more records are between 60 and 90 years, and can be explained by the increase of diseases in these ages and he only specialty where children up to 18 years predominate is ENT.

CONCLUSION

With the increasing expansion of health information systems, the Electronic Health Record (EHR) has become one of the most important sources of clinical information in the context of digital health. So, our main objective was to take advantage of this information in order to analyze the waiting lists for surgery in Portugal, analyzing data on several patients, which were later processed through the ETL process, part of the business intelligence process, with the consequent creation of indicators.

The realization of the theoretical introduction represented a time-consuming challenge requiring exhaustive and careful bibliographical research in order to collect information essential for the planning and development of the project. Other difficulties, technical and during use of the tool (Power BI), emerged in the course of this project. However, these difficulties were overcome with some research and practice.

The development of the indicators was performed successfully, allowing a comparison with the statistical data regarding the state of waiting lists for surgery in Portugal.

In conclusion, once the barriers have been overcome, the application of Business Intelligence to support the Management of the Enrollment Lists for Surgery in Continental Portugal has been successfully developed and may constitute a relevant support in the monitoring and management of the scheduled surgical activity in the hospital from which the data were extracted.

REFERENCES

ACSS. (2016). *Relatório síntese da atividade cirúrgica programada.* Retrieved from http://www.acss.min-saude.pt/wp-content/uploads/2016/10/UGA-20160927-RelSint_Ativ_Cir_2015-VE3.pdf

Barrento, M., Neto, M., Maria, M., & Dias, S. (2010). Sistemas de Business Intelligence Aplicados à Saúde. In E. U. F. Pessoa (Ed.), *Sistemas e tecnologias de informação na saúde* (pp. 77–91). Porto: Edições Universidade Fernando Pessoa.

Barros, P. P. (2008). *As listas de espera para intervenção cirúrgica em Portugal.* Retrieved from https://momentoseconomicos.files.wordpress.com/2011/06/listas_de_espera.pdf

Blumenthal, D., & Glaser, J. (2007). Information technology comes to medicine. *The New England Journal of Medicine*, *356*(24), 2527–2534. doi:10.1056/NEJMhpr066212 PMID:17568035

Caldeira, C. P. (2012). Data Warehousing - Conceitos e Modelos (2nd ed.). Academic Press.

Cardoso, L., Marins, F., Quintas, C., Portela, F., Santos, M., Abelha, A., & Machado, J. (2014). Interoperability in Healthcare. *Cloud Computing Applications for Quality Health Care Delivery*, 78-101.

De Mul, M., Alons, P., Van der Velde, P., Konings, I., Bakker, J., & Hazelzet, J. (2012). Development of a clinical data warehouse from an intensive care clinical information system. *Computer Methods and Programs in Biomedicine*, *105*(1), 22–30. doi:10.1016/j.cmpb.2010.07.002 PMID:20728956

El-Sappagh, S. H. A., Hendawi, A. M. A., & El Bastawissy, A. H. (2011). A proposed model for data warehouse ETL processes. *Journal of King Saud University-Computer and Information Sciences*, *23*(2), 91–104. doi:10.1016/j.jksuci.2011.05.005

Fayyad, U., Piatetsky-Shapiro, G., Smyth, P., & Uturusamy, R. (1996). *Advances in knowledge discovery and data mining*. Cambridge, MA: The MIT Press.

Fernandes, A., Perelman, J., & Mateus, C. (2010). *Health and Healthcare in Portugal: Does Gender Matter?*. Lisboa, Portugal: Instituto Nacional Ricardo Jorge.

Ferreira, J., Miranda, M., Abelha, A., & Machado, J. (2010). O processo ETL em sistemas data warehouse. In *INForum 2010* (pp. 757–765). II Simpósio de Informática.

Khan, A., Ehsan, N., Mirza, E., & Sarwar, S. (2012). *Integration between customer relationship management (CRM) and data warehousing*. Procedia Technology.

Kimball, R., & Ross, M. (2002). The Data Warehouse Toolkit (2nd ed.). Robert Ipsen.

Luís, T. (2013, November). *Business Intelligence para apoio à Gestão das Listas de Inscritos para Cirurgia em Portugal Continental*. Lisboa: Universidade Nova.

Majchrzak, T., Jansen, T., & Kuchen, H. (2011, March 21-25). Efficiency evaluation of open source etl tools. *SAC*, *11*, 287–294.

Marins, F., Cardoso, L., Portela, F., Santos, M., Abelha, A., & Mahado, J. (2014). Improving High Availability and Reliability of Health Interoperability Systems. In *Advances in Intelligent Systems and Computing* (Vol. 275). Springer. doi:10.1007/978-3-319-05948-8_20

Martins, M. (2011). *Processo Clínico Eletrónico - Levantamentos de Processos no Hospital da Prelada* (Master Thesis). Faculdade de Engenharia da Universidade do Porto, Portugal.

Mendes, R., & Rodrigues, P. (2010). *Main Barriers for Quality Data Collection in EHR - A Review*. Porto: Universidade do Porto.

Microsoft. (2017). *O que é Power BI?*. Retrieved April 1, 2017, retrieved from https://powerbi.microsoft.com/pt-br/what-is-power-bi/

Miranda, M., Duarte, J., Abelha, A., Machado, J., & Neves, J. (2010). Interoperability in healthcare. In *European Simulation and Modelling Conference*. Hasselt, Belgium: ESM.

Oliveira, O. (2012). *Extração de Conhecimento nas Listas de Espera para Consulta e Cirurgia*. Braga, Portugal: Dissertação de Mestrado, Universidade do Minho.

OPSS Observatório Português dos Sistemas de Saúde. (2003). Saúde: que rupturas?. *Relatório de Primavera*, 1 – 124.

Peixoto, H., Machado, J., Neves, J., & Abelha, A. (2010). Semantic Interoperability and Health Records. *1st IMIA/IFIP Joint Symposium, E-Health 2010, IMIA; IFIP, E-HEALTH, IFIP Advances in Information and Communication Technology, 335.*

Portela, F., Gago, P., Santos, M. F., Silva, A., Rua, F., Machado, J., & Neves, J. (2011). Knowledge Discovery For Pervasive And Real-Time Intelligent Knowledge Discovery for Pervasive and Real-time Intelligent Decision Support in Intensive Care Medicine. *Proceedings of KMIS 2011 – International Conference on Knowledge Management and Information Sharing.*

Reed, S., Na, D., Mayo, T., Shapiro, L., Duty, B., Conklin, J., & Brown, D. (2010). Implementing and analyzing a data mart for the arlington county initiative to manage domestic violence offenders. *Proceedings of the 2010 IEEE Systems and Information Engineering Design Symposium.* doi:10.1109/SIEDS.2010.5469673

Romero, O., & Abelló, A. (2010). A framework for multidimensional design of data warehouses from ontologies. *Data & Knowledge Engineering*, *69*(11), 1138–1157. doi:10.1016/j.datak.2010.07.007

Sezões, C., Oliveira, J., & Baptista, M. (2006). Business Intelligence. S.S. P. d. Inovação Ed. Porto.

Siciliani, L., & Hurst, J. (2005). Tackling excessive waiting times for elective surgery: A comparative analysis of policies in 12 OECD countries. *Health Policy (Amsterdam)*, *72*(2), 201–215. doi:10.1016/j.healthpol.2004.07.003 PMID:15802155

Thalhammer, T., Schrefl, M., & Mohania, M. (2001). Active data warehouses: Complementing olap with analysis rules. *Data & Knowledge Engineering*, *39*(3), 241–269. doi:10.1016/S0169-023X(01)00042-8

Vatovec, E. (2011). *Intelligent Value Chain Networks: Business Intelligence and Other ICT Tools and Technologies in Supply/Demand Chains.* Supply Chain Management - New Perspectives.

Wieder, B., & Ossimitz, M. (2015). The impact of Business Intelligence on the quality of decision making – a mediation model. *Procedia Computer Science Conference*, *64*, 1163 – 1171.

Zhang, J., & Walji, M. (2011). TURF: Toward a unified framework of EHR usability. *Journal of Biomedical Informatics*, *44*(6), 1056–1067. doi:10.1016/j.jbi.2011.08.005 PMID:21867774

Chapter 12
Pervasive Business Intelligence Platform to Support the Decision-Making Process in Waiting Lists

Marisa Esteves
University of Minho, Portugal

Filipe Miranda
University of Minho, Portugal

António Abelha
University of Minho, Portugal

ABSTRACT

In recent years, the increase of average waiting times in waiting lists is an issue that has been felt in health institutions. Thus, the implementation of new administrative measures to improve the management of these organizations may be required. Hereupon, the aim of this present work is to support the decision-making process in appointments and surgeries waiting lists in a hospital located in the north of Portugal, through a pervasive Business Intelligence platform that can be accessed anywhere and anytime by any device connected within the hospital's private network. By representing information that facilitate the analysis of information and knowledge extraction, the Web tool allows the identification in real-time of average waiting times outside the outlined patterns. Thereby, the developed platform permits their identification, enabling their further understanding in order to take the necessary measures. Thus, the main purpose is to enable the reduction of average waiting times through the analysis of information in order to, subsequently, ensure the satisfaction of patients.

DOI: 10.4018/978-1-5225-2851-7.ch012

INTRODUCTION

Over the past few years, the Business Intelligence (BI) technology has been increasingly a major interest to health professionals and Information Technology (IT) professionals due to its applicability in the Electronic Health Record (EHR) (Bonney, 2013). In short, BI is a process of extraction, collection, storage, processing, analysis and access to information and data from information systems in order to support and improve the decision-making process (Chaudhuri, Dayal, & Narasayya, 2011; Hočevar & Jaklič, 2010a).

On the other hand, the increase of average waiting times is an issue that has been recently felt in health institutions (Ballini et al., 2015; Barros, 2008; Miyanji et al., 2015; Moscelli, Siciliani, & Tonei, 2016; Odorico, 2014). Thus, the implementation of new administrative measures to improve the management of these organizations may be required. One of the main problems caused by delays lies in the possibility of causing serious adverse consequences to patients' health (Ballini et al., 2015; Barros, 2008; Miyanji et al., 2015; Moscelli et al., 2016; Odorico, 2014).

Thus, due to the current needs of generating clinical and performance indicators of waiting lists (appointments and surgeries) in a hospital located in the north of Portugal, allied to the benefits of using the BI technology, this study was carried out. A clinical decision support system (CDSS) was designed and developed to support the decision-making process regarding waiting lists, namely a pervasive BI platform, for the scheduled appointments and surgeries in the hospital units of the health institution.

The realization of this project included the Extract, Transform and Load (ETL) of the data from information systems, followed by the construction of a data warehouse (DW). It also involved the creation of clinical and performance indicators, and their subsequent integration into the Web application developed.

The next section of this chapter presents the state of the art associated with this study (section "State of the Art"). After that, in section "Research Methodologies", the research methodologies adopted are briefly described. The section "Case Study" explains succinctly the problem and main motivations behind this project, and the key steps followed throughout its realization. Thereafter, the results are presented and discussed in section "Results and Discussion". This section is followed by the "Proof of Concept" section, which consists essentially of a strengths, weaknesses, opportunities and threats (SWOT) analysis. The conclusion and future work conclude this chapter (section "Conclusion and Future Work").

STATE OF THE ART

This section intends to highlight briefly the main theoretical topics addressed throughout this chapter, namely clinical decision support systems (CDSSs) and Business Intelligence (BI) and clinical information, including the Extract, Transform and Load (ETL) process, and data warehousing.

Clinical Decision Support Systems

In recent years, the recognition of the importance of CDSSs as practical tools has increased exponentially (Castaneda et al., 2015; Marins, Cardoso, Esteves, Machado, & Abelha, 2017; Musen, Middleton, & A.Greenes, 2014). This promising trend is largely due to the inexorable growth in the complexity and unnecessary costs associated with the delivery of healthcare services, the rising challenges of offering personalized medical services to each patient (according to his/her needs), the increasingly felt pressure to adopt Electronic Health Record (EHR) processes in health institutions, as well as the increasingly frequent introduction of mandatory requirements regarding the implementation of this type of computing tools in the healthcare industry (Butler et al., 2015; Loya, Kawamoto, Chatwin, & Huser, 2014; Mattila, Koikkalainen, Virkki, Van Gils, & Lötjönen, 2012; Musen et al., 2014; Sayyad Shirabad, Wilk, Michalowski, & Farion, 2012).

Conceptually, CDSSs allow not only the retrieval of relevant information, but they also permit the distribution and communication of information in the clinical context, thus providing specific information and recommendations. Thereby, these systems provide fundamental knowledge and analysis needed in order to assist decision-makers, including healthcare organizations and professionals, in the delivery of medical services (Butler et al., 2015; Loya et al., 2014; Musen et al., 2014).

Thus, CDSSs can use information from the current clinical context to retrieve relevant documents, create and send alerts or recommendations to patients and/or healthcare professionals, or even organize and present the information available in dashboards, graphics and tables, and documents and reports, in order to facilitate, speed up and improve the decision-making process (Castaneda et al., 2015; Musen et al., 2014).

Hence, the main objective of CDSSs is to assist, rather than replace, health professionals in their day-to-day work, thus consisting of computing tools to support the decision-making process in order to reduce the frequency of medical errors, improve the quality of services delivered to patients, as well as to reduce the unnecessary costs and waste associated with the delivery of medical services (Butler et al., 2015; Loya et al., 2014; Musen et al., 2014).

Business Intelligence and Clinical Information

The concept of BI refers to the process of collecting, transforming, organizing, analyzing and distributing data from various external sources of information to improve the business decision-making process (Mettler & Vimarlund, 2009). Thus, it corresponds to a set of theories, methodologies, processes, structures and decision support technologies that allows grouping data in order to make a more informed decision (Bonney, 2013; Trujillo & Maté, 2012). In this way, based on past experiences, BI transforms a large amount of raw data into useful information for a strategic decision-making process.

Over the past few years, the number of services and products that use the concept of BI in its development has increased exponentially (Alpuim, Esteves, Pereira, & Santos, 2016; Brandão et al., 2014, 2016; Chaudhuri et al., 2011; Chen, Chiang, & Storey, 2012; Esteves, 2016; Trujillo & Maté, 2012). BI technologies are now used globally to obtain useful real-time knowledge with the aim of improving the decision-making process in the most diverse scientific areas. The BI technology transforms information into knowledge and presents the ability to put the right information, in the right hands, at the right time, in order to support the decision-making process (Bonney, 2013).

BI systems correspond to one of the components of the architecture of an information system of an organization to support the decision-making process by analyzing the data of a business (Mettler & Vimarlund, 2009).

Its greatest advantage is the standardization of information that is dispersed by several sources of information, to which it is impossible to access through queries for multidimensional data analysis. In this way, using the BI technology, it is guaranteed that everyone works with the same reality, facilitating the decision-making process. Its standardization also allows a faster access to information as well as greater reliability in data, thus generating significant gains in work efficiency and a considerable reduction in time wastes (Bonney, 2013; Hočevar & Jaklič, 2010b; Raghupathi & Raghupathi, 2014).

In the healthcare industry, more and more large amounts of data have been generated, mostly due to the increasingly more demanding mandatory requirements to be fulfilled in healthcare services, thus leading to a better maintenance and management of clinical records (Mettler & Vimarlund, 2009; Raghupathi & Raghupathi, 2014).

Thereby, these large datasets, called “Big Data”, present the potential to improve the quality of healthcare delivery and to reduce the costs and waste associated by being able to support a wide range of functions in the healthcare industry, including the development of CDSSs and their applicability in the EHR (Bonney, 2013; Raghupathi & Raghupathi, 2014).

Tools that resort to BI technologies include the application of several processes including the ETL process that handles the extraction, cleanup, normalization and loading of data, the construction of data warehouses (DWs) for structuring the data in order to facilitate its analysis (data warehousing) and, finally, the visualization, analysis and interpretation of the information represented by the data (Bonney, 2013; Chaudhuri et al., 2011; Hočevar & Jaklič, 2010b).

Extract, Transform and Load

In short, ETL is a set of processes that involves extracting data from external data sources that can come in various formats, transforming it to fit business needs and, ultimately, loading it into a target data structure such a data mart or DW, being typically associated with data warehousing. The ETL processes are schematized in Figure 1.

The database functions are described as follows (El-Sappagh et al., 2011; Ferreira, Miranda, Abelha, & Machado, 2010; Gour, Sarangdevot, Tanwar, & Sharma, 2010; Morris et al., 2008):

- **Extract:** The process of reading data from specified external data sources and extracting a desired subset of data. The data is then propagated to the data staging area (DSA) where it is transformed and cleaned (*transform step*) before loaded to a repository (*load step*);

Figure 1. A general framework for extract, transform, and load processes
Adapted from El-Sappagh, Hendawi, and El Bastawissy (2011)

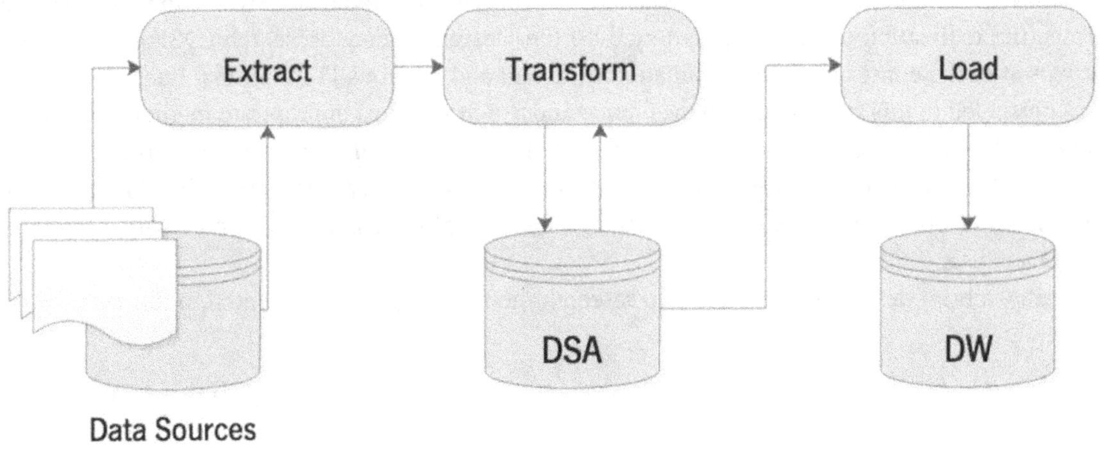

- **Transform:** Transforms the extracted/acquired data by storing it in the proper format or structure for the purposes of querying and analysis, i.e., cleaning it up and formatting it uniformly. Nonetheless, some data does not require any transformation at all;
- **Load:** Loads the transformed data into the target multidimensional structure, e.g., data mart or data warehouse.

Thus, ETL is a key set of processes in order to bring all the data together in a standard homogenous environment, i.e., by reshaping the relevant data from the data sources into useful information to be store into the target data structure.

Data Warehousing

A DW is a repository of all the data that an organization's collects, supporting the decision-making process. Warehoused data must be stored in a manner that is secure, reliable, easy to retrieve and to manage, i.e., the information must be stored into an optimized structure for those tasks (March & Hevner, 2007).

Generally, a data mart is a subset of the DW that it is usually oriented to a specific department or line of business, i.e., it is basically a small slice of the DW. Data marts usually contain data required for specific business processes or specific departments. Thus, it serves the same role as a DW, but it is intentionally limited in scope (March & Hevner, 2007).

Data warehousing emphasizes the collection of data from diverse heterogeneous sources in order to usefully analysis and access data (Cuzzocrea, 2015; Cuzzocrea, Bellatreche, & Song, 2013).

In short, while data marts are limited for use of a specific department only, data warehousing applies to an entire organization. Nonetheless, data marts are sometimes complete individual data warehouses that are usually smaller than the data warehouse itself.

RESEARCH METHODOLOGIES

The realization of any study in the field of Information Technologies (ITs) includes the scrutinized research and analysis of the set of methodologies and technologies available and feasible in the design of the defined IT solutions. The choice of the most appropriate methods and tools is mostly based on the advantages pointed out, as well as on associated limitations and compliance issues with related systems.

Thus, the realization of this study is based on the Design Science Research (DSR) methodology, mostly used in the construction and evaluation of useful and rigorous IT solutions. Each of the design phases presented in this study included the choice and use of the most appropriate methodologies, technologies and tools for the definition and elaboration of the desired solution. Finally, a Proof of Concept (PoC) was also carried out corroborating the viability and usefulness of the pervasive BI platform designed and developed, which consisted essentially of a strengths, weaknesses, opportunities and threats (SWOT) analysis.

Thereby, a brief description of these two research methodologies are presented in this section.

Design Science Research Methodology

In the area of ITs, the main objective of the use of the DSR methodology is the construction and evaluation of objects, also called "artefacts", that allow professionals to process organizational information and develop actions to solve a problem (Bilandzic & Venable, 2011; March & Storey, 2008).

Thus, the methodology that drove the realization of this project is the DSR. It consists of a rigorous method of scientific research used to develop successful artefacts (Peffers, Tuunanen, Rothenberger, & Chatterjee, 2007). It focuses on the IT artefact with a high priority in its relevancy in its application domain. Thus, in the context of solving real-world business problems, it is critical to try to improve the relevance and usefulness of the artefact (A. R. Hevner & Chatterjee, 2004; a. R. Hevner, March, & Park, 2004). The designed appliance must correspond to a viable technological solution for solving important and relevant business problems, and its usefulness, quality and effectiveness must be rigorously demonstrated through well-executed evaluation methods. In addition, research should provide clear and verifiable contributions, and should be based on the application of rigorous methods in its construction and evaluation process (A. R. Hevner & Chatterjee, 2004; a. R. Hevner et al., 2004).

In Figure 2, the DSR methodology is outlined, that is, its different interconnected steps that synthesize the steps to be followed through the DSR in the construction of scientific IT artefacts, namely the steps of "Identify Problem & Motivate", "Define Objectives of a Solution", "Design & Development", "Demonstration", "Evaluation" and "Communication". These are the phases adopted in the design of this study.

In short, in the first steps, the problem and the motivation are defined, as well as the objectives of the solution found. Then the artefact is designed and developed, directed to an important business problem to be solved that must be relevant to the solution of the same. Its development must follow a rigorous scientific process based on the knowledge and the theory already explored. Finally, the solution must be demonstrated, evaluated, communicated and propagated efficiently to the target audience (March & Storey, 2008; Vaishnavi & Kuechler, 2015).

Figure 2. Schematic representation of the design science research methodology
Adapted from Peffers et al. (2007)

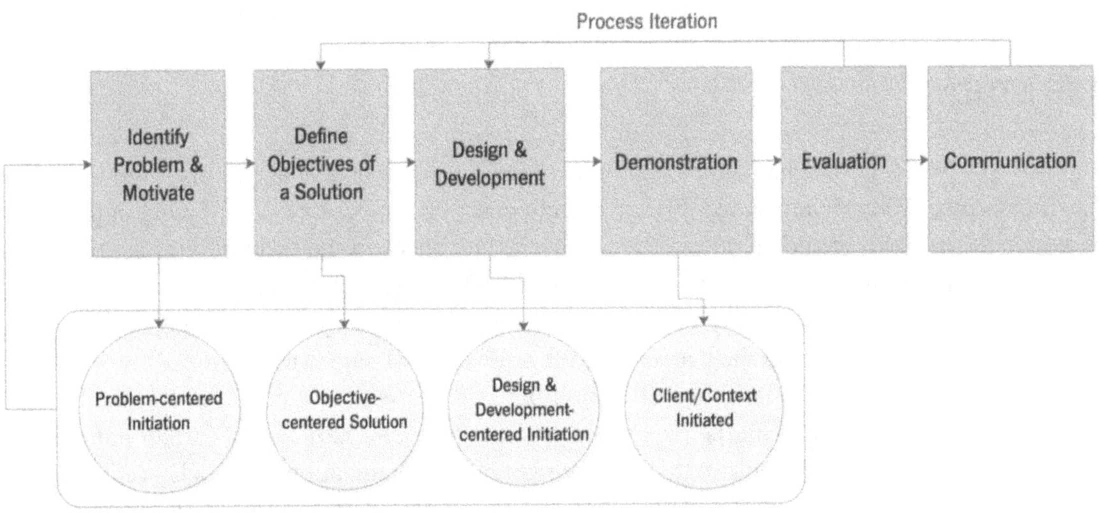

Thus, the study described in this chapter follows the DSR research methodology because the IT solution defined meets the needs of health professionals of the health institution, that is, a new pervasive Business Intelligence (BI) platform to support them in the decision-making process, meeting the challenges currently existing at the hospital facilities regarding waiting lists of appointments and surgeries.

Therefore, it provides the health institution with an appropriate and well-founded solution, based on methods and technologies that have already been explored and adapted to solve the problem in question, and stimulate new knowledge for the organization and the scientific community. Thus, the development of this project also included the dissemination of the IT artifact to the professionals of the hospital, as well as the writing of scientific papers.

Finally, it is important to note that the Web application developed was duly evaluated through a SWOT analysis. It should also be pointed out that the application of the PoC research methodology to prove the feasibility, usefulness and usability of the tool, which included a SWOT analysis, is briefly described in section "Proof of Concept" of this chapter.

Proof of Concept Methodology

The PoC research methodology consists of a practical model that can prove or validate the concept established through analysis or even technical articles. Thus, it goes on to verify whether a concept or theory is successful and feasible and, on the other hand, is thus susceptible of being exploited in a useful way (Sergey, Alexandr, & Sergey, 2015).

Therefore, a PoC is often pointed out as one of the most important steps in the design, development, implementation and proposal process of a prototype of a IT solution, mainly to establish if an IT solution fulfills its purpose, that is, it meets the requirements and defined objectives for which it was originally designed. On the other hand, it also allows the identification of potential failures or errors in the IT solution developed (Schmidt, 2006).

Summarizing, a PoC allows to demonstrate in practice the concepts, methodologies and technologies involved in the elaboration of a given project and thus validate the proposed solution by proving its feasibility and usefulness for the purpose for which it is intended by defending its potential.

In this study, the defense of the viability and usefulness of the BI platform went through the application of the PoC methodology. Thus, a SWOT analysis was carried out for the Web application.

CASE STUDY

Over the past few years, there has been a steady increase of waiting lists in health institutions (Ballini et al., 2015; Barros, 2008; Miyanji et al., 2015; Moscelli et al., 2016; Odorico, 2014). One of the possible reasons for this increase could be due to the significant advances in the technologies associated with surgeries, namely the anesthesia procedures (Barros, 2008). These advances have greatly improved the safety and efficiency of the surgical procedures offered by healthcare systems and, consequently, there have been important increases in the demand for the realization of surgeries.

The existence of waiting lists in health institutions can be seen as a result of an inability of the healthcare system to respond to all the requests of patients (Oliveira, 2012), and further administrative measures may be necessary to improve the management of the organization since delays can cause serious adverse consequences to patients' health (Ballini et al., 2015; Barros, 2008; Miyanji et al., 2015; Moscelli et al., 2016; Odorico, 2014).

In this hospital located in the north of Portugal, there was no clinical decision support system (CDSS) that could use the clinical data resulting from the records of waiting lists (appointments and surgeries), and that could thereafter transform those records into useful knowledge for the decision-making process, i.e. clinical and performance indicators through the Business Intelligence (BI) technology.

Thus, after a succinct analysis of the clinical data, and meetings with health professionals and Information Technology (IT) professionals of the health institution, a pervasive BI platform was designed and developed. The choice of all its modules, components and functionalities was based on these meetings, particularly regarding the technical requirements. Its design and development also included the construction of a data warehouse (DW) of waiting lists with the data stored into the information systems of the hospital. Then, the indicators were created from those records and integrated into the Web application.

The core module of the BI platform consists of the Business Intelligence module that enables the generation and visualization of clinical and performance indicators. Therefore, from this module it is possible to visualize several indicators that can assist in the evaluation of a healthcare process, and monitor and evaluate the quality of clinical management and medical services delivered to patients. It can also alert its users and guide them through the monitoring, evaluation and improvement of the medical services provided to patients.

Finally, this work was based entirely on the Design Science Research (DSR) methodology, described in section "Research Methodologies". Then, a Proof of Concept (PoC) was carried out through the PoC methodology, described in the same section of this chapter, to corroborate the viability and usefulness of the Web tool designed and developed, which consisted essentially of a strengths, weaknesses, opportunities and threats (SWOT) analysis.

RESULTS AND DISCUSSION

In this section, the main results of this study are presented and briefly discussed, namely regarding the architecture of the pervasive Business Intelligence (BI) platform that was designed and developed, and its application to support the decision-making process in appointments and surgeries waiting lists in a hospital in the north of Portugal.

Architecture of the Pervasive Business Intelligence Platform

The BI platform is currently implemented in a production machine Ubuntu in the hospital.

It should be noted that all the research methodologies associated with its development are briefly described in section "Research Methodologies" of this chapter. In summary, the BI platform was developed using the AngularJS framework in JavaScript, HTML and CSS, which supports the development of single-page applications (SPAs) that can be accessed via a Web browser. The programming languages PHP and SQL were also used, but to develop the CRUD RESTful PHP Web services and to make requests (SQL queries) to the database, namely an Oracle database. Lastly, Apache corresponds to the Web server that supports the Web application.

On the other hand, the BI platform is divided into five distinct modules, namely Home, Data Warehouse, Business Intelligence, Data Mining and User Area. Thereafter, each of the Web tool modules are briefly described:

- **Home:** Includes a dashboard with the key indicators;
- **Data Warehouse:** Provides an overview of all the tables of the data warehouse (DW);
- **Business Intelligence:** Allows the visualization of the clinical and performance indicators generated by submodule, namely the Appointments and Surgeries submodules;
- **Data Mining:** A module for the future addition of predictive data mining models;
- **User Area:** Includes the management of users and notifications, as well as forms for the questionnaire and suggestions, and a visualization of the number of accesses to the Web application.

Its main innovative features, as well as a brief description, are presented and described in Table 1.

Table 1. Key innovative features of the pervasive business intelligence platform

Innovative Feature	Description
Scalable architecture	The architecture of the computer tool is easy to maintain, and it is relatively simple to expand its functionalities
User-friendly	Highly intuitive and easy to use
Interactive data visualization	The BI platform enables the interactivity between its users and the graphics and tables (clinical and performance indicators). Thus, it facilitates the understanding of the information available
Pervasive	It is not necessary to install the BI platform on all the computers of the hospital. When it is installed on a production machine (server), the Web application is thus distributed to all the users connected to the Intranet, that is within the private network of the health institution, and it can be easily accessed through a Web browser
Interoperability	It enables the communication and sharing of information between different systems, that is, connecting the application to the data
Real-time	It is possible to access the BI platform and the information provided in real-time, that is, to consult actual and current data in the decision-making process
Ubiquity	The Web application will be gradually disseminated by the hospital healthcare facilities and, on the other hand, it is constantly available
Installation of plugins	By using the AngularJS framework to support the development of the BI platform, it is possible to add new functionalities to the Web tool by installing plugins. The installation of plugins is possible through Bower, that is, a tool to install and uninstall packages in AngularJS
Mobile support	It is possible to access the Web application by means other than a computer, namely using mobile devices

Support in the Decision-Making Process in Appointments and Surgeries Waiting Lists

After meetings with health professionals and Information Technology (IT) professionals of the health institution, it was decided to divide the clinical data related to the waiting lists into two different data marts, namely Appointments and Surgeries. Thus, data were extracted from the information systems of the hospital, and a dimensional model was designed according to the star schema. The DW was constructed through the Extract, Transform and Load (ETL) process. The data of the DW, which is constituted by two data marts (Appointments and Surgeries), is stored into an Oracle database.

In this way, the BI module of the Web application is divided into two different submodules, from which it is possible to visualize the clinical and performance indicators generated in each one. The parameters evaluated include date, specialty, pathology, surgical intervention and healthcare professional, which are parameters that were chosen because they hypothetically influence the values of the indicators. In the Appointments submodule, indicators related to the scheduled appointments were generated with the data stored into the information systems of the health institution. Indicators regarding the scheduled surgeries are presented in the Surgeries submodule. Both submodules are then divided into three different tabs, namely:

- **Number of Appointments/Surgeries (Depending on the Submodule):** Indicators related to the number of appointments/surgeries scheduled this current year are presented, including the number of appointments/surgeries by date, day of the week, month and specialty;
- **Average Waiting Time:** Indicators related to the average waiting times (in days) of appointments/surgeries this current year are presented, including the average waiting time by specialty, pathology, surgical intervention and healthcare professional;
- **Temporal Evolution:** Indicators related with the temporal evolution of appointments/surgeries scheduled over the last years in the hospital are presented, including the number of appointments/surgeries scheduled by year and the average waiting time by year.

Approximately 40 clinical and performance indicators were generated, divided into the Appointments and Surgeries submodules.

Discussion

The main advantage of the application of this type of BI system in a health institution lies in the possibility of supporting health professionals with the power in the decision-making process within the organization through the availability and access to information. Thus, the decision-making process is improved with the analysis of data.

Thereby, approximately 40 clinical and performance indicators were generated, divided into the Appointments and Surgeries submodules, which were posteriorly integrated into the BI platform. The defined indicators are divided into three different tabs, namely Number of Appointments/Surgeries, Average Waiting Time and Temporal Evolution, for both submodules.

Briefly, the Number of Appointments/Surgeries tab lets the user measure the flow of scheduled appointments and surgeries in the hospital during the current year. On the other hand, analyzing the indicators in the Average Waiting Time tab allows the identification in real-time of average waiting times outside the outlined patterns. Thereby, the BI platform permits their identification, enabling their further understanding in order to take the necessary measures. Through the Temporal Evolution tab, it is also possible to visualize the temporal evolution of the appointments and surgeries registered in recent years in the health institution.

Thus, this BI system allows its users to critically interpret the generated data, making it possible to identify easily and quickly inconsistencies. By analyzing the data effectively, health professionals can get the answers they need to create strategies such as taking new administrative measures to improve the management of the organization. Therefore, they can make efficient decisions in order to decrease the average waiting times in waiting lists for appointments and surgeries. That is, if any average waiting time in a waiting list is detected outside the outlined patterns, such as for a specialty in one of the hospital units, solutions must be found and followed quickly in order to correct this type of situation.

Finally, allowing the access to quality information in the decision-making process in the context of waiting lists, a better understanding of the internal and external reality of the organization, the identification and further correction of potential risks, and driving innovation, are some benefits that this BI system brings to the health organization.

PROOF OF CONCEPT

To test the viability, utility, quality and efficiency of the Web application, a Proof of Concept (PoC) was necessary, which consisted essentially of a SWOT analysis. This analysis allowed the identification of the strengths, weaknesses, opportunities and threats of the application.

Thus, after several tests and evaluations of the pervasive Business Intelligence (BI) platform, the strengths, weaknesses, opportunities and threats associated with the Web tool were identified.

Regarding the strengths, the following points were identified:

- Allowing the access to quality information in the decision-making process in the context of waiting lists (appointments and surgeries);
- A better understanding of the internal and external reality of the organization;
- The identification and further correction of potential risks;
- High scalability;
- Easily adaptable to different case studies;
- High usability, i.e., it is an intuitive and user-friendly Web tool;
- Unlike many other BI systems, it does not require other external applications to be active by using directives from the AngularJS framework for the interactive visualization of data (graphics and tables).

On the other hand, the weaknesses of the system were also identified:

- Requires Intranet connection.

Regarding the opportunities, which correspond to the external factors that positively influence the BI platform:

- Reducing medical errors;
- The expansion of the clinical data stored into the Hospital Information Systems (HISs) in order to generate more clinical and performance indicators;
- The implementation of new modules, components and functionalities;
- The application and use of the BI platform in more case studies.

Finally, it is possible to highlight the following possible threats to the system:

- The lack of acceptance to resort to new technologies by health professionals;
- Potential problems associated with the network connectivity to the Intranet.

CONCLUSION AND FUTURE WORK

Within the scope of this study, clinical and performance indicators were generated for which, until now, information was available in the Electronic Health Record (EHR) of the health institution in the context of waiting lists, namely regarding appointments and surgeries. The main motivations behind the realization of this project were to support health professionals in the decision-making process, and the possibility of implementing new administrative measures in the future in order to improve the management of the organization. It is intended, therefore, to limit possible adverse consequences on patients' health by reducing the average waiting time in waiting lists.

Thus, the development of this case study was based on the need to treat large amounts of clinical data from waiting lists produced daily by the EHR of the health institution, and the feasibility of acquiring knowledge with sufficient value to support the medical services provided by health professionals.

As future work, it is intended to generate more clinical and performance indicators regarding waiting lists of appointments and surgeries. Thus, the enrichment of the Business Intelligence (BI) module with a wider range of indicators for interactive data visualization, and their subsequent analysis, is projected to strengthen the decision support for health professionals.

On the other hand, the development and integration of predictive data mining models in the Data Mining module of the Web application is also foreseen. Predictive models that can predict the average waiting time (in days) in waiting lists of appointments and surgeries, according to attributes that will be defined after analyses as factors that may influence the outcome, are examples of possible data mining models that may be integrated soon into the BI system.

Finally, regarding the architecture of the pervasive BI platform, it is intended to expand its modules, components and functionalities, as well as to apply it to more case studies in order to encourage its continuous growth. In the future, the implementation and configuration of user roles and access permissions is also one of the main objectives to fulfill.

In this way, it is confirmed the continuous maintenance, growth and expansion of the innovative solution implemented in the health institution.

ACKNOWLEDGMENT

This work has been supported by Compete POCI-01-0145-FEDER-007043 and FCT - *Fundação para a Ciência e Tecnologia* within the Project Scope UID/CEC/00319/2013.

REFERENCES

Alpuim, A., Esteves, M., Pereira, S., & Santos, M. F. (2016). Monitoring Time Consumption in Complementary Diagnostic and Therapeutic Procedure Requests. In *Applying Business Intelligence to Clinical and Healthcare Organizations* (pp. 208–240). IGI Global. doi:10.4018/978-1-4666-9882-6.ch011

Ballini, L., Negro, A., Maltoni, S., Vignatelli, L., Flodgren, G., & Simera, I. ... Grilli, R. (2015). Interventions to Reduce Waiting Times for Elective Procedures. *The Cochrane Database of Systematic Reviews, 2*(2). https://doi.org/10.1002/14651858.CD005610.pub2

Barros, P. P. (2008, March). As Listas de Espera para Intervenção Cirúrgica em Portugal. *Iprisverbis, 4*.

Bilandzic, M., & Venable, J. (2011). Towards Participatory Action Design Research: Adapting Action Research and Design Science Research Methods for Urban Informatics. *The Journal of Community Informatics*, *7*(3). Retrieved from http://ci-journal.net/index.php/ciej/article/view/786/804

Bonney, W. (2013). Applicability of Business Intelligence in Electronic Health Record. *Procedia: Social and Behavioral Sciences*, *73*, 257–262. doi:10.1016/j.sbspro.2013.02.050

Brandão, A., Pereira, E., Esteves, M., Portela, F., Santos, M., Abelha, A., & Machado, J. (2016). A Benchmarking Analysis of Open-Source Business Intelligence Tools in Healthcare Environments. *Information, 7*(4), 57. https://doi.org/10.3390/info7040057

Brandão, A., Pereira, E., Portela, F., Santos, M., Abelha, A., & Machado, J. (2014). Real-time Business Intelligence Platform to Maternity Care. In *IEEE Conference on Biomedical Engineering and Sciences* (pp. 379–384). IEEE. doi:10.1109/IECBES.2014.7047525

Butler, C. E., Noel, S., Hibbs, S. P., Miles, D., Staves, J., Mohaghegh, P., ... Murphy, M. F. (2015). Implementation of a Clinical Decision Support System Improves Compliance with Restrictive Transfusion Policies in Hematology Patients. *Transfusion, 55*(8), 1964–1971. https://doi.org/10.1111/trf.13075

Castaneda, C., Nalley, K., Mannion, C., Bhattacharyya, P., Blake, P., & Pecora, A. ... Suh, K. S. (2015). Clinical Decision Support Systems for Improving Diagnostic Accuracy and Achieving Precision Medicine. *Journal of Clinical Bioinformatics, 5*(4), 1–16. https://doi.org/10.1186/s13336-015-0019-3

Chaudhuri, S., Dayal, U., & Narasayya, V. (2011). An Overview of Business Intelligence Technology. *Communications of the ACM*, *54*(8), 88. doi:10.1145/1978542.1978562

Chen, H., Chiang, R. H. L., & Storey, V. C. (2012). Business Intelligence and Analytics: From Big Data to Big Impact. *Management Information Systems Quarterly, 36*(4), 1165–1188. https://doi.org/10.1145/2463676.2463712

Cuzzocrea, A. (2015). Data Warehousing and OLAP over Big Data: A Survey of the State-of-the-art, Open Problems and Future Challenges. *Int. J. Business Process Integration and Management, 7*(4), 372–377. doi:10.1504/IJBPIM.2015.073665

Cuzzocrea, A., Bellatreche, L., & Song, I.-Y. (2013). Data Warehousing and OLAP over Big Data: Current Challenges and Future Research Directions. *DOLAP '13 Proceedings of the Sixteenth International Workshop on Data Warehousing and OLAP*, 67–70. https://doi.org/10.1145/2513190.2517828

El-Sappagh, S. H. A., Hendawi, A. M. A., & El Bastawissy, A. H. (2011). A Proposed Model for Data Warehouse ETL Processes. *Journal of King Saud University - Computer and Information Sciences, 23*(2), 91–104. https://doi.org/10.1016/j.jksuci.2011.05.005

Esteves, M. (2016). *Desenvolvimento e Exploração de uma Nova Geração de Ferramentas de Business Intelligence para o Apoio à Decisão e a Prática Clínica em Unidades Hospitalares*. Universidade do Minho.

Ferreira, J., Miranda, M., Abelha, A., & Machado, J. (2010). O Processo ETL em Sistemas Data Warehouse. *INForum 2010 - II Simpósio de Informática*, 757–765.

Gour, V., Sarangdevot, S. S., Tanwar, G. S., & Sharma, A. (2010). Improve Performance of Extract, Transform and Load (ETL) in Data Warehouse. *International Journal on Computer Science and Engineering, 1*(3), 786–789.

Hevner, A. R., & Chatterjee, S. (2004). Design Research in Information Systems. *Design Research in Information Systems, 28*, 75–105. https://doi.org/10.1007/978-1-4419-5653-8

Hevner, R., March, S. T., & Park, J. (2004). Design Science in Information Systems Research. *Management Information Systems Quarterly, 28*(1), 75–105. https://doi.org/10.2307/25148625

Hočevar, B., & Jaklič, J. (2010). Assessing Benefits of Business Intelligence Systems – A Case Study. *Management, 15*(1), 87–119.

Loya, S. R., Kawamoto, K., Chatwin, C., & Huser, V. (2014). Service Oriented Architecture for Clinical Decision Support: A Systematic Review and Future Directions. *Journal of Medical Systems, 38*(12), 1–22. doi:10.1007/s10916-014-0140-z PMID:25325996

March, S. T., & Hevner, A. R. (2007). Integrated Decision Support Systems: A Data Warehousing Perspective. *Decision Support Systems, 43*(3), 1031–1043. doi:10.1016/j.dss.2005.05.029

March, S. T., & Storey, V. C. (2008). Design Science in the Information Systems discipline: An introduction to the special issue on Design Science Research. *MIS Quartly, 32*(4), 725–730.

Marins, F., Cardoso, L., Esteves, M., Machado, J., & Abelha, A. (2017). An Agent-Based RFID Monitoring System for Healthcare. In *Advances in Intelligent Systems and Computing (AISC)* (pp. 407–416). Springer. https://doi.org/10.1007/978-3-319-56541-5_42

Mattila, J., Koikkalainen, J., Virkki, A., Van Gils, M., & Lötjönen, J. (2012). Design and Application of a Generic Clinical Decision Support System for Multiscale Data. *IEEE Transactions on Bio-Medical Engineering*, *59*(1), 234–240. doi:10.1109/TBME.2011.2170986 PMID:21990325

Mettler, T., & Vimarlund, V. (2009). Understanding Business Intelligence in the Context of Healthcare. *Health Informatics Journal*, *15*(3), 254–264. doi:10.1177/1460458209337446 PMID:19713399

Miyanji, F. O., Newton, P., Samdani, A. F. A., Shah, S., Varghese, R. A., Reilly, C. W., & Mulpuri, K. (2015). The Impact of Surgical Waitlist Times on Scoliosis Surgery: The Surgeons Perspective. *The Spine Journal*, *40*(11), 823–828. doi:10.1097/BRS.0000000000000205 PMID:24430712

Morris, H., Liao, H., Padmanabhan, S., Srinivasan, S., Lau, P., Shan, J., & Wisnesky, R. (2008). Bringing Business Objects into Extract-transform-load (ETL) Technology. *IEEE International Conference on e-Business Engineering 2008*, 709–714. https://doi.org/10.1109/ICEBE.2008.72

Moscelli, G., Siciliani, L., & Tonei, V. (2016). Do Waiting Times affect Health Outcomes? Evidence from Coronary Bypass. *Social Science & Medicine*, *161*, 151–159. doi:10.1016/j.socscimed.2016.05.043 PMID:27299977

Musen, M. A., Middleton, B., & Greenes, A. R. (2014). Clinical Decision-Support Systems. In *Biomedical Informatics* (pp. 643–674). Springer-Verlag London. https://doi.org/10.1001/jama.296.21.2624

Odorico, J. S. (2014). Waiting List Management for Pancreas and Islet Transplantation. In A. D. Kirk, S. J. Knechtle, C. P. Larsen, J. C. Madsen, T. C. Pearson, & S. A. Webber (Eds.), *Textbook of Organ Transplantation* (1st ed.; pp. 482–488). John Wiley & Sons, Ltd. doi:10.1002/9781118873434.ch41

Oliveira, O. R. F. (2012). *Extração de Conhecimento nas Listas de Espera para Consulta e Cirurgia*. Universidade do Minho. Retrieved from http://repositorium.sdum.uminho.pt/handle/1822/23504

Peffers, K., Tuunanen, T., Rothenberger, M. A., & Chatterjee, S. (2007). A Design Science Research Methodology for Information Systems Research. *Journal of Management Information Systems*, *24*(3), 45–77. doi:10.2753/MIS0742-1222240302

Raghupathi, W., & Raghupathi, V. (2014). Big Data Analytics in Healthcare: Promise and Potential. *Health Information Science and Systems*, *2*, 3. https://doi.org/10.1186/2047-2501-2-3

Sayyad Shirabad, J., Wilk, S., Michalowski, W., & Farion, K. (2012). Implementing an Integrative Multi-agent Clinical Decision Support System with Open Source Software. *Journal of Medical Systems*, *36*(1), 123–137. doi:10.1007/s10916-010-9452-9 PMID:20703742

Schmidt, B. (2006). Proof of Principle Studies. *Epilepsy Research*, *68*(1), 48–52. doi:10.1016/j.eplepsyres.2005.09.019 PMID:16377153

Sergey, A. B., Alexandr, D. B., & Sergey, A. T. (2015). Proof of Concept Center — A Promising Tool for Innovative Development at Entrepreneurial Universities. *Procedia - Social and Behavioral Sciences, 166*, 240–245. https://doi.org/10.1016/j.sbspro.2014.12.518

Trujillo, J., & Maté, A. (2012). Business Intelligence 2.0: A General Overview. *Lecture Notes in Business Information Processing, 96*, 98–116. https://doi.org/10.1007/978-3-642-27358-2_5

Vaishnavi, V. K., & Kuechler, W. (2015). *Design Science Research Methods and Patterns: Innovating Information and Communication Technology* (2nd ed.). CRC Press. Retrieved from https://books.google.pt/books?hl=pt-PT&lr=&id=OOE_CQAAQBAJ&oi=fnd&pg=PP1&dq=Design+science+research+methods+and+patterns:+innovating+information+and+communication+technology&ots=ZFBpZsW9gs&sig=wGD5o_q96t1Z_xZqHKYxjOOUSpo&redir_esc=y#v=onepage&q=Designsci

ADDITIONAL READING

Alpuim, A., Esteves, M., Pereira, S., & Santos, M. F. (2016). Monitoring Time Consumption in Complementary Diagnostic and Therapeutic Procedure Requests. In *Applying Business Intelligence to Clinical and Healthcare Organizations* (pp. 208–240). IGI Global. doi:10.4018/978-1-4666-9882-6.ch011

Brandão, A., Pereira, E., Esteves, M., Portela, F., Santos, M., Abelha, A., & Machado, J. (2016). A Benchmarking Analysis of Open-Source Business Intelligence Tools in Healthcare Environments. *Information, 7*(4), 57. https://doi.org/10.3390/info7040057

Brandão, A., Pereira, E., Portela, F., Santos, M., Abelha, A., & Machado, J. (2014). Real-time Business Intelligence Platform to Maternity Care. In *IEEE Conference on Biomedical Engineering and Sciences* (pp. 379–384). IEEE. doi:10.1109/IECBES.2014.7047525

Esteves, M. (2016). *Desenvolvimento e Exploração de uma Nova Geração de Ferramentas de Business Intelligence para o Apoio à Decisão e a Prática Clínica em Unidades Hospitalares*. Universidade do Minho.

Ferreira, J., Miranda, M., Abelha, A., & Machado, J. (2010). O Processo ETL em Sistemas Data Warehouse. *INForum 2010 - II Simpósio de Informática*, 757–765.

Oliveira, O. R. F. (2012). *Extração de Conhecimento nas Listas de Espera para Consulta e Cirurgia*. Universidade do Minho. Retrieved from http://repositorium.sdum.uminho.pt/handle/1822/23504

KEY TERMS AND DEFINITIONS

Dashboard: It consists of the visual presentation of the most important and essential information and data. It is basically a way for managers and decision makers to quickly identify the data that is important to them.

Data Mart: It is a subset of data from a data warehouse (DW). Thus, they meet the needs of specific business units, while a DW involves the entire organization.

Electronic Health Record (EHR): It consists of the collection and registration of a set of clinical data of an individual, including information about its current state of health, medical history, previous appointments and surgeries, among others, in digital format.

Indicators: They correspond to a way of simplifying and synthesizing complex information through its quantification (parameter, measure or value).

Intranet: It is a network of computers like the Internet, but it is of exclusive use of a certain organization, that is, it can only be used by the machines belonging to its private network.

Plugin: It is an extension module used to add functions to other larger programs in order to add more functionalities to them.

Queries: They are requests of information or data to a database or a set of tables.

User-Friendly: Defines applications, tools, systems or processes that are highly intuitive and easy to use.

Web: It consists of a system of Web pages interconnected and executed in the Internet.

Web Browser: It is a computer program developed to enable browsing through the Web, including accessing and interpreting files in the HTML, CSS and JavaScript formats.

Chapter 13
Business Intelligence for Nutrition Therapy

Rita Reis
University of Minho, Portugal

Ana Mendonça
University of Minho, Portugal

Diana Lisandra Azevedo Ferreira
University of Minho, Portugal

Hugo Peixoto
University of Minho, Portugal

José Machado
University of Minho, Portugal

ABSTRACT

The assessment of health status in communities throughout the world is a massive information technology challenge. Data warehousing provides a flexible environment to support the business management and serve as an integrated repository for data. With the addition of models and analytic tools that have the potential to provide actionable information resources and support effective problem identification, critical decision-making, and strategy formulation, implementation, and evaluation. Of particular interest are the factors of influence like the patient's height or weight and its impact on processes and results. A multidimensional process is a way to discover health care processes according to certain factors of influence. This study aims to implement a data warehousing environment for decision support, in the context of nutrition evaluation, to integrate data obtained from a health care facility. This paper highlights the implementation of Business Intelligence in health care settings allows searching and interpreting stored information to support decisions concerning people's life.

DOI: 10.4018/978-1-5225-2851-7.ch013

INTRODUCTION

Identifying the risk of malnutrition in patients from predictive variables is the first step towards an adequate nutritional control. Given its prevalence, the traceability and monitoring of nutritional status should be available in the hospital environment to prevent, treat and improve its prognosis. With this, morbidity, mortality, as well as hospitalization time and hospital costs will be reduced, enhancing the quality of life. Given this reality, the nutritionist plays a crucial role, since it's able to identify early cases of nutritional risk. In this way, the nutritionist can interfere with the control of patient's clinical status and, consequently, prevent and control its malnutrition, as well as infer the improvement of its clinical state. Thus, each health institution should identify the most common nutritional risk factors that affect the population and develop its instrument of nutritional tracking.

Malnutrition refers to both overnutrition and undernutrition. People are malnourished if their diet doesn't provide enough calories and protein for growth and maintenance or they are incapable of utilizing the food they eat due to illness (undernutrition). They are also malnourished if they consume too many calories (overnutrition) (UNICEF, 2006).

According to the World Health Organization (WHO), undernutrition is an individual nutritional status characterized by the insufficient intake of energy and nutrients, the body's inability to absorb nutrients or the abnormal body loss of nutrients. This results from the complex interaction between diet, health status, and, socioeconomic and social conditions in which the individual lives, being a common health problem in hospital admission (Amaro et al., 2016). Everyone is vulnerable to undernutrition, but certain groups of people are at greater risk. This is the case of the elderly, children, pregnant women and individuals who are sick. Examples of the most common symptoms observed in undernourished individuals are the loss of body fat, reduced appetite, fatigue and poor concentration (Correia et al., 2014).

Overnutrition is defined as the overconsumption of nutrients and food owing to the unlimited amounts of food available to eat. Most of the industrialized and prosperous communities have a great percentage of individuals that eat too much, to the point at which health is adversely affected. Overnutrition can be developed into obesity, which increases the risk of serious health conditions, including cardiovascular disease, hypertension, cancer and type-2 diabetes (White et al., 2012).

Malnutrition in children can be classified into three types: stunted, wasted and overweight. Stunting refers to a child who is too short for his age, and it's related to the failure of growing both physically and cognitively. It results of chronic or recurrent malnutrition. Wasting, or acute malnutrition, refers to a child who is too thin for his height, and it's related to a rapid weight loss or to the failure to gain weight. Overweight refers to a child who is too heavy for his height due to the consumption of too many calories that enhances the risk of diseases later in life (UNICEF, WHO, & The World Bank Group, 2016).

All around the world, disease-related malnutrition is common and costly. The hospitalization itself is often associated with the risk of worsening the patient's nutritional status which, in turn, can lead to delayed recovery and functional decline. Although several clinical guidelines specify care processes, malnutrition is still overlooked and undertreated (Aquino & Philippi, 2011).

Through the statistics presented in Figure 1, it is possible to note that, in 2015, Africa and Asia had the greatest share of all forms of children's malnutrition.

Over the last years, health organizations have been developing new means of response for citizens and, new ways of communication and information transmission, supported by technological systems. Business intelligence tools are now used in public health fields for financial and administrative purposes,

Figure 1. Global percentage of stunted, overweight, and wasted children under 5 in 2015
UNICEF et al. (2016)

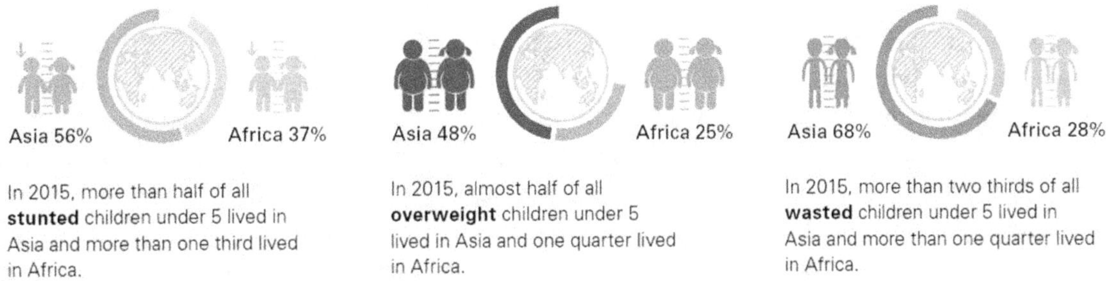

for diagnosing and treating patients and for evaluating alternative treatments based on outcomes analysis (Jinpon et al., 2011).

In this sense, and based on a BI methodology, it is presented a data warehouse system for the use of evidence-based medicine in the context of nutrition evaluation.

The accomplishment of this project presupposed the execution of a certain set of steps. In the first section was carried out research related to health information systems and to what extent concepts such as interoperability and usability influence it. Fundamental concepts, namely, business intelligence, data warehouse, extract-transform-load, and OLAP were discussed in subsequent sections. Along with these concepts, the project phases were described: the construction of a multidimensional model (identifying facts and dimensions), data extraction, transformation, cleaning, and loading into a data warehouse and the construction of health indicators. As the construction of indicators presupposes the availability of data, the results and conclusions may not be entirely accurate because there were missing values in the population and this was a case study in one particular hospital. Besides that, constructed indicators present nutritional data in a clear and objective manner and may generate positive outcomes in the nutritional field.

HEALTH INFORMATION SYSTEMS

The quality of information provided by information systems must be as reliable as possible to deliver quality services (Marins et al., 2015; Neves et al., 2016). To enable the various health activities carried out by the numerous health professionals in different places, multiple information on the patient's condition must be accessible (Portela et al., 2015). With this, different data sources are generated that, consequently, give rise to different information that not assure data accuracy and quality. The quality of information is vital since data will be organized to produce a health system that supports decision making. If there is no data quality control, erroneous support decision making may be returned, that in a health context reflect devastating results (Machado et al., 2010). Furthermore, validation of data accuracy and consistency are also significant problems for many health organizations. The result can be a disaster for a data warehouse that depends on such systems for its content. For this reason, data quality is a primary concern (March & Hevner, 2007).

Clinical data extracted from several sources and used for multiple purposes have heterogeneity as a dominant characteristic, often not suitable for traditional information systems, where integration is not always privileged. The predominance in most countries is a fragmented system that doesn't always have integration and interoperability characteristics (Peixoto et al., 2012; Rodrigues et al., 2013).

Basic interoperability is achieved through the standard exchange of messages between systems. The adoption of interoperability standards in the health sector has become increasingly indispensable due to the existence of a vast conceptual diversity of hardware and software platforms, the need to search and communicate clinical and administrative information in real time and, the viability to use increasingly sophisticated decision support systems. There has been a need to ensure the overall process's flow, which should be based on interoperability standards and good practices. Functional interoperability requires that information is readable to humans. Additionally, it describes an interaction of two or more systems to exchange information according to a defined set of rules. Semantic interoperability is translated into the ability of several systems to share information that is conceptually compatible with each other (Peixoto, H., 2010). In other words, systems have a formal agreement on the concepts involved in the exchanges and presuppose the usage of standardized vocabulary in messages. Thus, to establish interoperability, these standards of registration, communication, and documentation should be implemented and adhered by the intervenient systems (Cavalini & Cook, 2012).

It is also important to note that each health professional has different information needs. Therefore, applications and user interfaces need to be easily understood and handled to ensure usability. Usability defends the assumption that the system should satisfy the user's needs. This depends on the circumstances in which a system is used, on users, tasks, equipment (hardware, software, and materials) and social and physical environment. Thus, usability helps to retain the user in a system by making it easy to learn and use, reduces redundancy, consistency errors and loss of system integrity, and also guarantees the system security (Pereira & Paiva, 2011).

METHODOLOGY

Health organizations collect significant volumes of data and have a lot of information to gather and process to be able to make the best decision as fast as possible. One solution that can improve the decision-making process is Business Intelligence (BI). BI tools help to transform raw data into smart information and knowledge. BI refers to methodologies and technologies for the collection, integration, analysis and presentation of all relevant information. There are many BI tools such as extract transform and load (ETL), data warehouse (DW), online analytical processing (OLAP), and dashboards (Jinpon et al.,2011).

The understanding of the presented case study implies the knowledge of the concept, architecture, and main steps to implement a DW solution. Data warehousing is a collection of decision support technologies, aimed at allowing the user to make better and faster decisions (Pereira & Paiva, 2011). Bill Inmon defined a DW as a subject-oriented, integrated, time-variant, and non-volatile collection of data in support of management's decision-making process (Inmon, 2005).

DW is targeted for decision support and distributed for load balancing, scalability, and higher availability. The data is stored and managed by one or more warehouse servers, which present multidimensional views of data to a variety of front-end tools: query tools, report writers, analysis tools, and data mining tools (Kimball & Ross, 2013).

The DW backstage includes many software modules responsible for data extraction from relevant sources, transformation, and preprocessing to produce useful integrated data and load it into the actual DW structures (Berndt, Hevner, & Studnicki, 2003). Those software modules are commonly known as Extract-Transform-Load (ETL) activities. The ETL process is quite complex, and it's considered the most time consuming and expensive portion of the DW development lifecycle, mostly due to the plethora and large volume of the different activities contained in such process (Vassiliadis, Simitsis, & Baikousi, 2009). Studies have shown that ETL and data cleaning tools consume one-third of the budget in a DW project and can, in terms of its development time, consume 80% of that value. Additionally, some studies mentioned that the ETL process has costs in the order of 55% of the project's total execution time (Inmon, 1997).

Despite this, the ETL activities have a substantial importance in the design and maintenance of the DW. Some common activities are data cleansing (such as correcting misspellings, dealing with missing elements, detecting duplicate data, and checking for integrity constraints violations), filters, groupers, assigning warehouse keys and so on (Vassiliadis et al., 2009).

Once the DW construction is completed, one of the most used tools for accessing and analyzing data is OLAP. This tool allows the treatment of data coming from different sources in real time, through faster and more efficient methods. It also allows the usage of a wide variety of data visualization tools and data organization using the desired selection criteria. However, the greatest advantage of OLAP is the ability to perform multidimensional data analysis, associated with complex calculations, trend analysis and modeling (Ferreira, Miranda, Abelha, & Machado, 2010).

Warehousing Architecture

The general structure of the ETL process is presented in Figure 2. The lower left layer represents the original data coming from several sources, which compound the raw material for the DW. This data is obtained by extraction routines and it's later propagated to the data staging area (DSA) for further manipulation (Ferreira et al., 2010).

The data staging area is both a storage area, as well as the place where data is subjected to cleaning, integration, and transformation procedures before being loaded into the DW. It is somehow analogous to the kitchen of a restaurant, where food products are transformed into a meal. In the DW, raw data is converted into a warehouse derivable fit for user query. In comparison to the restaurant's kitchen, the backroom data staging area is available only to skilled professionals (Kimball & Ross, 2013).

The data loading into the DW structures is performed through load activities, represented in the upper right portion of the figure, and organized into an appropriate model which is called the multidimensional model (Ferreira et al., 2010).

A DW project comprises a set of tasks for the implementation of each component described in Figure 2. There are several methodological approaches that define a sequence of steps essential for accomplishing these tasks. The methodology used included the following steps: 1) construction of the multidimensional model, identifying dimensions and facts; 2) data extraction from the source (Excel); 3) data transformation and cleaning; 4) loading data into MySQL database structure; 5) building indicators through PowerBI.

Figure 2. Illustration of the ETL process in data warehouse systems

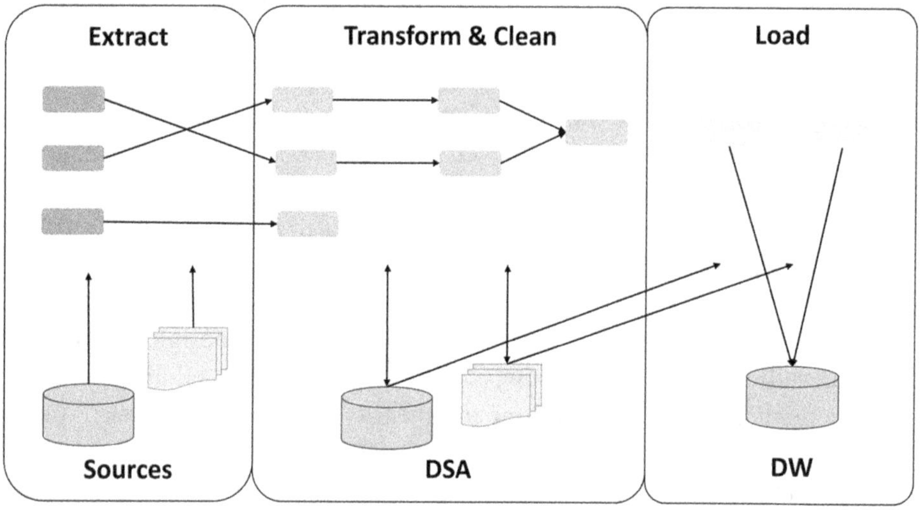

Back End Activities

Data warehousing systems use a variety of data extraction and cleaning tools as well as load and refresh utilities for populating warehouses. Extraction is the first step in the process of getting data into the DW environment. Since a DW is used for decision making, it's vital to ensure its reliability (Chaudhuri & Dayal, 1997). The data used in this project consists of clinical records – referring to one year of evaluation records of nutrition episodes – extracted from a Portugal hospital and consequently filled by health professionals. The lack of standards and rules for filling these records lead to a high probability of errors and irregularities. Not surprisingly, data entry fields had significant inconsistent data. Therefore, it was necessary to process data through cleaning and transformation procedures. Such procedures comprised: transformation of dates to standardized formats; dealing with duplicate data; assigning warehouse keys; standardize units of measure; rename doctors and nutritionists to ensure their privacy; rectify inconsistent value assignments; removal of irregular characters; parsing into standard formats; assign descriptions to values in order to facilitate their understanding; creating new data through functions that relate one or more attributes. Note that patient identification data were disregarded at this project, allowing total anonymity.

It is also important to note that the extracted data for this project was in two different data files: XML and Excel. For this reason, it was required to convert data from both Excel and XML to MySQL.

After extracting, cleaning and transforming, data were loaded into the DW. Additional preprocessing was still required: checking integrity constraints, sorting, aggregation and other computation to build the derived tables stored in the warehouse. A load utility must provide the system administrator to monitor status, to suspend, cancel and resume a load, as well as to restart after failure with no loss of data integrity (Chaudhuri & Dayal, 1997). With this in mind, the tool used was MySQL Workbench 6.3, which is a unified visual tool for database developers that provides data modeling, SQL development, and comprehensive administration tools for server configuration, user administration, and backup. MySQL Workbench also enables a developer to visually design, model, generate, and manage databases (MySQL, 2016).

Database Design Methodology

The data presentation area is where data is stored, organized, and available for direct querying by users. Since the backroom staging area is out of reach, the presentation area is the DW as far as the business community is concerned (Kimball & Ross, 2013).

Dimensional modeling is the ablest to succeed technique for delivering data to DW users. Dimensional modeling is different from third-normal-form (3NF) modeling – sometimes referred as entity-relationship (ER) models – which is a design technique that removes data redundancies. The use of ER models in the DW presentation area defeats the purpose of data warehousing, namely, intuitive and high-performance retrieval of data (Kimball & Ross, 2013). In this sense, ER diagrams are unsuitable for decision support systems where efficiency in querying and in loading data are necessary. The multidimensional view of data in the warehouse is a conceptual model that influences the database design, the front-end tools, and the query engines for OLAP. In this sense, to facilitate sophisticated analyses and visualization, the data in the warehouse was modeled multidimensionally (Chaudhuri & Dayal, 1997).

In a multidimensional data model, the objects of analysis are the set of numeric measures. In nutritional context, examples of such measures are the patient's age, weight, height and BMI. Time is a measure of particular significance to decision support systems (e.g., trend analysis). Every numeric measure depends on a set of dimensions, which provide the context for the measure. For instance, the dimensions associated with the answer processing time are the service and the doctor that made the request, the nutritionist, and the answer state. The dimensions together are assumed to determine the measure uniquely. Each dimension is described by a set of attributes. For example, the doctor dimension consists of two attributes: id and name. Along with those attributes could be many other characteristics considered relevant according to the context (Chaudhuri & Dayal, 1997).

The star schema was the shape used to represent the multidimensional data model since it's easy to design, configure, and implement. It also has been recognized as an effective structure for organizing data, has a quick query response, and can be understood by a typical user. The star schema is characterized by a single center fact table and a single table for each dimension (Berndt et al, 2003).

Each tuple in the fact table consists of a pointer (foreign key) to every dimension that provides its multidimensional coordinates and stores the numeric measures for those coordinates (Chaudhuri & Dayal, 1997). The most relevant facts are additive numeric data items that can be averaged, summed or combined in other ways to create summary statistics. The only way to compress data and produce a reasonably sized answer set is to present some mathematical summarization. No one wants thousands, let alone millions, of items in answer to their queries (Berndt et al, 2003). As Kimball points out ''the best and most useful facts are numeric, continuously valued, and additive.'' (Chaudhuri & Dayal, 1997). It is theoretically possible for a measured fact to be textual. In most cases, a textual measurement is a description of something and is drawn from a discrete list of values. However, a text fact is rare in a DW because of its unpredictable content that makes it nearly impossible to analyze. The fact table usually has its primary key made up of a subset of the foreign keys. This key is called a composite or concatenated key (Kimball & Ross, 2013).

In this case, the fact table refers to the nutritional episode's evaluation and it's composed by its primary key - the episode's id -, by the foreign keys that relate the table of facts with all the dimensions, and also by the measures, namely, the patient's age, weight, height and BMI as well as the request and answer dates, the answer processing time and whether or not the patient follows nutrition.

The set of dimensions consists of many categorical or textual attributes. The dimensions determine the query environment, the richer the set of dimensions the more ways the data can be accessed via queries. Every dimension table consists of columns that correspond to the dimensions' attributes (Chaudhuri & Dayal, 1997). The multidimensional model created has seven dimensions: *gender* referring to the patient's gender; *doctor* and *servrequest* concerning the doctor and the service demanding the request; *nutritionist* and *answer_state* who refer, respectively, to the nutritionist responsible for the request analysis and the status of his/her response; *age_classification* and *nutrition_classification* regarding the classification of the patient's age and nutritional status.

Star schemas have a simple and understandable dimensional structure that supports a large and useful universe of queries. Users benefit from the dimensional schema's simplicity and symmetry, not only because it provides them an easier way to understand and navigate through data, but also because of its ability to accommodate change (Kimball & Ross, 2013).

Indicators

BI uses dashboards in the presentation step to deliver the information to end users. The dashboard is used to summarize key metrics and help with management and decision-making so that one can see the most salient information at a glance. In healthcare, dashboards are used to diagnose problem areas and drive management related to just about any hospital activity. A clinical dashboard will contain locally defined clinical indicators, which can help improve a clinical team's ability to focus on improving the quality of care with immediate effect (Jinpon et al.,2011).

An indicator is an instrument that measures quality in a quantitative way. It measures the degree of fulfillment of the criterion when compared with the considered standard. Indicators can assess the program's effects, assist planning and resource allocation decisions, measure and compare results and evaluate trends evolution over time (Magalhães, 2013).

There are several definitions for a health indicator. The Dictionary of Epidemiology defines health indicator as "a variable that can be measured directly and reflects the health status of people in a community." A health indicator is useful for quantification, monitorization, and evaluation of health and its determinants (Dias et al., 2007).

The construction of an indicator presupposes the availability of data. These original sources of data are almost always integrated into information systems whose overall quality is fundamental to the indicators quality. Thus, the quality of an indicator depends to a large extent on the quality of its original components (Dias et al., 2007).

Through indicators, a health professional should be able to identify a health problem (e.g.: excess of cardiovascular disease in a population) and health needs (e.g.: reduce the proportion of obese people). Then, transform these needs into services (e.g.: diagnosis and control of obesity, availability of equipment for physical activity) that verify and guarantee effectiveness, whether close to their delivery (effect, or favorable change in health needs), or, more remotely (impact on health level state) (Dias et al., 2007).

In the context of this paper, the purpose of constructing nutrition-related indicators is to explore the available data, to contribute to a comparative statistical analysis, over time, and to improve the quality of health services in organizations.

The indicators were built using Power BI which is a suite of business analytics tools to create dashboards to report and analyze data. Power BI dashboards provide a 360-degree view for users with the most relevant metrics in one place, updated in real time (Power BI, 2017). It was made a connection between Power BI and MySQL Workbench to gather all the data needed to the construction of health indicators.

RESULTS

In 2013, 588 patients with nutritional needs were evaluated in a hospital in Portugal. There were teenagers between the ages of 10 to 18 years old, adults between the ages of 19 to 65 years old and elderly people, aged over 65 years old.

According to Table 1 and Figure 3, 322 patients (54.76%) were elderly people, of which 151 were female individuals and 171 were male individuals, 249 (42.35%) were adults, of which 87 were female individuals and 162 males were male individuals, 17 (2.89%) teenagers, 8 of them female individuals and 9 of them male individuals. The majority of the population in this case study was elderly population. Furthermore, and in this case study, there were more men (58,16%) than women (41,84%) evaluated.

During the same year, there were 693 nutrition episodes, i.e., 693 requests from doctors to follow-up patients in nutrition. As observed in Table 2 and Figure 4, 650 (93.80%) of nutritionists' answers were not published, 12 (1.73%) were published, and 31 (4.47%) of the requests have not been answered.

Figure 5 shows the number of nutrition episodes, the number of patients and percentage who followed nutrition, per month and in 2013. Of the total number of episodes (694), 31 of them had no associated dates. The months with the majority of nutrition episodes were August (73) and October (73) and with fewer episodes was January (38). The patients who followed nutrition were in greater number in October

Table 1. Population characterization

Age Category	Female	Male	Total
Adult	87	162	**249**
Elderly	151	171	**322**
Teenager	8	9	**17**
Total	**246**	**342**	**588**

Figure 3. Population characterization (%) by age category and gender

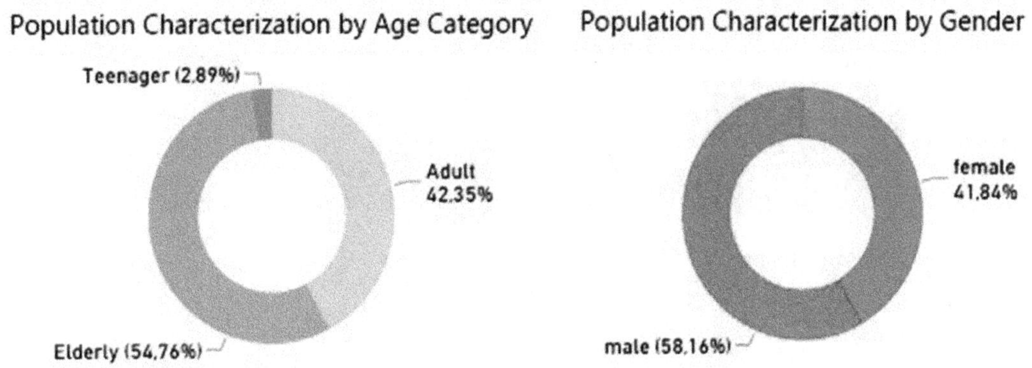

Table 2. Number of doctors' requests per state of the nutritionists' answer

State of the Answer	Number Episodes
Not published	650
Published	23
Without answer	31
Total	**693**

Figure 4. Percentage of doctors' requests per state of the nutritionists' answer

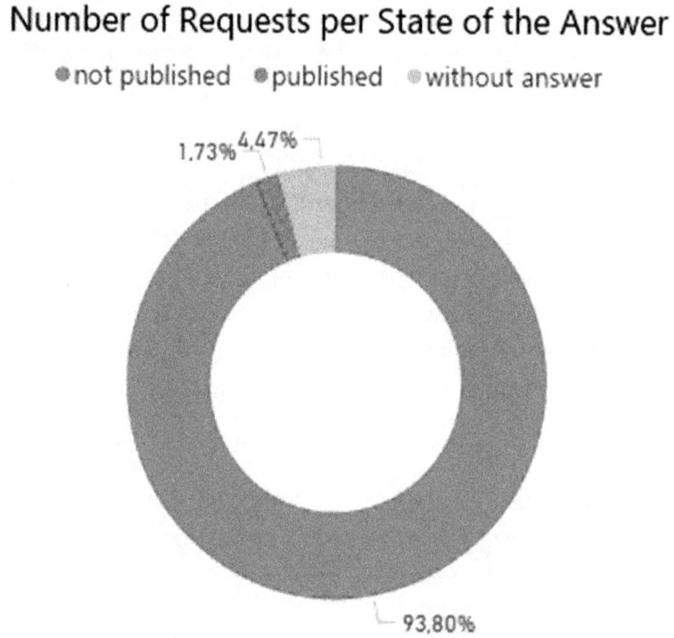

Figure 5. Number of nutrition episodes, patients following nutrition (n, %) by month

Month	Number of Episodes	Number of Patients Following Nutrition	% Patients Following Nutrition
January	38	37	97,37
February	39	35	89,74
March	53	48	90,57
April	47	42	89,36
May	67	62	92,54
June	59	52	88,14
July	63	60	95,24
August	73	69	94,52
September	57	55	96,49
October	73	72	98,63
November	53	52	98,11
December	40	40	100,00
Total	**662**	**624**	**94,26**

(72) and smaller number in February (35). December had a percentage of 100% for patients following nutrition (40) concerning the number of nutrition episodes (40) in that month. In contrast, June, obtained the lowest percentage (88.14%), with 59 nutrition episodes and 52 patients following nutrition. Overall, 94.26% of the patients in 2013 followed nutrition.

Figure 6 shows the maximum and minimum process times between the request made by the physician and the response given by the nutritionist. The first was approximately 7 days and 20 hours and the second was approximately 2 minutes.

According to the criteria recommended by WHO (World Health Organization), Figure 7 shows the proportion of individuals by category in this case study, classified through BMI calculation.

Body mass index (BMI) is a measure for indicating nutritional status in adults. It is defined as an individual's weight in kilograms divided by the square of the person's height in meters (kg/m2). For adults over 19 years old, BMI falls into one of the following categories: below 18,5 – underweight; between 18,5 and 24,9 – normal weight; between 25,0 and 29,9 – pre-obesity; between 30,0 and 34,9 – obesity class I; between 35,0 and 39,9 – obesity class II; above 40 – obesity class III (WHO, 2017).

The BMI ranges are based on the effect excessive body fat has on illness and death and are reasonably well related to adiposity. BMI is a risk indicator of disease and as it increases, so does the risk for some diseases. BMI is also recommended for use in adolescents and children. In children, BMI is calculated as for adults and then compared with z-scores or percentiles. During adolescence and childhood, the ratio between height and weight varies with age and sex, so the cut-off values that determine the nutritional status are gender and age-specific (WHO, 2017).

Analyzing Figure 7, it can be verified that 44.81% of the patients had a normal weight and 29.55% were undernourished.

It is also important to mention that these percentages are not related to the entire population in this case study since 280 patients presented null values of weight and height, which did not allow BMI calculation and, consequently, to attribute them to a category.

In order to observe the relationship between nutritional status and age classification, a graph showing the number of adult and elderly patients classified according to WHO criteria is shown in Figure 8. Since there was a low number of teenagers in the population with nutritional information (only 3 individuals had height and weight defined), these were not considered.

There were 49 of 152 adults integrated into the underweight category, higher number compared to the elderly population, which had 40 cases of undernutrition out of 153. There were 61 adults and 76 elders with a normal weight. For the pre-obesity category, 23 adults and 23 older adults were included in it. In the three remaining categories, obesity class I, II and III, 11 adults and 7 elders integrated the first one, 5 adults and 3 elders integrated the second and finally 3 adults and 4 elders integrated the third one.

Figure 9 shows the number of patients integrated into obesity class I, II and III categories, normal weight category (healthy patients) and underweight category, by gender. There were 21 women and 12

Figure 6. Maximum and minimum process times between request and answer

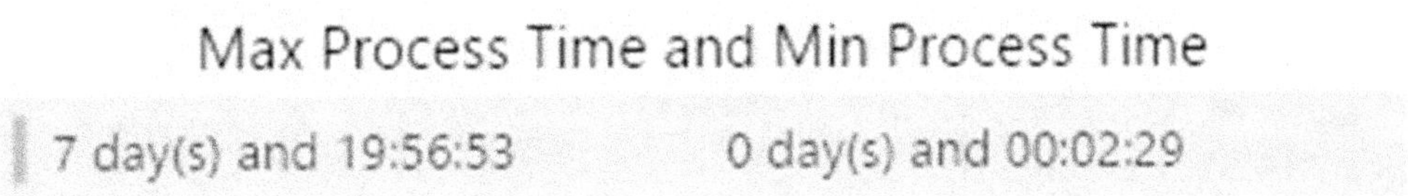

Figure 7. Percentage of patients by nutrition classification

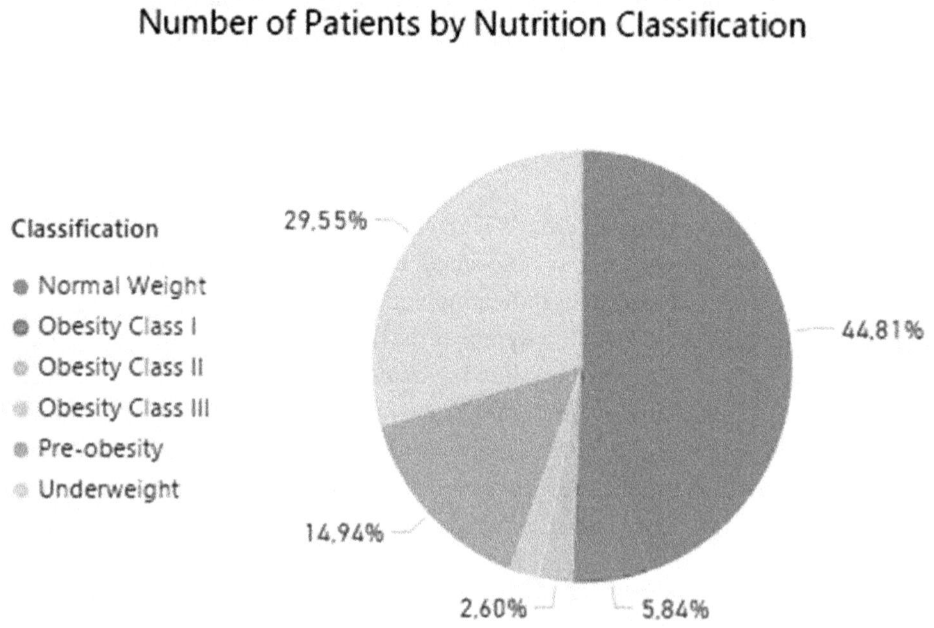

Figure 8. Number of patients by age and nutrition classification

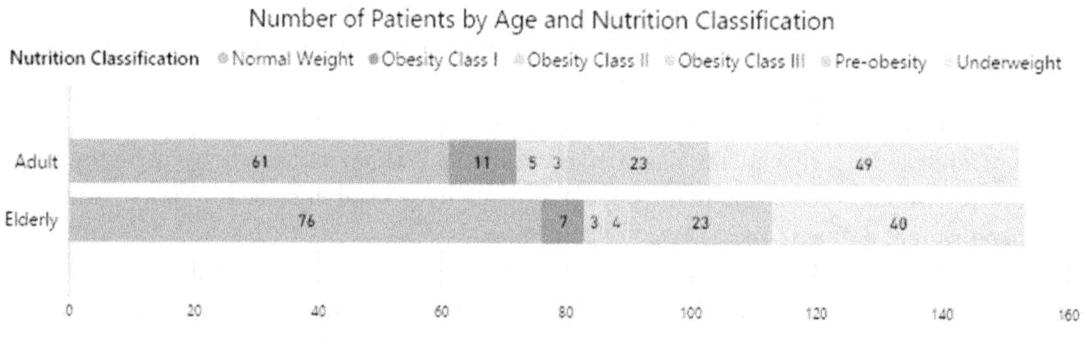

Figure 9. Number of obese patients, healthy patients, and underweight patients by gender

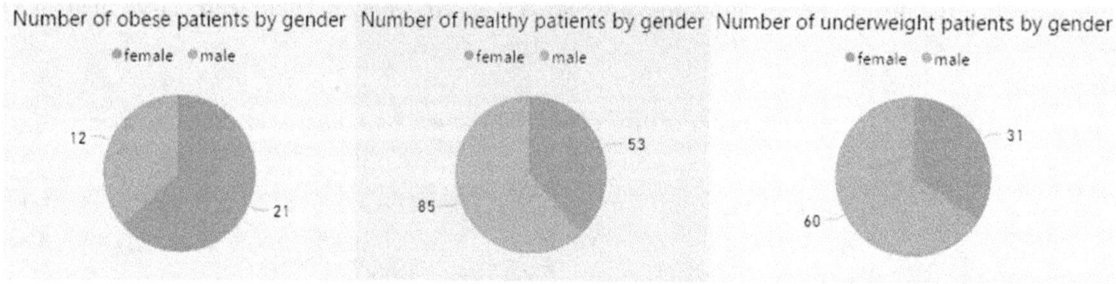

men who suffered from obesity problems, 85 men and 53 women that were healthy and 60 men and 31 women that were undernourished.

DISCUSSION

Nutritional status allows us to assess the health status of a population and to understand the extent to which health programs can be adjusted to better monitor patients at risk.

Of the evaluated population in this case study, more than half was elderly and a substantial proportion of the rest was adult. There were evaluated more men than women.

From the results presented, it is worth noting the high number of unpublished answers by nutritionists. Only about 2% of the total number of requests in 2013 was published, which is extremely low. However, only 5% of the total number of requests did not receive an answer from nutritionists, which was considered a good result.

Almost all the episodes evaluated demonstrated that the patient needed to be followed by a nutrition specialist. It should also be noted that the maximum processing time between a request made by a physician and a response by a nutritionist was approximately 7 days, which means that the patient didn't have to wait for a long period of time to know the results and the need for a possible treatment. The minimum processing time was a couple of minutes which is an extremely low value.

BMI, being a combination of weight and height measurements, is the most frequently used parameter to track changes in the nutritional status of adults and elders.

The majority of the studied population presented normal BMI values, the second largest group was the undernourished population, the third the pre-obese population and finally the population belonging to obesity class I, obesity class II and obesity class III categories, respectively. More adults were suffering from undernutrition than seniors that had the highest number of individuals with BMI values considered normal. Regarding the three categories defined by WHO on obesity, adults and elders had almost the same values. However, there were more obese adults than obese older adults.

The prevalence of obesity in adults has been increasing. In 2009, and at a global level, the percentage of men and women considered obese was 9.1% and 13.2%, respectively. In 2013, this percentage increased in the same proportion for both sexes, rising to 10.4% for men and to 14.5% for women. In Portugal, and in 2013, 19,5% of the female population and 18,9% of the male population were obese (WHO, 2016).

In the population of this case study, there were also obese adults and statistical differences between genders. The statistics mentioned above are in line with those of the population studied, since there were more obese women than obese men.

To conclude, and as the construction of indicators presupposes the availability of data, the results and conclusions may not be entirely accurate because there were missing values in the population and this was a case study in one particular hospital. Besides that, constructed indicators are easily understood and useful to its users as well as consistent and relevant, providing information that advances the understanding of the bridges between doctors and nutritionists and patients nutritional status.

CONCLUSION

In this paper, it's shown the role of data warehousing for the use of evidence-based medicine in the context of nutrition evaluation. Regardless of data origin or its form of extraction and transformation, data must be presented and serve the end users in a proper and useful way, without the need of interpreters. Business intelligence is used as a tool for the collection, integration, and analysis of all relevant nutritional information for the purpose of better decision-making.

The actions of intervention on population's health are today, guided by the best available evidence, and integrated with the best practice. Health indicators are no more than attempts to capture the enormous diversity of levels and dimensions of reality to bring man closer to his health control. It's essential to use indicators that measure the quality and quantity of what is done concerning health programs and services and that they cover all of its components such as structures, processes, and results. It remains to emphasize the need for a storage system that allows the assembly of historical series that provide comparisons with other institutions or with themselves when analysed over time.

In this sense, there were created health indicators that are vital for the construction of clinical scenarios which, when well used, support the healthcare providers to generate positive outcomes in the context of nutrition evaluation. Additionally, and as health indicators have the ability to generate positive outcomes, they must be created and used not only in the context of nutrition evaluation but on the wide diversity of services that health professionals could provide to their community. Those indicators have the potential to make strong contributions to outcomes and performance, especially in the data-intensive environment of healthcare planning assessment and review.

REFERENCES

Amaro, J. D. S., Correia, A. C., & Pereira, C. (2016). Avaliação do Risco de Desnutrição num Serviço de Medicina do Hospital Distrital de Santarém (Medicina IV). *Acta Portuguesa de Nutrição, 06-09*(4).

Aquino, R. D. C., & Philippi, S. T. (2011). Identificação de fatores de risco de desnutrição em pacientes internados. *Revista da Associação Médica Brasileira, 57*(6), 637–643. doi:10.1590/S0104-42302011000600009 PMID:22249542

Berndt, D. J., Hevner, A. R., & Studnicki, J. (2003). The Catch data warehouse: Support for community health care decision-making. *Decision Support Systems, 35*(3), 367–384. doi:10.1016/S0167-9236(02)00114-8

Cavalini, L. T., & Cook, T. W. (2012). Knowledge engineering of healthcare applications based on minimalist multilevel models. In *e-Health Networking, Applications and Services (Healthcom), 2012 IEEE 14th International Conference on* (pp. 431-434). IEEE. doi:10.1109/HealthCom.2012.6379454

Chaudhuri, S., & Dayal, U. (1997). An overview of data warehousing and OLAP technology. *SIGMOD Record, 26*(1), 65–74. doi:10.1145/248603.248616

Correia, M. I. T., Hegazi, R. A., Higashiguchi, T., Michel, J. P., Reddy, B. R., Tappenden, K. A., & Muscaritoli, M. (2014). Evidence-based recommendations for addressing malnutrition in health care: An updated strategy from the feedM. E. Global Study Group. *Journal of the American Medical Directors Association*, *15*(8), 544–550. doi:10.1016/j.jamda.2014.05.011 PMID:24997720

Dias, C. M., Freitas, M., & Briz, T. (2007). Indicadores de saúde: Uma visão de Saúde Pública, com interesse em Medicina Geral e Familiar. *Revista Portuguesa de Medicina Geral e Familiar*, *23*(4), 439–450.

Ferreira, J., Miranda, M., Abelha, A., & Machado, J. (2010). O processo etl em sistemas data warehouse. INForum, 757-765.

Inmon, B. (1997, January). The data warehouse budget. *DM Review Magazine*. doi:10.1145/1651291.1651297

Inmon, W. H. (2005). *Building the data warehouse*. John Wiley & Sons.

Jinpon, P., Jaroensutasinee, M., & Jaroensutasinee, K. (2011). Business intelligence and its applications in the public healthcare system. *Walailak Journal of Science and Technology*, *8*(2), 97–110.

Kimball, R., & Ross, M. (2013). *The data warehouse toolkit: The definitive guide to dimensional modeling*. John Wiley & Sons.

Machado, J., Abelha, A., Novais, P., Neves, J., & Neves, J. (2010). Quality of service in healthcare units. *International Journal of Computer Aided Engineering and Technology*, *2*(4), 436–449. doi:10.1504/IJCAET.2010.035396

Magalhães, A. S. C. (2013). *Indicadores de Qualidade na Emergência Médica Pré-hospitalar*. Retrieved from RUN - Repositório Universidade Nova: https://run.unl.pt/bitstream/10362/15233/1/RUN%20-%20Trabalho%20Final%20CEAH%20-%20Ana%20Sofia%20Carvalho%20de%20Magalhaes.pdf

March, S. T., & Hevner, A. R. (2007). Integrated decision support systems: A data warehousing perspective. *Decision Support Systems*, *43*(3), 1031–1043. doi:10.1016/j.dss.2005.05.029

Marins, F., Cardoso, L., Portela, F., Santos, M. F., Abelha, A., & Machado, J. (2014). Improving High Availability and Reliability of Health Interoperability Systems. In New Perspectives in Information Systems and Technologies (vol. 2, pp. 207-216). Springer International Publishing. doi:10.1007/978-3-319-05948-8_20

MySQL. (2016). *MySQL Enterprise Edition*. Retrieved from https://www.mysql.com/products/enterprise/mysql-datasheet.en.pdf

Neves, J., Abelha, V., Vicente, H., Neves, J., & Machado, J. (2016). Length of Hospital Stay and Quality of Care. In Knowledge, Information and Creativity Support Systems (pp. 273-287). Springer International Publishing. doi:10.1007/978-3-319-27478-2_19

Peixoto, H., Machado, J., Neves, J., & Abelha, A. (2010). Semantic interoperability and health records. In *E-Health* (pp. 236–237). Springer Berlin Heidelberg. doi:10.1007/978-3-642-15515-4_30

Peixoto, H., Santos, M., Abelha, A., & Machado, J. (2012, December). Intelligence in Interoperability with AIDA. In *International Symposium on Methodologies for Intelligent Systems* (pp. 264-273). Springer Berlin Heidelberg.

Pereira, S. R., & Paiva, P. B. (2011). A importância da Engenharia da Usabilidade para a Segurança de Sistemas Informatizados em Saúde. *Journal of Health Informatics*, *3*(3).

Portela, F., Oliveira, S., Santos, M., Machado, J., & Abelha, A. (2015, December). A real-time intelligent system for tracking patient condition. In *Ambient Intelligence for Health* (pp. 91–97). Springer International Publishing. doi:10.1007/978-3-319-26508-7_9

Power, B. I. (2017). *Guided Learning for Power BI*. Retrieved from https://powerbi.microsoft.com/en-us/documentation/powerbi-learning-0-0-what-is-power-bi/

Rodrigues, F., Pereira, D., Nascimento, J. C., Ribeiro, J., Barros, P., Correia, R., . . . Gomes, R. (2013). *Interoperabilidade na Saúde - Onde Estamos?*. Retrieved from http://www.apdsi.pt/uploads/news/id719/Estudo_APDSI_Interoperabilidade_Sa%C3%BAde_completo.pdf

UNICEF. (2006). *Nutrition, survival and development*. Retrieved from https://www.unicef.org/progressforchildren/2006n4/index_undernutrition.html

UNICEF, WHO, & The World Bank Group. (2016). *Levels and trends in child Malnutrition*. Retrieved from http://www.who.int/nutgrowthdb/jme_brochure2016.pdf?ua=1

Vassiliadis, P., Simitsis, A., & Baikousi, E. (2009). A taxonomy of ETL activities. In *Proceedings of the ACM twelfth international workshop on Data warehousing and OLAP* (pp. 25-32). ACM.

White, J. V., Guenter, P., Jensen, G., Malone, A., & Schofield, M. (2012). Consensus statement of the Academy of Nutrition and Dietetics/American Society for Parenteral and Enteral Nutrition: Characteristics recommended for the identification and documentation of adult malnutrition (undernutrition). *Journal of the Academy of Nutrition and Dietetics*, *112*(5), 730–738. doi:10.1016/j.jand.2012.03.012 PMID:22709779

WHO. (2016). *Global Health Observatory indicator views*. Retrieved from http://apps.who.int/gho/data/node.imr.NCD_BMI_30A?lang=en

WHO. (2017). *Body mass index - BMI*. Retrieved from http://www.euro.who.int/en/health-topics/disease-prevention/nutrition/a-healthy-lifestyle/body-mass-index-bmi

Chapter 14
Indian Healthcare Service Management Through Data Mining:
Datamining for Healthcare Services

Manaswini Pradhan
Fakir Mohan University, India

ABSTRACT

The main intention of our method is to provide better Healthcare services over the rural areas in terms of prediction of the chief hospitals with required basic facilities around that particular area. Accordingly, a Questionnaire survey is made for collecting the relevant hospital data around the Odisha region. Then, the concept of data mining is utilized in order to extract the data from the Questionnaire. Further, Incremental Spanning algorithm is introduced here for the mining of data from the Questionnaire. In the Questionnaire, appropriate score values were assigned for each category based on the requirement. Moreover, the hospital satisfying all the required components within the Questionnaire have to be determined for predicting the better hospitals. The Genetic Algorithm is introduced so as to determine the maximum of the score values obtaining for the input hospital data. Finally, the ranking of first five supreme hospitals is determined around the Odisha region.

1. INTRODUCTION

Health care services in India have undergone a vast change over the last few decades and encompass the entire nation. India's health care system was carefully structured so that it can provide primary, preventative, and curative health care within a reasonable distance of the population even in remote, rural areas. Delivering affordable health care to India's billion plus people presents enormous challenges and opportunities for the medical community (Aliman & Mohamad, 2016; Silas & Rajsingh, 2016).

DOI: 10.4018/978-1-5225-2851-7.ch014

The World Health Organization (1997) defined healthcare sector reform as a sustained process of fundamental change in policy and institutional arrangements of the healthcare sector, usually guided by the government. It is designed to identify the functioning and performance of the healthcare service provided by each hospital to the people. In spite of the fact that the Indian healthcare industry is rapidly expanding, healthcare infrastructure in India is very poor (Kaushik & Raman, 2015; Sharma & Reimer-Kirkhamb, 2015). A noticeable percentage of India suffers from poor standard of healthcare services. Most of the healthcare facilities of India provided by the various healthcare services are limited and of low standard. In order to understand the current status of the healthcare services in India, it is important to know about the healthcare services found in the country (Yeha et al., 2011; Sung et al., 2015).

Healthcare industry today generates large amounts of complex data about doctor qualification, hospitals resources, disease diagnosis, electronic patient records, medical devices etc. These large amounts of data are a key resource to be processed and analyzed for knowledge extraction that enables support for cost savings and decision making. Data mining is a technology that is used to transform the mounds of data into useful information and helps in decision making that benefits in providing healthcare services to patients (Ngai et al., 2011; Chen et al., 2016).

Gathering the information from hospitals allows us to put academic effort and practical usage side by side and conclude on actual DM usage, and to understand if there is a gap between data analysis experts' community and healthcare practitioners and scientists. Data Mining is one of the most vital and motivating area of research with the objective of finding meaningful information from huge data sets (Chen et al., 2016; Lin et al., 2015). In present era, Data Mining is becoming popular in healthcare field because there is a need of efficient analytical methodology for detecting unknown and valuable information in health data. In this paper, an efficient algorithm, called IncSpan, is developed, for incremental mining over multiple database increments. In order to reduce the using time in mining incremental sequences, the algorithm used semi frequent patterns for incremental mining (Deshmukh, 2016).

The GA is applied over the problem domain where the outcome is very unpredictable and the process of outcome contains complex inter related modules. Also GA is very apt for such class of problem where problem specification is very difficult to formulate. During the last few decades, computer science has seen huge advancements in demands and its implementation. As per now heavy cross demands are in fire and hence implementation and analytics is becoming more and more chaos. The situation is very apt for applying genetics and getting optimal results (Bessant, 2014; Yin, 2016).

2. RELATED WORKS

Yuehong Yin et al. (2016) have explained a method for healthcare systems. Extensive research had been dedicated to the exploration of various technologies such as information technologies (IT) in complementing and strengthening existing healthcare services. In particular, the Internet of Things (IoT) had been widely applied to interconnect available medical resources and provide reliable, effective and smart healthcare service to the elderly and patients with a chronic illness. The aim was to summarize the applications of IoT in the health care industry and identify the intelligentization trend and directions of future research in this field. The advancement of IoT in healthcare systems had been examined from the perspectives of enabling technologies and methodologies, IoT-based smart devices and systems, and diverse applications of IoT in the healthcare industries.

Nagesh Shukla et al. (2014) have stated a Variations in service delivery it had been identified as a major challenge to the success of process improvement studies in service departments of hospital such as radiology. Largely, these variations were due to inherent system level factors, i.e., system variations such as unavailability of resources (nurse, bed, doctors, and equipment). These system variations were largely unnecessary/unwarranted and mostly lead to longer waiting times, delays, and lowered productivity of the service units. There was limited research on identifying system variations and modelling them for service improvements within hospital. Therefore, they used a modelling methodology to model system variations in radiology based on real time locating system (RTLS) tracking data. The methodology employs concepts from graph theory to identify and represent system variations. In particular, edge coloured directed multi-graphs (ECDMs) were used to model system variations which were reflected in paths adopted by staff, i.e., sequence of rooms/areas traversed while delivering services. The main steps of the methodology were: (1) identifying the most standard path followed by staff for service delivery; (2) filtering the redundant events in RTLS tracking database for analysis; (3) identifying rooms/areas of hospital site involved in the service delivery; (4) determining patterns of paths adopted by staff from filtered tracking database; and, (5) representation of patterns in graph based model called as edge coloured directed multigraphs (ECDMs) of a role.

Shin-Horng Chen et al. (2014) have proposed a current understanding of systemic service innovations by making intensive inquiries into the issue of how to formulate a commercially viable business concept for e-healthcare. Business models as key to success in service innovations require formulating and articulating a good and meaningful business concept right from the beginning. Taking into account the systemic nature of e-healthcare services, a conceptual framework had been developed and four cases were gathered from Taiwan's innovative e-healthcare programs to unveil the key ingredients of the business concept required for innovative e-healthcare services. Quite often, demand for e-healthcare services was associated with the healthcare and wellbeing need of the elderly and/or people with chronic diseases. In fact, such a view may be oversimplified. Instead, when paying attention to a distinction between direct demand and "derived" demand, one may better deal with an important issue of who was to pay. In addition, for e-healthcare to develop into commercially viable service innovation, the timing and location aspects, apart from those of people and information, had become relevant and crucial. The results of our case studies suggest that the needs of the cared may had different shades of meanings, in terms of value proposition. They introduce a few terms "nice-to-have", "had-better-have" and "must-have" to differentiate value to customers. Differences between these terms had implications for issues such as how crucial the service was to the users and customers and their willingness to pay. With no intention to play down the patient-centered view used by experts from other disciplines, they suggest that the service organization of e-healthcare needs to take a broad view towards customer space and service benefit, especially when it comes to the formation of a commercially viable business concept. In addition, e-healthcare services were not just means of promoting healthcare service quality and health interest of the service recipients, but may bring about a substantial impact on the cost and revenue structure of the service organization. It was therefore essential for the manager in the hospital to consider e-healthcare services as an integral part of medical care operations, when evaluating the cost-effectiveness of e-healthcare.

Tsung-Han Chang et al. (2014) have explained a framework based on the concept of fuzzy sets theory and the VIKOR method to provide a rational, scientific and systematic process for evaluating the hospital service quality under a fuzzy environment where the uncertainty, subjectivity and vagueness were address with linguistic variables parameterized by triangular fuzzy numbers. This study applies the fuzzy multi-criteria decision making approach to determine the importance weights of evaluation criteria and the VIKOR method was taken to consolidate the service quality performance ratings of the feasible alternatives. An empirical case involving evaluation criteria, 2 public and 3 private medical centers in Taiwan assessed by 18 evaluators from various fields of medical industry was solicited to demonstrate it. The service quality of private hospitals was better than public hospitals because the private hospitals were rarely subsidized by government alagencies. These private hospitals had to fend themselves to retain existing patients or attract patients to ensue sustainable survival.

Niels Ketelhöhn et al. (2016) have explained a JBR special section, and relates these cases to the management priorities in the healthcare industry in Latin America. It was based on a review of the literature on healthcare management, a survey of hospital managers in Latin America and the analysis of cases included in this special section. This special section includes ten teaching cases of healthcare institutions from six countries that were designed to address nine of the ten most relevant management issues in the sector. The most important management issues among healthcare institutions in Latin America were common to public and private hospitals, relating to the areas of strategy, management training, healthcare informatics and organizational change. Generally, private hospitals suffer from problems of underutilized capacity, so their managers were concerned with issues of marketing, pricing and demand forecasting. Conversely, public hospitals were overwhelmed with patients and need to better manage capacity, inventories, waiting lines, and working capital. The cases included in this special section address most of the problems in these three categories.

Rashedur M. Rahman et al. (2011) have stated a decision tree induction algorithm on Hospital Surveillance data to classify admitted patients according to their critical condition. Three class labels, low, medium and high, were used to distinguish the criticality of the admitted patients. Several decision tree models are developed, evaluated, and compared with different performance metrics. Finally an efficient classifier was developed to classify records and make decision/predictions on some input parameters. The models developed in this research could be helpful during epidemic when huge number of patients arrive daily. Due to rush of duty doctors and scarcity of required number of physicians, it was hard to diagnose every patient. Any computer application could be helpful to diagnose and measure the criticality of the newly arrived patient with the help of the historical data kept in the surveillance database. The application would ask few questions on physical condition and on history of disease of the patient and accordingly determines the critical condition of the patient as low, medium or high.

Hayden Wimmer et al. (2016) have described an evidence-based medicine. It was the modern standard for clinical decision making where the use of medical evidence combined with clinical expertise and research was leveraged for clinical decisions. Supporting evidence-based medicine (EBM) and clinical decision making (CDM) requires access to accurate predictive models and a multidimensional patient view that was aggregated from multiple sources in a multitude of configurations. Data sharing in healthcare remains a challenge due to widespread privacy concerns. Despite abundant research in privacy preserving data mining, healthcare organizations were unwilling to release their medical data on account of the Health Insurance Portability and Accountability Act (HIPAA) requires protecting the confidentiality and security of healthcare data. Further, sensitive data spanning multiple organizations result in not only the data syntax and semantic heterogeneity but also diverse privacy requirements, posing additional challenges to data sharing and integration. In overcoming these challenges, a multi-agent approach was a viable alternative. Despite its potential for addressing the aforementioned issues, little research had been conducted in integrating a multi-agent architecture with privacy preserving data mining in big healthcare data spanning multiple organizations. This research proposes a multi-agent architecture coupled with privacy preserving techniques to facilitate data sharing while preserving privacy. our design artifact was capable of overcoming the aforementioned challenges, thereby facilitating data sharing for knowledge discovery in healthcare and supporting evidence based medicine and clinical decision making via improving predictive models.

3. PROBLEM DESCRIPTION

The data generated by the healthcare organizations is very vast and complex due to which it is difficult to analyze the data in order to make important decision regarding which hospital providing best healthcare service. This data contains details regarding hospitals facilities, patients, medical claims, treatment cost etc. So, there is a need to generate a powerful tool for analyzing and extracting important information from this complex data for recognizing the best hospital.

4. PROPOSED METHODOLOGY

A huge amount of hospital related data is generated and stored by various healthcare organizations. But there are various challenges related to data stored by various hospitals which may play serious hurdles in the making proper decisions. The major challenge is format of hospital data being stored is different in different healthcare organizations. Till date there is no standard format is laid down for data being stored. In epidemic situations, this lack of standard format can make the epidemic situations even more badly. Patients' satisfaction is the basic objective for healthcare service provider as this satisfaction is directly related to quality of services provided by hospitals. In recent year, the healthcare industry has reorganized its service system. The reformation has focused on finding effective ways to meet the needs and desires of the patients.

Healthcare reveals the perfect storm for predictive analytics of hospitals facilities related data. The digitalization of the hospitals facilities records offers vast quantities of information. Innovations in data management permit unstructured hospitals data to be structured into compelling set ups. A growing number of technologists understand the nuances of how to manage and organize data and workflow so that creating and integrating estimations into healthcare workflow is becoming increasingly simple. Finally, we discover that major healthcare providing hospitals and technology distributors often partner together to create predictive solutions for healthcare services in rural areas.

The proposed method architecture to find the Indian Healthcare Service Providence through Data Mining Technique associated with Incremental Spanning and Genetic Algorithm is shown in Figure 1. In order to identify which hospital providing best service to the patients a collection of Odisha region hospitals is chosen in our experiment. A collection of questionnaire corresponding to hospitals facilities is created and forwarded to data mining stage; its patterns are extracted. The score values are assigned depending on their satisfaction to certain predefined conditions. Incspan algorithm helps to incremental mining of sequential patterns. Using genetic algorithm optimal patterns are identified it helps to recognize the best hospitals.

The steps used in proposed method Architecture is as follows:

Figure 1. Architecture of the proposed methodology

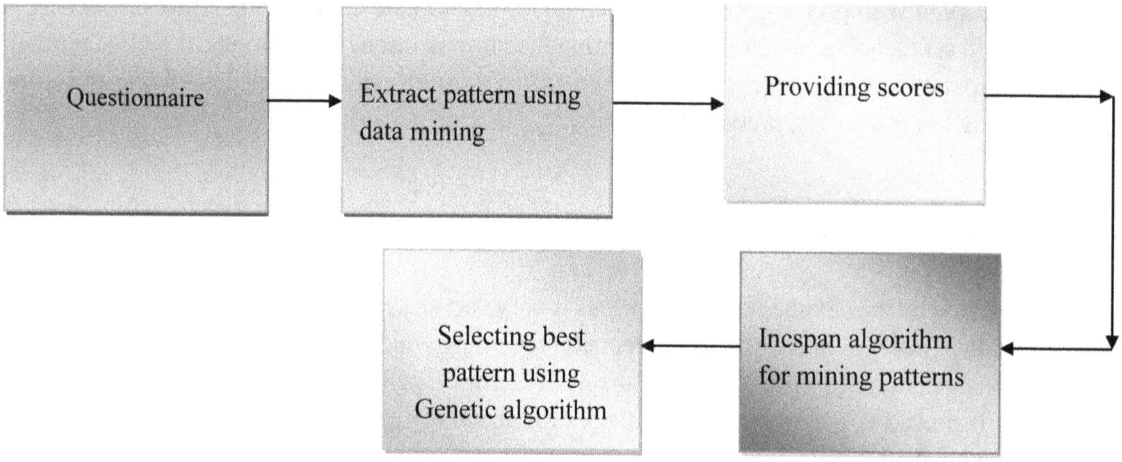

1. Questionnaire
2. Data mining
3. Score allocation
4. Incspan algorithm
5. Genetic algorithm

1. Questionnaire

A questionnaire is simply a 'tool' for collecting information about a particular issue of interest. We conduct an online survey and present questionnaire about the service problem facilities of various hospitals in order to measure the satisfaction of patients with an Indian Healthcare Service Providence the questionnaires related to Odisha region hospital is used in our experiment.

2. Data Mining

The questionnaires regarding to various hospital facilities is given as input to Data Mining step its target is to finding important information from huge data sets. In present time, Data Mining is becoming popular in healthcare field as there is a need of efficient conditional methodology for detecting unfamiliar and valuable information in healthcare Service Providence data. Data mining represents the process of analyzing raw data with the aid of computer and extraction of their meaning. It is frequently defined as discovering previously unknown and potentially useful information from large volume of data. It is possible to predict trends in hospital and thus provide the quality services to patients. Data mining uses a variety of techniques to find hidden patterns and relationships in large pools of data and infer from them that can predict future behaviors and guide in decision making.

3. Score Allocation

According to their valuable response collected from various hospitals score values are provided it is denoted from 1-5. If the response for the questionnaires is very good then it get the score 5 but if the response is good only then it get the score 4.Like that if the response is moderate then it get the score3. The response for the questionnaires is poor then it get the score2 while if the response is very poor then it get the score 1.

4. Incremental Spanning

IncSpan algorithms obtain the score allocated patterns and then mine them. It is an extension of PrefixSpan algorithm. IncSpan algorithm uses the concept of a projected-database to recursively mine sequential patterns. Unfortunately, IncSpan algorithms only address the insertion of transactions into the pre-existing user sequences. Generally, the change on a sequential database can be categorized as 1) deleting records, 2) inserting new records, and 3) appending new items on the existing records.

The semi-frequent patterns are buffered using this algorithm it can be considered as a statistics-based approach. The strategy lower the min sup rate by a buffer ratio $\mu <= 1$ and keep a set SFS in the original database G. This is because the sequences in SFS are "almost frequent", most of the frequent sub sequences in the appended database will either come from SFS or they may be already frequent in the original database. With a minor update to the original database, it is expected that only a small fraction of sub sequences which were occasional previously would become recurrent.

Items consist of n distinct literals is denoted as:

$$X = \{x_1, x_2 \ldots x_n\}$$

Item set is a subset of X. Each pattern consist of set of items .A sequence $m = < r_1, r_2, \ldots, r_s > (r_i \subseteq X)$ is an ordered list. Without loss of generality, we assume that the items in each item set are sorted in certain order such as alphabetic order (a, b, c …).

For an original database G, an appended database G', a threshold min sup, a buffer ratio μ, a set of frequent sequences FS and a set of semi-frequent sequences SFS, we want to discover the set of frequent sequences FS' in G'. The set of frequent sequences in G' is denoted as FS'. As a result, we have the following formula.

$$G' = G + gb = (ODB + NDB) + gb = (ODB + gb) + NDB = LDB + NDB.$$

Where $G = \{m_1, m_2, \ldots, m_n\}$

LDB - set of sequences in G' which are appended with items/itemsets.
ODB - set of sequences in G which are appended with items/itemsets in G'
NDB - set of sequences in G is not appended with items/item sets in G'.

The basic ideas of algorithm are described as follows.

Step 1: Initially we scan single items in LDB.
Step 2: Then we check each pattern in FS and SFS in LDB to adjust the support of those patterns.
Step 2.1: Frequent pattern becomes, add into FS'.

Then check whether it meets the projection condition. If so, use it as prefix to project database.

Step 2.2: Semi-frequent pattern becomes, add into SFS'.

Algorithm Outline: IncSpan(G', min_sup, μ, FS, SFS)
Input: An appended database G', min_sup, FS and SFS in G
Output: FS' in G'

Method:

1. FS' = ϕ; SFS' = ϕ;
2. Scan the LDB for new single items
3. Add new frequent items into FS'
4. Add new semi-frequent items into SFS'
5. For each new item x in FS' do
6. PrefixSpan(i, G'|x, μ * min_sup, FS', SFS')
7. For every pattern R in FS or SFS do
8. Check Δsup (R) = sup gb(R)
9. If sup G' (R) = sup G (R) + Δsup (R) $\geq$ min_sup
10. Insert (FS', R)
11. If supLDB(p) $\geq$ (1 - μ) * min_sup
12. PrefixSpan(R, G'|R, μ * min_sup, FS', SFS')
13. Else
14. Insert (SFS', R)
15. Return;

IncSpan outperforms the non-incremental algorithm PrefixSpan and an incremental mining algorithm ISM. IncSpan is a promising algorithm to solve practical problems with many real applications. Its cost is low and its processing also very fast.

5. Genetic Algorithms

The mined patterns are given as input to Genetic algorithms stage it select the optimal patterns from the mined patterns for identifying best hospitals healthcare Service Providence. The principle of Genetic algorithm is genetic modification, mutation and natural selection. These are generally algorithmic optimization strategies encouraged by the principles discovered in natural evolution. The genetic algorithm creates a number of random strategies to the problem. All these solutions might not exactly be good, a group of solutions can be skipped entirely, and it can come down to the overlapping solutions. Poor solutions are discarded, and the good ones maintained. Good solutions are then being hybridized, and then the whole process is repeated. Finally, similar to the means of natural selection, only the best alternatives solutions remain. So, from the set of potential solutions to the problems those remain competitive with one another, the best solutions are chosen and combined with each other in order to obtain a universal solution from the pair of solutions that will become better and better, similar to the means of evolution of organisms.

Genetic Algorithm Procedure

- Select the initial population of individuals
- Find each individual fitness value in that population
- Do it again on this generation until termination condition is reached (time limit, sufficient fitness achieved, etc.):
- Select the best-fit individuals for reproduction is selected
- The birth to offspring happen when we breed new individuals through crossover and mutation operations
- Measure the specific fitness of new individuals
- Then replace least-fit population with new individuals

The initial population chosen by this algorithm is denoted as T_i. Initial population is consisting of M_t chromosomes. It is randomly generated then Crossover and mutations are responsible for generation of new population. In crossover process two members of a population T_j are utilized as input and two new members of the next population T_{j+1} are generated. Thus genetic information from the predecessors is included in new chromosomes. Genetic information of a chromosome incorporated in T_j is transformed to generate a new chromosome T_{j+1} of with help of mutation process.

GA is formulated on five basic principles:

1. Initialization

The initial step in GA is to create a set consist of whole sample points (the entire population). Database tables must be present in Sample points or population it is a direct input of real life scenarios. The later principles changes accordingly. In case of database tables, the semantic analytics are type casted into statistical theorem using random number generators creating density functions. In case of real time data, the whole process shapes as natural language parsing, then statistics is deployed.

$$F(x) = w_1 f_1(x_1) + w_2 f_2(x_2) + \ldots + w_n f_n(x_n)$$

2. Selection

A set is obtained from previous step then for that subset is created. This subset is just a way to categorize data. This idea of Selection pivots is based on the Darwin's theory of survival of the fittest. They may contain data that seems to be logically related at a particular instant of time or otherwise. They may contain multiple sets, each having specific domain data like, data relating to Doctors their qualification, experience, hospital facilities etc.

3. Cross Over/Recombination

During crossover the gene, an individual member of a particular set, is crossed over with a gene of another set. This cross over results in exchange of behavior and trends over different sets creating logical relation between set and reducing degree of randomness among sets. At any instant cross over is done only between two respective genes, leaving all other unaltered.

4. Mutation

The prior idea of mutation is to generate genetic diversity. In cross over, the properties and trends of other genes are taken which may result in suppression of one's own properties (alleles), thus mutation is important way to maintain individuality. Mutation may also result in generation of important alleles via combination of different genes.

5. Acceptance

If mutation process is over then the new offspring get created and it replaces the place of worst offspring, i.e. hospitals for next level of iteration are selected. The hospitals with good score are selected while the hospitals with low score get eliminated. During this elimination round we calculate the percentage of acceptable features for a single hospital. Those hospitals that cross that cut off mark are forwarded to next level population. This whole process continues till change between two successive level hospitals is negligibly small.

5. RESULT AND DISCUSSION

All the simulations were performed on a 2.80 GHz Pentium(R) 4 PC dual core CPU E5400 with 1 GB of main memory, running Windows 7. All the algorithms were implemented in JAVA.

5.1. Performance Evaluation

The following parameters are used to evaluate the performance of proposed method they are Sensitivity, Specificity, and Accuracy. There are several terms that are commonly used along with the description of sensitivity, specificity and accuracy. They are true positive (TP), true negative (TN), false negative (FN), and false positive (FP). True positive (TP): hospitals that are correctly identified as best hospital. False positive (FP): hospitals that are incorrectly identified as best hospital True negative (TN): hospitals that are correctly rejected as worst hospital. False negative (FN): hospitals that are incorrectly rejected as worst hospital.

Sensitivity

Sensitivity is a statistical metric that measures the fraction of actual positives that are correctly identified as such. It is calculated using the following equation:

Sensitivity = TP / (TP + FN)

Specificity

Specificity is a statistical metric that measures the fraction of negatives that are correctly identified as such. It is calculated using the following equation:

Specificity = TN / (TN + FP)

Accuracy

Accuracy is the fraction of correct predictions regardless of being positives or negatives. This metric may not be enough for measuring the performance, especially when negative cases are much higher that positive ones. So, other metrics described above are needed to measure the performance from different aspects. Accuracy is calculated using the following equation:

Accuracy = (TP + TN) / (P + N)

The Performance Measure calculated for various hospitals in providing the best quality of service is listed in Table 1.

Hospital provided best quality service is determined using sensitivity parameter and it is shown in Figure 2.

Hospital provided worst quality service is determined using sensitivity parameter and it is shown in Figure 3.

Accuracy measure helps to identifying quality of service provided by various hospitals is shown in Figure 4.

CONCLUSION

The hospital facilities related data collected by Questionnaire survey from odisha region is used in this experiment. For this information its patterns are extracted using data mining technique. The score values are allocated then extacted patterns are minned using incspan algorithm. Genetic algorithm will choose the best hospitals from the minned pattern. The implementation of proposed method is done in java platform it helps to strongly identifying which hospitals providing best quality of service. In future we can use other algorithm for pattern mining and optimization so that we can more effectively identify the best hospitals.

Table 1. Performance measure

Threshold	TP	TN	FP	FN	Sensitivity	Specificity	Accuracy
0.001	45	29	12	12	0.789474	0.707317	0.755102
0.002	43	28	14	13	0.767857	0.666667	0.72449
0.003	43	28	14	13	0.767857	0.666667	0.72449
0.004	40	26	17	15	0.727273	0.604651	0.673469

Figure 2. Proposed method sensitivity

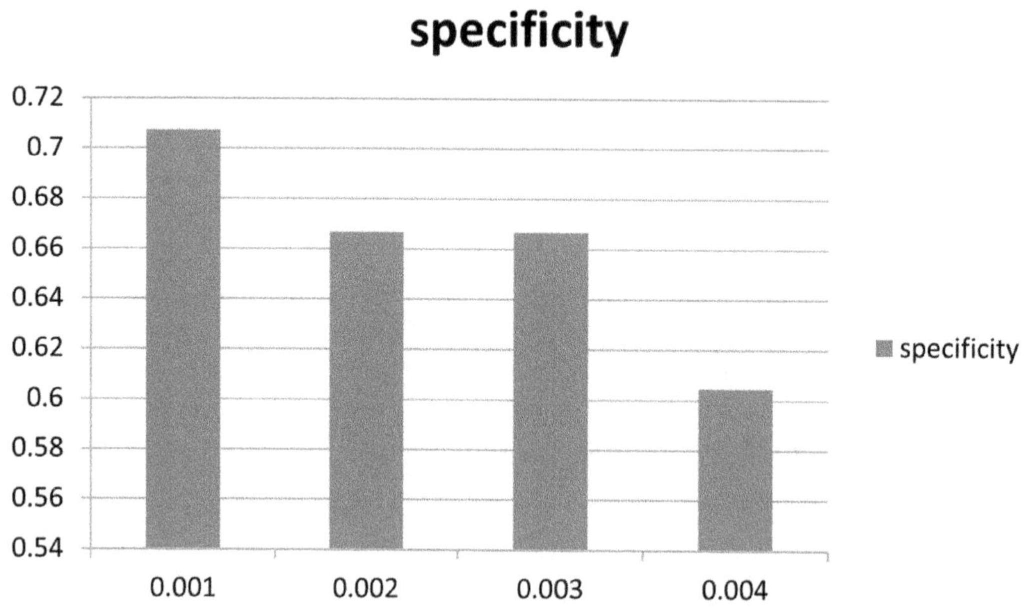

Figure 3. Proposed method specificity

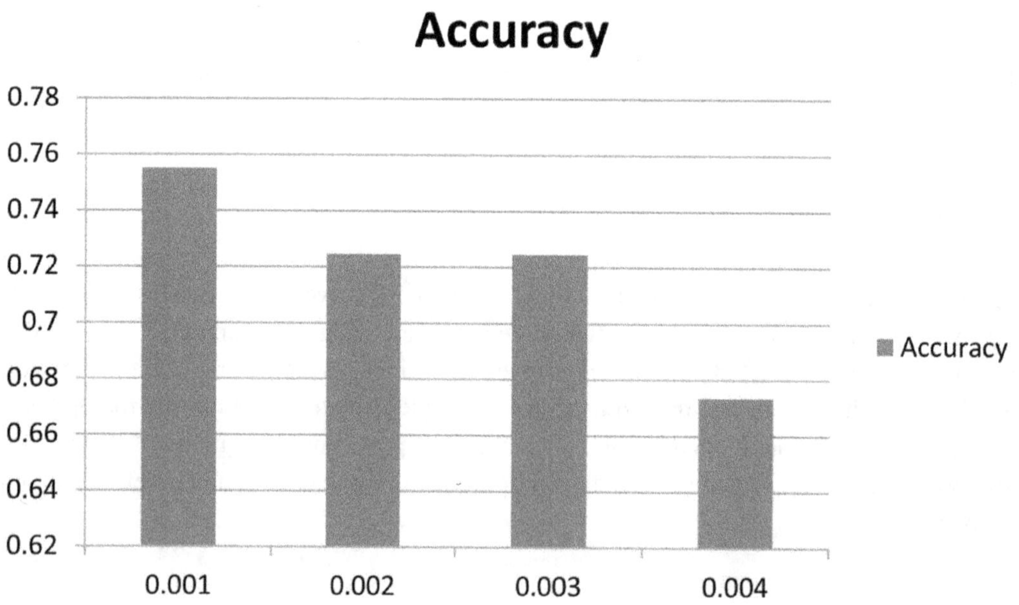

Figure 4. Proposed method accuracy

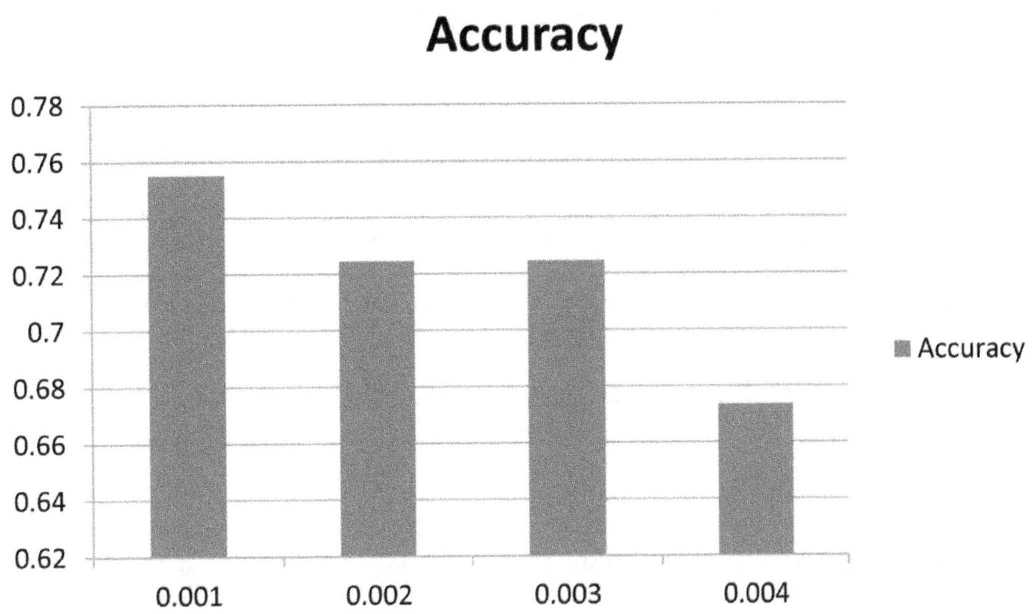

ACKNOWLEDGMENT

The author acknowledges Science and Engineering Research Board (SERB), Department of Science and Technology (DST), New Delhi, India for research support for the on-going research study.

The preparation of the chapter/manuscript and the subsequent finishing touches have taken a great deal of work by many individuals besides me. I am grateful to my friends and fellow members of the teaching staff at the Fakir Mohan University, Balasore. My special thanks would always go to my parents. My sincere thanks go to my students for their inspiration in writing this book chapter. Finally, I would like to acknowledge the technical assistance for sparing his precious time to help me design and test the programs. Last but not the least, my acknowledgements will remain incomplete if I do not thank the IGI Global Publisher, for supporting my creative writing activities over the past few months/year. Some errors might have unwittingly crept in. I shall be grateful if same are brought to my notice. Suggestions for further improvement of the book chapter will be thankfully acknowledged. I wish the readers success and many accomplishments.

REFERENCES

Aliman, N. K., & Mohamad, W. N. (2016). Linking Service Quality, Patients Satisfaction and Behavioral Intentions: An Investigation on Private Healthcare in Malaysia. *Procedia: Social and Behavioral Sciences*, *224*, 141–148. doi:10.1016/j.sbspro.2016.05.419

Bessant, J. (2014). *Service Productivity in the Healthcare Sector*. Management for Professionals.

Chang, T.-H. (2014). Fuzzy VIKOR method: A case study of the hospital service evaluation in Taiwan. *Information Sciences*, *271*, 196–212. doi:10.1016/j.ins.2014.02.118

Chen, S.-H., Wen, P.-C., & Yang, C.-K. (2014). Business concepts of systemic service innovations in e-Healthcare. *Technovation*, *34*(9), 513–524. doi:10.1016/j.technovation.2014.03.002

Chen, X., Wang, L., Ding, J., & Thomas, N. (2016). Patient Flow Scheduling and Capacity Planning in a Smart Hospital Environment. *IEEE Access*, *4*, 135–148. doi:10.1109/ACCESS.2015.2509013

Deshmukh. (2016). Design of cloud security in the EHR for Indian healthcare services. *Journal of King Saud University - Computer and Information Sciences*.

Kaushik, A., & Raman, A. (2015). The new data-driven enterprise architecture for e-healthcare: Lessons from the Indian public sector. *Government Information Quarterly*, *32*(1), 63–74. doi:10.1016/j.giq.2014.11.002

Ketelhöhn, N., & Sanz, L. (2016). Healthcare management priorities in Latin America: Framework and responses. *Journal of Business Research*, *69*(9), 3835–3838. doi:10.1016/j.jbusres.2016.04.008

Khambete, P., Athavankar, U., Doke, P., Shinde, R., Roy, D., Devkar, S., . . . Chaudhary, S. (2014). A Case Study in Participatory Service Design for Rural Healthcare System in India Using a Pattern Language. ICoRD'15 – Research Into Design Across Boundaries, 1, 3-13.

Lin, J. C.-W., Gan, W., Hong, T.-P., & Vincent, S. (2015). Efficient algorithms for mining up-to-date high-utility patterns. *Advanced Engineering Informatics*, *29*(3), 648–661. doi:10.1016/j.aei.2015.06.002

Manaswini, P. (2017). Status and Challenges on Adaptation for Indian Healthcare Services with Data Mining Technique. In Innovative Healthcare Systems for the 21st Century. Springer.

Ngai, E. W. T., & Yong Hu, Y. H. (2011). The application of data mining techniques in financial fraud detection: A classification framework and an academic review of literature. *Decision Support Systems*, *50*(3), 559–569. doi:10.1016/j.dss.2010.08.006

Rahman, R. M., & Md, F. R. (2011). Using and comparing different decision tree classification techniques for mining ICDDR,B Hospital Surveillance data. *Expert Systems with Applications*, *38*(9), 11421–11436. doi:10.1016/j.eswa.2011.03.015

Ren, Y., Werner, R., Pazzi, N., & Boukerche, A. (2010). Monitoring patients via a secure and mobile healthcare system. *IEEE Wireless Commun.*, *17*(1), 59–65. doi:10.1109/MWC.2010.5416351

Sharmaa, S., & Reimer-Kirkhamb, S. (2015). Faith as social capital: Diasporic women negotiating religion in secularized healthcare services. *Womens Studies International Forum*, *49*, 34–42. doi:10.1016/j.wsif.2015.01.005

Shukla, N., Keast, J., & Ceglarek, D. (2014). Modelling variations in hospital service delivery based on real time locating information. *Applied Mathematical Modelling*, *38*(3), 878–893. doi:10.1016/j.apm.2013.07.024

Silas, S., & Rajsingh, E. B. (2016). Performance analysis on algorithms for selection of desired healthcare services. *Perspectives on Science*, *8*, 107–109. doi:10.1016/j.pisc.2016.04.009

Sung, S.-F., Hsieh, C.-Y., Yang, Y.-H. K., Lin, H.-J., Chen, C.-H., Chen, Y.-W., & Hu, Y.-H. (2015). Developing a stroke severity index based on administrative data was feasible using data mining techniques. *Journal of Clinical Epidemiology*, *68*(11), 1292–1300. doi:10.1016/j.jclinepi.2015.01.009 PMID:25700940

Wimmer, H., Yoon, V. Y., & Sugumaran, V. (2016). A multi-agent system to support evidence based medicine and clinical decision making via data sharing and data privacy. *Decision Support Systems*, *88*, 51–66. doi:10.1016/j.dss.2016.05.008

Yeha, J.-Y., Wub, T.-H., & Tsaoa, C.-W. (2011). Using data mining techniques to predict hospitalization of hemodialysis patients. *Decision Support Systems*, *50*(2), 439–448. doi:10.1016/j.dss.2010.11.001

Yuehong, Y. I. N. (2016). The internet of things in healthcare: An overview. *Journal of Industrial Information Integration*, *1*, 3–13. doi:10.1016/j.jii.2016.03.004

Compilation of References

Abinaya, V. K., Kumar, V., & Swathika, . (2015). Ontology Based Public Healthcare System in Internet of Things (IoT). *Procedia Computer Science, 50*, 99–102. doi:10.1016/j.procs.2015.04.067

Abuidhail, J. (2009). Women's health and health informatics: Perinatal care health education. In D. Parry & E. Parry (Eds.), *Medical informatics in obstetrics and gynecology* (pp. 263–277). Hershey, PA: IGI Global. doi:10.4018/978-1-60566-078-3.ch013

ACSS. (2016). *Relatório síntese da atividade cirúrgica programada.* Retrieved from http://www.acss.min-saude.pt/wp-content/uploads/2016/10/UGA-20160927-RelSint_Ativ_Cir_2015-VE3.pdf

Advantages, T. (2016). *The Advantages and Disadvantages of BYOD.* Retrieved from http://www.businesszone.co.uk/community-voice/blogs/scott-drayton/the-advantages-and-disadvantages-of-byod

Aehlert, B. (2011). *ACLS Advanced Cardiac Life Support, Study Guide* (4th ed.). Mosby.

Agarwal, S., Perry, H. B., Long, L. A., & Labrique, A. B. (2015). Evidence on feasibility and effective use of mHealth strategies by frontline health workers in developing countries: Systematic review. *Tropical Medicine & International Health, 20*(8), 1003–1014. doi:10.1111/tmi.12525 PMID:25881735

Aggarwal, R., & Das, M. L. (2012). RFID security in the context of internet of things. In *Proceedings of the First International Conference on Security of Internet of Things* (pp. 51-56). ACM. doi:10.1145/2490428.2490435

Agrawal, R., & Srikant, R. (1994). Fast algorithms for mining association rules. *Proc. 20th int. conf. very large data bases, VLDB*, 487-499.

Airinei, D., & Homocianu, D. (2009). DSS vs. business intelligence. *Revista Economica.*

Akaichi, J., & Mhadhbi, L. (2016). A clinical decision support system: Ontology-driven approach for effective emergency management. In J. Moon & M. Galea (Eds.), *Improving health management through clinical decision support systems* (pp. 270–294). Hershey, PA: IGI Global. doi:10.4018/978-1-4666-9432-3.ch013

Akerkar, R. (2016). Towards an intelligent integrated approach for clinical decision support. In A. Aggarwal (Ed.), *Managing big data integration in the public sector* (pp. 187–205). Hershey, PA: IGI Global. doi:10.4018/978-1-4666-9649-5.ch011

Akujuobi, C. M. (2017). Nanotechnology applications in biomedical engineering. In Oncology: Breakthroughs in research and practice (pp. 352–365). Hershey, PA: IGI Global. doi:10.4018/978-1-5225-0549-5.ch012

Akyildiz, I. F., Su, W., Sankarasubramaniam, Y., & Cayirci, E. (2002). Wireless sensor networks: A survey. *Computer Networks, 38*(4), 393–422. doi:10.1016/S1389-1286(01)00302-4

Al Ameen, M., Liu, J., & Kwak, K. (2012). Security and privacy issues in wireless sensor networks for healthcare applications. *Journal of Medical Systems, 36*(1), 93–101. doi:10.1007/s10916-010-9449-4 PMID:20703745

Alavi, M., & Leidner, D. E. (2005). Review: Knowledge management and knowledge management systems: conceptual foundations and research issues. *Knowledge Management: Critical Perspectives on Business and Management*, 163.

Alemdar, H., & Ersoy, C. (2010). C. E. (2010). Wireless Sensor Networks for Healthcare: A Survey. *Computer Networks*, *54*(15), 2688–2710. doi:10.1016/j.comnet.2010.05.003

Al-Hyari, A. Y., Al-Taee, A. M., & Al-Taee, M. A. (2014). Diagnosis and classification of chronic renal failure utilising intelligent data mining classifiers. *International Journal of Information Technology and Web Engineering*, *9*(4), 1–12. doi:10.4018/ijitwe.2014100101

Aliman, N. K., & Mohamad, W. N. (2016). Linking Service Quality, Patients Satisfaction and Behavioral Intentions: An Investigation on Private Healthcare in Malaysia. *Procedia: Social and Behavioral Sciences*, *224*, 141–148. doi:10.1016/j.sbspro.2016.05.419

Ali, O. T., Nassif, A. B., & Capretz, L. F. (2013). Business intelligence solutions in healthcare a case study: Transforming OLTP system to BI solution. *Communications and Information Technology (ICCIT), 2013 Third International Conference* (pp. 209-214). IEEE.

Ali, S. M., Giordano, R., Lakhani, S., & Walker, D. M. (2016). A review of randomized controlled trials of medical record powered clinical decision support system to improve quality of diabetes care. *International Journal of Medical Informatics*, *87*, 91–100. doi:10.1016/j.ijmedinf.2015.12.017 PMID:26806716

Al-Jumeily, D., Hussain, A., Mallucci, C., & Oliver, C. (2015). *Applied Computing in Medicine and Health*. Morgan Kaufmann.

Al-Khasawneh, A., & Hijazi, H. (2014). A predictive e-health information system: Diagnosing diabetes mellitus using neural network based decision support system. *International Journal of Decision Support System Technology*, *6*(4), 31–48. doi:10.4018/ijdsst.2014100103

Al-Khudairy, S. (2014). Caring for our aging population: Using CPOE and telehomecare systems as a response to health policy concerns. In C. El Morr (Ed.), *Research perspectives on the role of informatics in health policy and management* (pp. 153–166). Hershey, PA: IGI Global. doi:10.4018/978-1-4666-4321-5.ch010

Almarri, A., & Bhatti, T. (2015). Consumers Attitude towards the Use of Mobile Health Apps: An Empirical Review. *Proceedings of Second International Conference on Electrical and Electronics Engineering, Clean Energy and Green Computing*, 56–61.

Almunawar, M. N., Anshari, M., & Younis, M. Z. (2015). Incorporating customer empowerment in mobile health. *Health Policy and Technology*, *4*(4), 312–319. doi:10.1016/j.hlpt.2015.08.008

Alpuim, A., Esteves, M., Pereira, S., & Santos, M. F. (2016). Monitoring Time Consumption in Complementary Diagnostic and Therapeutic Procedure Requests. In *Applying Business Intelligence to Clinical and Healthcare Organizations* (pp. 208–240). IGI Global. doi:10.4018/978-1-4666-9882-6.ch011

Alyass, A., Turcotte, M., & Meyre, D. (2015). From big data analysis to personalized medicine for all: Challenges and opportunities. *BMC Medical Genomics*, *8*(1), 33. doi:10.1186/s12920-015-0108-y PMID:26112054

Amaro, J. D. S., Correia, A. C., & Pereira, C. (2016). Avaliação do Risco de Desnutrição num Serviço de Medicina do Hospital Distrital de Santarém (Medicina IV). *Acta Portuguesa de Nutrição*, *06-09*(4).

American Diabetes Association. (2016). *Checking Your Blood Glucose*. Retrieved September 14, 2016, from http://www.diabetes.org/living-with-diabetes/treatment-and-care/blood-glucose-control/checking-your-blood-glucose.html

American Heart Association. (2016). *Understanding Blood Pressure Readings*. Retrieved September 14, 2016, from http://www.heart.org/HEARTORG/Conditions/HighBloodPressure/AboutHighBloodPressure/Understanding-Blood-Pressure-Readings_UCM_301764_Article.jsp

Ammenwerth, E., Schnell-Inderst, P., Machan, C., & Siebert, U. (2008). The effect of electronic prescribing on medication errors and adverse drug events: A systematic review. *Journal of the American Medical Informatics Association, 15*(5), 585–600. doi:10.1197/jamia.M2667 PMID:18579832

AMPY. (2016). *AMPY Mov Live charged.* Retrieved August 8, 2016, from http://www.getampy.com/

Andreolini, M., Colajanni, M., Pietri, M., & Tosi, S. (2015). Adaptive, scalable and reliable monitoring of big data on clouds. *Journal of Parallel and Distributed Computing, 79*, 67–79. doi:10.1016/j.jpdc.2014.08.007

Angelidis, P. (2009). Mobile telemonitoring insights. In J. Tan (Ed.), *Medical informatics: Concepts, methodologies, tools, and applications* (pp. 107–112). Hershey, PA: IGI Global. doi:10.4018/978-1-60566-050-9.ch010

Angius, G., & Raffo, L. (2008). A Sleep Apnoea Keeper in a Wearable Device for Continuous Detection and Screening during Daily Life. *Computers in Cardiology, 35*, 433–436.

Anogianakis, G., Maglavera, S., Pomportsis, A., Bountzioukas, S., Beltrame, F., & Orsi, G. (1998). Medical emergency aid through telematics: Design, implementation guidelines and analysis of user requirements for the MERMAID project. *International Journal of Medical Informatics, 52*(1–3), 93–103. doi:10.1016/S1386-5056(98)00128-2 PMID:9848406

Anshari, M., & Almunawar, M. N. (2015). Mobile health (mHealth). In M. Khosrow-Pour (Ed.), *Encyclopedia of information science and technology* (3rd ed.; pp. 5607–5614). Hershey, PA: IGI Global. doi:10.4018/978-1-4666-5888-2.ch553

Aquino, R. D. C., & Philippi, S. T. (2011). Identificação de fatores de risco de desnutrição em pacientes internados. *Revista da Associação Médica Brasileira, 57*(6), 637–643. doi:10.1590/S0104-42302011000600009 PMID:22249542

Archer, N. (2010). Mobile e-health: Making the case. In K. Khoumbati, Y. Dwivedi, A. Srivastava, & B. Lal (Eds.), *Handbook of research on advances in health informatics and electronic healthcare applications: Global adoption and impact of information communication technologies* (pp. 446–457). Hershey, PA: IGI Global. doi:10.4018/978-1-60566-030-1.ch027

Arunasalam, U. S. a. B. (2013). Leveraging Big Data Analytics to Reduce Healthcare Costs. *IT Pro*, 21-28.

Atzori, L., Iera, A., & Morabito, G. (2010). The internet of things: A survey. *Computer Networks, 54*(15), 2787–2805. doi:10.1016/j.comnet.2010.05.010

Avinash, G., Liu, R., & Roehm, S. (2005). *System and method for integrated learning and understanding of healthcare informatics*. Google Patents.

Azar, A. T. (2013). Overview of biomedical engineering. In *Bioinformatics: Concepts, methodologies, tools, and applications* (pp. 1–28). Hershey, PA: IGI Global. doi:10.4018/978-1-4666-3604-0.ch001

Babu, B. S., Srikanth, K., Ramanjaneyulu, T., & Narayana, I. L. (2016). IoT for Healthcare. *International Journal of Science and Research, 5*(2).

Badiali, G., Ferrari, V., Cutolo, F., Freschi, C., Caramella, D., Bianchi, A., & Marchetti, C. (2014). Augmented reality as an aid in maxillofacial surgery: Validation of a wearable system allowing maxillary repositioning. *Journal of Cranio-Maxillo-Facial Surgery, 42*(8), 1970–1976. doi:10.1016/j.jcms.2014.09.001 PMID:25441867

Baecker, R. M. (2014). *Readings in Human-Computer Interaction: toward the year 2000.* Morgan Kaufmann.

Bais, A. (2016). *Security Risks associated with BYOD.* Academic Press.

Balas, E. A., Weingarten, S., Garb, C. T., Blumenthal, D., Boren, S. A., & Brown, G. B. (2000). Improving preventive care by prompting physicians. *Archives of Internal Medicine*, *160*(3), 301–308. doi:10.1001/archinte.160.3.301 PMID:10668831

Ballini, L., Negro, A., Maltoni, S., Vignatelli, L., Flodgren, G., & Simera, I. … Grilli, R. (2015). Interventions to Reduce Waiting Times for Elective Procedures. *The Cochrane Database of Systematic Reviews, 2*(2). https://doi.org/10.1002/14651858.CD005610.pub2

Bamigboye, A. (2012). Mobile healthcare: Challenges and opportunities. In B. Ciaramitaro (Ed.), *Mobile technology consumption: Opportunities and challenges* (pp. 77–98). Hershey, PA: IGI Global. doi:10.4018/978-1-61350-150-4.ch006

Bâra, A., & Lungu, I. (2012). *Improving Decision Support Systems with Data Mining Techniques*. INTECH Open Access Publisher. doi:10.5772/47788

Bardram, J. E., Frost, M., Szántó, K., Faurholt-Jepsen, M., Vinberg, M., & Kessing, L. V. (2013). Designing mobile health technology for bipolar disorder: a field trial of the monarca system. *Proceedings of the SIGCHI Conference on Human Factors in Computing Systems*. doi:10.1145/2470654.2481364

Barfield, W. (Ed.). (2015). *Fundamentals of wearable computers and augmented reality*. CRC Press. doi:10.1201/b18703

Barrento, M., Neto, M., Maria, M., & Dias, S. (2010). Sistemas de Business Intelligence Aplicados à Saúde. In E. U. F. Pessoa (Ed.), *Sistemas e tecnologias de informação na saúde* (pp. 77–91). Porto: Edições Universidade Fernando Pessoa.

Barros, P. P. (2008). *As listas de espera para intervenção cirúrgica em Portugal*. Retrieved from https://momentoseconomicos.files.wordpress.com/2011/06/listas_de_espera.pdf

Barros, P. P. (2008, March). As Listas de Espera para Intervenção Cirúrgica em Portugal. *Iprisverbis, 4*.

Bates, D. W., Saria, S., Ohno-Machado, L., Shah, A., & Escobar, G. (2014). Big data in health care: Using analytics to identify and manage high-risk and high-cost patients. *Health Affairs*, *33*(7), 1123–1131. doi:10.1377/hlthaff.2014.0041 PMID:25006137

Bazerbashi, H., Merriman, K. W., Toale, K. M., Chaftari, P., Carreras, M. T. C., Henderson, J. D., & Rice, T. W. et al. (2014). Low tissue oxygen saturation at emergency center triage is predictive of intensive care unit admission. *Journal of Critical Care*, *29*(5), 775–779. doi:10.1016/j.jcrc.2014.05.006 PMID:24973103

Beaudoin, M., Kabanza, F., Nault, V., & Valiquette, L. (2016). Evaluation of a machine learning capability for a clinical decision support system to enhance antimicrobial stewardship programs. *Artificial Intelligence in Medicine*, *68*, 29–36. doi:10.1016/j.artmed.2016.02.001 PMID:26947174

Bello Garba, A., Armarego, J., & Murray, D. (2015). A Policy-Based Framework for Managing Information Security and Privacy Risks in BYOD Environments. *International Journal of Emerging Trends & Technology in Computer Science*, *4*(2), 10.

Bello Garba, A., Armarego, J., Murray, D., & Kenworthy, W. (2015). Review of the Information Security and Privacy Challenges in Bring Your Own Device (BYOD) Environments. *Journal of Information Privacy and Security*, *11*(1), 38–54. doi:10.1080/15536548.2015.1010985

Benlamri, R., & Docksteader, L. (2010). MORF: A mobile health-monitoring platform. *IT Professional*, *3*(3), 18–25. doi:10.1109/MITP.2010.3

Ben-Zeev, D., Kaiser, S. M., Brenner, C. J., Begale, M., Duffecy, J., & Mohr, D. C. (2013). Development and usability testing of FOCUS: A smartphone system for self-management of schizophrenia. *Psychiatric Rehabilitation Journal*, *36*(4), 289–296. doi:10.1037/prj0000019 PMID:24015913

Berndt, D. J., Hevner, A. R., & Studnicki, J. (2003). The Catch data warehouse: Support for community health care decision-making. *Decision Support Systems, 35*(3), 367–384. doi:10.1016/S0167-9236(02)00114-8

Berner, E. S. (2009). *Clinical decision support systems: state of the art.* AHRQ Publication.

Bessant, J. (2014). *Service Productivity in the Healthcare Sector.* Management for Professionals.

Bhuyan, S. S., Zhu, H., Chandak, A., Kim, J., & Stimpson, J. P. (2014). Do service innovations influence the adoption of electronic health records in long-term care organizations? Results from the U.S. national survey of residential care facilities. *International Journal of Medical Informatics, 83*(12), 975–982. doi:10.1016/j.ijmedinf.2014.09.007 PMID:25453201

Bilandzic, M., & Venable, J. (2011). Towards Participatory Action Design Research: Adapting Action Research and Design Science Research Methods for Urban Informatics. *The Journal of Community Informatics, 7*(3). Retrieved from http://ci-journal.net/index.php/ciej/article/view/786/804

Billinghurst, M., Clark, A., & Lee, G. (2015). A survey of augmented reality. *Foundations and Trends® Human–Computer Interaction, 8*(2-3), 73-272.

Billsus, D., Brunk, C., Evans, C., Gladish, B., & Pazzani, M. (2002). Adaptive Interfaces for Ubiquitous Web Access: Allowing mobile users to access any information at any time from any location. *Communications of the ACM, 45*(5), 34–38. doi:10.1145/506218.506240

Bircher, N. G. (2010). The electronic patient record: A practicing physician's perspective. In S. Kabene (Ed.), *Healthcare and the effect of technology: Developments, challenges and advancements* (pp. 84–100). Hershey, PA: IGI Global. doi:10.4018/978-1-61520-733-6.ch006

Bizer, C., Boncz, P., Brodie, M. L., & Erling, O. (2012). The meaningful use of big data: Four perspectivesfour challenges. *SIGMOD Record, 40*(4), 56–60. doi:10.1145/2094114.2094129

Blizzard, S. (2015). Coming full circle: Are there benefits to BYOD? *Computer Fraud & Security, 2015*(2), 18–20. doi:10.1016/S1361-3723(15)30010-5

Blumenthal, D. (2009). Stimulating the adoption of health information technology. *The New England Journal of Medicine, 360*(15), 1477–1479. doi:10.1056/NEJMp0901592 PMID:19321856

Blumenthal, D., & Glaser, J. (2007). Information technology comes to medicine. *The New England Journal of Medicine, 356*(24), 2527–2534. doi:10.1056/NEJMhpr066212 PMID:17568035

Bolinder, J., et al. (in press). Novel glucose-sensing technology and hypoglycaemia in type 1 diabetes: a multicentre, non-masked, randomised controlled trial. *Lancet.*

Bonney, W. (2013). Applicability of Business Intelligence in Electronic Health Record. *Procedia: Social and Behavioral Sciences, 73*, 257–262. doi:10.1016/j.sbspro.2013.02.050

Bradley, T. (2011). *Pros and cons of byod bring your own device.* Retrieved February 22, 2017, from http://www.pcworld.com/article/246760/pros_and_cons_of_byod_bring_your_own_device_.html

Braga, A., Portela, F., Santos, M. F., Machado, J., Abelha, A., Silva, Á., & Rua, F. (2016). *Pervasive Patient Timeline for Intensive Care Units* (pp. 527–536). Cham: Springer. doi:10.1007/978-3-319-31307-8_55

Brandão, A., Pereira, E., Esteves, M., Portela, F., Santos, M., Abelha, A., & Machado, J. (2016). A Benchmarking Analysis of Open-Source Business Intelligence Tools in Healthcare Environments. *Information, 7*(4), 57. https://doi.org/10.3390/info7040057

Brandão, A., Pereira, E., Portela, F., Santos, M., Abelha, A., & Machado, J. (2014). Real-time Business Intelligence Platform to Maternity Care. In *IEEE Conference on Biomedical Engineering and Sciences* (pp. 379–384). IEEE. doi:10.1109/IECBES.2014.7047525

Brasil. (2013). *Ministério da Saúde. Secretaria de Atenção à Saúde. Departamento de Atenção Especializada. Manual instrutivo da Rede de Atenção às Urgências e Emergências no Sistema Único de Saúde (SUS).* Brasília, DF: Editora do Ministério da Saúde.

Brear, M. (2010). Organizational factors: Their role in health informatics implementation. In J. Rodrigues (Ed.), *Health information systems: Concepts, methodologies, tools, and applications* (pp. 1295–1303). Hershey, PA: IGI Global. doi:10.4018/978-1-60566-988-5.ch081

Brennan, T. (2010). Gestão da doença para promover o controle da pressão arterial entre os afro-americanos. *Popul Manag Saúde, 13*(2), 65–72.

Bright, T. J., Wong, A., Dhurjati, R., Bristow, E., Bastian, L., Coeytaux, R. R., & Musty, M. D. et al. (2012). Effect of clinical decision-support systems: A systematic review. *Annals of Internal Medicine, 157*(1), 29–43. doi:10.7326/0003-4819-157-1-201207030-00450 PMID:22751758

Bring Your Own Device. (n.d.). Retrieved March 22, 2017, from http://www.deeptech.com.au/solutions/byot/

Broberg, C. S., Mitchell, J., Rehel, S., Grant, A., Gianola, A., Beninato, P., & Sahn, D. J. et al. (2015). Electronic medical record integration with a database for adult congenital heart disease: Early experience and progress in automating multicenter data collection. *International Journal of Cardiology, 196*, 178–182. doi:10.1016/j.ijcard.2015.05.140 PMID:26142077

Brownstein, J. S., Freifeld, C. C., & Madoff, L. C. (2009). Digital disease detection—harnessing the Web for public health surveillance. *The New England Journal of Medicine, 360*(21), 2153–2157. doi:10.1056/NEJMp0900702 PMID:19423867

Bruder, P. (2014). Gadgets Go to School: The Benefits and Risks of BYOD (Bring Your Own Device). *Education Digest, 80*(3), 15–18. Retrieved from http://navigator-iup.passhe.edu/login?url=http://search.ebscohost.com/login.aspx?direct=true&db=eue&AN=99173566&site=ehost-live

Brusic, V., & Zeleznikow, J. (1999). Knowledge discovery and data mining in biological databases. *The Knowledge Engineering Review, 14*(3), 257–277. doi:10.1017/S0269888999003069

Budak, J. (2012). Should you bring your own mobile device to work?. *Canadian Business, 85*(8), 79. Retrieved from http://www.canadianbusiness.com/lifestyle/should-you-bring-your-own-mobile-device-to-work/

Butler, C. E., Noel, S., Hibbs, S. P., Miles, D., Staves, J., Mohaghegh, P., … Murphy, M. F. (2015). Implementation of a Clinical Decision Support System Improves Compliance with Restrictive Transfusion Policies in Hematology Patients. *Transfusion, 55*(8), 1964–1971. https://doi.org/10.1111/trf.13075

Cabrilo, I., Schaller, K., & Bijlenga, P. (2014). Augmented Reality-Assisted Bypass Surgery: Embracing Minimal Invasiveness. *World Neurosurgery, 83*(4), 596–602. https://doi.org/10.1016/j.wneu.2014.12.020

Cahill, T. J., & Prendergast, B. D. (2016). Infective endocarditis. *Lancet, 387*(10021), 882–893. doi:10.1016/S0140-6736(15)00067-7 PMID:26341945

Caldeira, C. P. (2012). Data Warehousing - Conceitos e Modelos (2nd ed.). Academic Press.

Calyam, P., Mishra, A., Antequera, R. B., Chemodanov, D., Berryman, A., Zhu, K., & Skubic, M. et al. (2016). Synchronous Big Data analytics for personalized and remote physical therapy. *Pervasive and Mobile Computing, 28*, 3–20. doi:10.1016/j.pmcj.2015.09.004

Camera Calibration and 3D Reconstruction — OpenCV 2. (n.d.). Retrieved from http://docs.opencv.org/2.4/modules/calib3d/doc/camera_calibration_and_3d_reconstruction.html

Campbell, A. T., Eisenman, S. B., Lane, N. D., Miluzzo, E., Peterson, R. A., Lu, H., & Ahn, G.-S. et al. (2008). The rise of people-centric sensing. *IEEE Internet Computing*, *12*(4), 12–21. doi:10.1109/MIC.2008.90

Cardoso, L., Marins, F., Portela, F., Abelha, A., & Machado, J. (2014). Healthcare interoperability through intelligent agent technology. *Procedia Technology*, 1334-1341.

Cardoso, L., Marins, F., Quintas, C., Portela, F., Santos, M., Abelha, A., & Machado, J. (2014). Interoperability in Healthcare. *Cloud Computing Applications for Quality Health Care Delivery*, 78-101.

Cardoso, L., Marins, F., Portela, F., Santos, M., Abelha, A., & Machado, J. (2014). The next generation of interoperability agents in healthcare. *International Journal of Environmental Research and Public Health*, *11*(5), 5349–5371. doi:10.3390/ijerph110505349 PMID:24840351

Carney, T. J., Weaver, M., McDaniel, A. M., Jones, J., & Haggstrom, D. A. (2016). Organizational factors influencing the use of clinical decision support for improving cancer screening within community health centers. In *E-health and telemedicine: Concepts, methodologies, tools, and applications* (pp. 118–148). Hershey, PA: IGI Global. doi:10.4018/978-1-4666-8756-1.ch007

Carspecken, C. W., Sharek, P. J., Longhurst, C., & Pageler, N. M. (2013). A clinical case of electronic health record drug alert fatigue: Consequences for patient outcome. *Pediatrics, 131*(6), e1970–e1973.

Castaneda, C., Nalley, K., Mannion, C., Bhattacharyya, P., Blake, P., & Pecora, A. … Suh, K. S. (2015). Clinical Decision Support Systems for Improving Diagnostic Accuracy and Achieving Precision Medicine. *Journal of Clinical Bioinformatics, 5*(4), 1–16. https://doi.org/10.1186/s13336-015-0019-3

Castillejo, P., Martinez, J. F., Rodriguez-Molina, J., & Cuerva, A. (2013). Integration of wearable devices in a wireless sensor network for an E-health application. *IEEE Wireless Communications*, *20*(4), 38–49. doi:10.1109/MWC.2013.6590049

Catapano, G., & Verkerke, G. J. (2011). Artificial organs. *International Journal of Biomaterials Research and Engineering*, *1*(2), 41–76. doi:10.4018/ijbre.2013070104

Cavalini, L. T., & Cook, T. W. (2012). Knowledge engineering of healthcare applications based on minimalist multilevel models. In *e-Health Networking, Applications and Services (Healthcom), 2012 IEEE 14th International Conference on* (pp. 431-434). IEEE. doi:10.1109/HealthCom.2012.6379454

Ceruti, M., Geninatti, S., & Siliquini, R. (2016). Use and reuse of electronic health records: Building information systems for improvement of health services. In *E-health and telemedicine: Concepts, methodologies, tools, and applications* (pp. 961–975). Hershey, PA: IGI Global. doi:10.4018/978-1-4666-8756-1.ch049

Chakraborty, B., & Yoshida, T. (2016). Design of a Framework for Wellness Determination and Subsequent Recommendation with Personal Informatics. *2016 AAAI Spring Symposium Series*, 332–336.

Chan, A. (2015). Big data interfaces and the problem of inclusion. *Media Culture & Society*, *37*(7), 1078–1083. doi:10.1177/0163443715594106

Chang, I. C., Hwang, H. G., Hung, W. F., & Li, Y. C. (2007). Physicians' acceptance of pharmacokinetics-based clinical decision support systems. *Expert Systems with Applications*, *33*(2), 296–303. doi:10.1016/j.eswa.2006.05.001

Chang, J. Y., Chen, L. K., & Chang, C. C. (2009). Perspectives and expectations for telemedicine opportunities from families of nursing home residents and caregivers in nursing homes. *International Journal of Medical Informatics*, *78*(7), 494–502. doi:10.1016/j.ijmedinf.2009.02.009 PMID:19345640

Chang, T.-H. (2014). Fuzzy VIKOR method: A case study of the hospital service evaluation in Taiwan. *Information Sciences, 271*, 196–212. doi:10.1016/j.ins.2014.02.118

Chapman, W. W., Bridewell, W., Hanbury, P., Cooper, G. F., & Buchanan, B. G. (2001). A simple algorithm for identifying negated findings and diseases in discharge summaries. *Journal of Biomedical Informatics, 34*(5), 301–310. doi:10.1006/jbin.2001.1029 PMID:12123149

Chapman, W. W., Chu, D., & Downling, J. N. (2007). Context: An algorithm for identifying contextual features from clinical text. *Proceedings of the Workshop on BioNLP 2007: Biological, Translational, and Clinical Language Processing*, 81-88. doi:10.3115/1572392.1572408

Chaudhry, B., Wang, J., Wu, S., Maglione, M., Mojica, W., Roth, E., & Shekelle, P. G. et al. (2006). Systematic review: Impact of health information technology on quality, efficiency, and costs of medical care. *Annals of Internal Medicine, 144*(10), 742–752. doi:10.7326/0003-4819-144-10-200605160-00125 PMID:16702590

Chaudhry, S. I., Mattera, J. A., Curtis, J. P., Spertus, J. A., Herrin, J., Lin, Z., & Krumholz, H. M. et al. (2010). Telemonitoring in patients with heart failure. *The New England Journal of Medicine, 363*(24), 2301–2309. doi:10.1056/NEJMoa1010029 PMID:21080835

Chaudhuri, S., & Dayal, U. (1997). An overview of data warehousing and OLAP technology. *SIGMOD Record, 26*(1), 65–74. doi:10.1145/248603.248616

Chaudhuri, S., Dayal, U., & Narasayya, V. (2011). An Overview of Business Intelligence Technology. *Communications of the ACM, 54*(8), 88. doi:10.1145/1978542.1978562

Chen, X., Xu, L., Wang, Y., Wang, H., Wang, F., Zeng, X., … Egger, J. (2015). Development of a surgical navigation system based on augmented reality using an optical see-through head-mounted display. *Journal of Biomedical Informatics, 55*, 124–131. https://doi.org/10.1016/j.jbi.2015.04.003

Chen, C., & Zhang, C.-Y. (2014). Data-intensive applications, challenges, techniques and technologies: A survey on Big Data. *Information Sciences, 275*, 314–347. doi:10.1016/j.ins.2014.01.015

Chen, H., Chiang, R. H. L., & Storey, V. C. (2012). Business Intelligence and Analytics: From Big Data to Big Impact. *Management Information Systems Quarterly, 36*(4), 1165–1188. https://doi.org/10.1145/2463676.2463712

Chen, H., Fuller, S. S., Friedman, C., & Hersh, W. (2006). *Medical informatics: knowledge management and data mining in biomedicine* (Vol. 8). Springer Science & Business Media.

Chen, L. M., Kennedy, E. H., Sales, A., & Hofer, T. P. (2013). Use of health IT for higher-value critical care. *The New England Journal of Medicine, 368*(7), 594–597. doi:10.1056/NEJMp1213273 PMID:23363474

Chen, S.-H., Wen, P.-C., & Yang, C.-K. (2014). Business concepts of systemic service innovations in e-Healthcare. *Technovation, 34*(9), 513–524. doi:10.1016/j.technovation.2014.03.002

Chen, X., Wang, L., Ding, J., & Thomas, N. (2016). Patient Flow Scheduling and Capacity Planning in a Smart Hospital Environment. *IEEE Access, 4*, 135–148. doi:10.1109/ACCESS.2015.2509013

Chen, Y., Lorenzi, N., Nyemba, S., Schildcrout, J. S., & Malin, B. (2014). We work with them? Health workers interpretation of organizational relations mined from electronic health records. *International Journal of Medical Informatics, 83*(7), 495–506. doi:10.1016/j.ijmedinf.2014.04.006 PMID:24845147

Chib, A. (2010). The Aceh Besar midwives with mobile phones project: Design and evaluation perspectives using the information and communication technologies for healthcare development model. *Journal of Computer-Mediated Communication, 15*(3), 500–525. doi:10.1111/j.1083-6101.2010.01515.x

Chiti, F., Fantacci, R., Loreti, M., & Pugliese, R. (2016). Context-aware wireless mobile autonomic computing and communications: Research trends and emerging applications. *IEEE Wireless Communications*, *23*(2), 86–92. doi:10.1109/MWC.2016.7462489

Chiuchisan, I., Costin, H. N., & Geman, O. (2014, October). Adopting the internet of things technologies in health care systems. In *Electrical and Power Engineering (EPE), 2014 International Conference and Exposition on* (pp. 532-535). IEEE. doi:10.1109/ICEPE.2014.6969965

Choi, S. H., Kang, S., & Jeon, Y. J. (2006). Personalized recommendation system based on product specification values. *Expert Systems with Applications*, *31*(3), 607–616. doi:10.1016/j.eswa.2005.09.074

Ciaramitaro, B. L., & Skrocki, M. (2012). mHealth: Mobile healthcare. In B. Ciaramitaro (Ed.), Mobile technology consumption: Opportunities and challenges (pp. 99–109). Hershey, PA: IGI Global. doi:10.4018/978-1-61350-150-4.ch007

Cifuentes, J. D. M. (2013). Context modelling for serendipitous discoveries in exploratory mobile search over social media. *Fifth BCS-IRSG Symposium on Future Directions in Information Access (FDIA 2013).*

Cinque, M., Coronato, A., & Testa, A. (2012). Dependable services for mobile health monitoring systems. *International Journal of Ambient Computing and Intelligence*, *4*(1), 1–15. doi:10.4018/jaci.2012010101

CMS.gov. (2016). *Centers for Medicare & Medicaid Services.* Retrieved September 15, 2016, from http://www.cms.gov/

Cody, W. F., Kreulen, J. T., Krishna, V., & Spangler, W. S. (2002). The integration of business intelligence and knowledge management. *IBM Systems Journal*, *41*(4), 697–713. doi:10.1147/sj.414.0697

Cohen, P., & Oviatt, S. (2000). Multimodal interfaces that process what comes naturally. *Communications of the ACM*, *43*(3), 45–33. doi:10.1145/330534.330538

Conrad, C., Fusaglia, M., Peterhans, M., Lu, H., Weber, S., & Gayet, B. (2016). Augmented Reality Navigation Surgery Facilitates Laparoscopic Rescue of Failed Portal Vein Embolization. *Journal of the American College of Surgeons*, *223*(4), e31–e34. doi:10.1016/j.jamcollsurg.2016.06.392 PMID:27450989

Constantinescu, L., Kim, J., & Feng, D. D. (2012). SparkMed: A framework for dynamic integration of multimedia medical data into distributed m-health systems. *IEEE Transactions on Information Technology in Biomedicine*, *16*(1), 40–52. doi:10.1109/TITB.2011.2174064 PMID:22049371

Cooper, D. (2016). *New wearable device analyses sweat to detect health problems.* Retrieved October 12, 2016, from http://www.abc.net.au/news/2016-01-28/new-wearable-device-measures-sweat-to-track-your-health/7118234

Correia, M. I. T., Hegazi, R. A., Higashiguchi, T., Michel, J. P., Reddy, B. R., Tappenden, K. A., & Muscaritoli, M. (2014). Evidence-based recommendations for addressing malnutrition in health care: An updated strategy from the feedM. E. Global Study Group. *Journal of the American Medical Directors Association*, *15*(8), 544–550. doi:10.1016/j.jamda.2014.05.011 PMID:24997720

Cortes, B. (2005). *Sistemas de suporte à decisão.* FCA-Editora Informática.

Costa, R., Novais, P., Machado, J., Alberto, C., & Neves, J. (2007). Inter-organization cooperation for care of the elderly. *Integration and Innovation Orient to E-Society*, *2*, 200–208.

Coulter, A. (2012). Patient engagement—what works? *The Journal of Ambulatory Care Management*, *35*(2), 80–89. doi:10.1097/JAC.0b013e318249e0fd PMID:22415281

Crossley, G. H., Boyle, A., Vitense, H., Chang, Y., & Mead, R. H. (2011). CONNECT Investigators. The CONNECT (Clinical Evaluation of Remote Notification to Reduce Time to Clinical Decision) trial: The value of wireless remote monitoring with automatic clinician alerts. *Journal of the American College of Cardiology, 57*(10), 1181–1189. doi:10.1016/j.jacc.2010.12.012 PMID:21255955

Curtis, L. H., Brown, J., & Platt, R. (2014). Four health data networks illustrate the potential for a shared national multipurpose big-data network. *Health Affairs, 33*(7), 1178–1186. doi:10.1377/hlthaff.2014.0121 PMID:25006144

Cuzzocrea, A., Bellatreche, L., & Song, I.-Y. (2013). Data Warehousing and OLAP over Big Data: Current Challenges and Future Research Directions. *DOLAP '13 Proceedings of the Sixteenth International Workshop on Data Warehousing and OLAP*, 67–70. https://doi.org/10.1145/2513190.2517828

Cuzzocrea, A. (2015). Data Warehousing and OLAP over Big Data: A Survey of the State-of-the-art, Open Problems and Future Challenges. *Int. J. Business Process Integration and Management, 7*(4), 372–377. doi:10.1504/IJBPIM.2015.073665

D'Abundo, M. L. (2013). Electronic health record implementation in the United States healthcare industry: Making the process of change manageable. In V. Wang (Ed.), *Handbook of research on technologies for improving the 21st century workforce: Tools for lifelong learning* (pp. 272–286). Hershey, PA: IGI Global. doi:10.4018/978-1-4666-2181-7.ch018

Dabbs, A. D., Myers, B. A., Mc Curry, K. R., Dunbar-Jacob, J., Hawkins, R. P., Begey, A., & Dew, M. A. (2009). User-centered design and interactive health technologies for patients. *Computers, Informatics, Nursing, 27*(3), 175–183. doi:10.1097/NCN.0b013e31819f7c7c PMID:19411947

Dalrymple, P. W. (2011). Data, information, knowledge: The emerging field of health informatics. *Bulletin of the Association for Information Science and Technology, 37*(5), 41–44. doi:10.1002/bult.2011.1720370512

Dao, T. H., Jeong, S. R., & Ahn, H. (2012). A novel recommendation model of location-based advertising: Context-Aware Collaborative Filtering using GA approach. *Expert Systems with Applications, 39*(3), 3731–3739. doi:10.1016/j.eswa.2011.09.070

Darji, A., & Waghela, D. (2014). Parallel Power Iteration Clustering for Big Data using MapReduce in Hadoop. *International Journal of Advanced Research in Computer Science and Software Engineering, 4*(6).

Darma Cushion. (2016). *Buy Darma Cushion now*. Retrieved August 23, 2016, from http://darma.co/Pages/DarmaInc.-Products.html

de la Torre Díez, I., Sánchez, R. H., Coronado, M. L., & López Gálvez, M. I. (2010). Electronic health records in a tele-ophthalmologic application with Oracle 10g. In A. Lazakidou (Ed.), *Biocomputation and biomedical informatics: Case studies and applications* (pp. 89–105). Hershey, PA: IGI Global. doi:10.4018/978-1-60566-768-3.ch005

De Mul, M., Alons, P., Van der Velde, P., Konings, I., Bakker, J., & Hazelzet, J. (2012). Development of a clinical data warehouse from an intensive care clinical information system. *Computer Methods and Programs in Biomedicine, 105*(1), 22–30. doi:10.1016/j.cmpb.2010.07.002 PMID:20728956

de Wit, H. A. J. M., Gonzalvo, C. M., Cardenas, J., Derijks, H. J., Janknegt, R., & van der Kuy, P. H. M. (2015). Evaluation of clinical rules in a standalone pharmacy based clinical decision support system for hospitalized and nursing home patients. *International Journal of Medical Informatics, 84*(6), 396–405. doi:10.1016/j.ijmedinf.2015.02.004 PMID:25746461

Delicato, F. C., Pires, P. F., & Batista, T. (2013). *Middleware solutions for the Internet of Things*. Springer London. doi:10.1007/978-1-4471-5481-5

Demirkan, H., & Delen, D. (2013). Leveraging the capabilities of service-oriented decision support systems: Putting analytics and big data in cloud. *Decision Support Systems, 99*(1), 412–421. doi:10.1016/j.dss.2012.05.048

Deng, Z., Mo, X., & Liu, S. (2014). Comparison of the middle-aged and older users' adoption of mobile health services in China. *International Journal of Medical Informatics*, *83*(3), 210–224. doi:10.1016/j.ijmedinf.2013.12.002 PMID:24388129

Department of Economic and Social Affairs of the United Nations. (2009). *World Population Ageing*. New York: United Nations.

DeRenzi, B., Borriello, G., Jackson, J., Kumar, V. S., Parikh, T. S., Virk, P., & Lesh, N. (2011). Mobile phone tools for field-based health care workers in low-income countries. *Mount Sinai Journal of Medicine: A Journal of Translational and Personalized Medicine, 78*(3), 406–418. doi:10.1002/msj.20256

Deshmukh. (2016). Design of cloud security in the EHR for Indian healthcare services. *Journal of King Saud University - Computer and Information Sciences.*

Devedzic, G., Ristic, B., Stefanovic, M., Cukovic, S., & Lukovic, T. (2012). Development of 3D parametric model of human spine and simulator for biomedical engineering education and scoliosis screening. *Computer Applications in Engineering Education*, *20*(3), 434–444. doi:10.1002/cae.20411

Dhingra, M. (2016). Legal Issues in Secure Implementation of Bring Your Own Device (BYOD). *Procedia Computer Science, 78*, 179–184. https://doi.org/10.1016/j.procs.2016.02.030

Dias, C. M., Freitas, M., & Briz, T. (2007). Indicadores de saúde: Uma visão de Saúde Pública, com interesse em Medicina Geral e Familiar. *Revista Portuguesa de Medicina Geral e Familiar*, *23*(4), 439–450.

Dias, C. M., Ribeiro, A. G., & Furtado, S. F. (2016). An overview about the use of healthcare applications on mobile devices. In M. Cruz-Cunha, I. Miranda, R. Martinho, & R. Rijo (Eds.), *Encyclopedia of e-health and telemedicine* (pp. 285–298). Hershey, PA: IGI Global. doi:10.4018/978-1-4666-9978-6.ch024

Dix, A. (2009). *Human-computer interaction.* Springer.

Domingo, M. C. (2012). An Overview of the Internet of Things for People with Disabilities. *Journal of Network and Computer Applications*, *35*(2), 584–59. doi:10.1016/j.jnca.2011.10.015

Douali, N., & Jaulent, M. (2013). Clinical practice guidelines formalization for personalized medicine. *International Journal of Applied Evolutionary Computation*, *4*(3), 26–33. doi:10.4018/jaec.2013070103

Duarte, J., Portela, C. F., Abelha, A., Machado, J., & Santos, M. F. (2011). Electronic health record in dermatology service. *International Conference on ENTERprise Information Systems*, 156-164.

Dwivedi, S. (2016). Reshaping Medical Practice and Care with Health Information Systems. In R. Misra (Ed.), *The Benefits and Challenges of Using Mobile-Based Tools in Self-Management and Care* (pp. 1–13). University of Hull. doi:10.4018/978-1-4666-9870-3

Dwivedi, Y. K., Shareef, M. A., Simintiras, A. C., Lal, B., & Weerakkody, V. (2016). A generalised adoption model for services: A cross-country comparison of mobile health (m-health). *Government Information Quarterly*, *33*(1), 174–187. doi:10.1016/j.giq.2015.06.003

Eberhardt, J., Bilchik, A., & Stojadinovic, A. (2012). Clinical decision support systems: Potential with pitfalls. *Journal of Surgical Oncology*, *105*(5), 502–510. doi:10.1002/jso.23053 PMID:22441903

Eckerson, W. (2003). *Smart companies in the 21st century: The secrets of creating successful business intelligence solutions*. Academic Press.

Edirisinghe, R., Stranieri, A., & Wickramasinghe, N. (2017). A taxonomy for mHealth. In N. Wickramasinghe (Ed.), *Handbook of research on healthcare administration and management* (pp. 596–615). Hershey, PA: IGI Global. doi:10.4018/978-1-5225-0920-2.ch036

Effler, P., Ching-Lee, M., Bogard, A., Ieong, M. C., Nekomoto, T., & Jernigan, D. (1999). Statewide system of electronic notifiable disease reporting from clinical laboratories: Comparing automated reporting with conventional methods. *Journal of the American Medical Association, 282*(19), 1845–1850. doi:10.1001/jama.282.19.1845 PMID:10573276

Eisenberg, D. M., Davis, R. B., Ettner, S. L., Appel, S., Wilkey, S., Van Rompay, M., & Kessler, R. C. (1998). Trends in alternative medicine use in the United States, 19901997: Results of a follow-up national survey. *Journal of the American Medical Association, 280*(18), 1569–1575. doi:10.1001/jama.280.18.1569 PMID:9820257

El Morr, C. (2014). *Research perspectives on the role of informatics in health policy and management*. Hershey, PA: IGI Global. doi:10.4018/978-1-4666-4321-5

El-Fakdi, A., Gamero, F., Melendez, J., Auffret, V., & Haigron, P. (2014). eXiTCDSS: A framework for a workflow-based CBR for interventional clinical decision support systems and its application to TAVI. *Expert Systems with Applications, 41*(2), 284–294. doi:10.1016/j.eswa.2013.05.067

El-Sappagh, S. H. A., Hendawi, A. M. A., & El Bastawissy, A. H. (2011). A Proposed Model for Data Warehouse ETL Processes. *Journal of King Saud University - Computer and Information Sciences, 23*(2), 91–104. https://doi.org/10.1016/j.jksuci.2011.05.005

El-Sappagh, S. H. A., Hendawi, A. M. A., & El Bastawissy, A. H. (2011). A proposed model for data warehouse ETL processes. *Journal of King Saud University-Computer and Information Sciences, 23*(2), 91–104. doi:10.1016/j.jksuci.2011.05.005

Emani, C. K., Cullot, N., & Nicolle, C. (2015). Understandable big data: A survey. *Computer Science Review, 17*, 70–81. doi:10.1016/j.cosrev.2015.05.002

Erwin, J., Kompanje, O., Jansen, N. E., & de Groot, Y. J. (2013). 'in plain language': Uniform criteria for organ donor recognition. *Intensive Care Medicine*.

Esteves, M. (2016). *Desenvolvimento e Exploração de uma Nova Geração de Ferramentas de Business Intelligence para o Apoio à Decisão e a Prática Clínica em Unidades Hospitalares*. Universidade do Minho.

Etheredge, L. M. (2014). Rapid learning: A breakthrough agenda. *Health Affairs, 33*(7), 1155–1162. doi:10.1377/hlthaff.2014.0043 PMID:25006141

Ettehad, D., Emdin, C. A., Kiran, A., Anderson, S. G., Callender, T., Emberson, J., & Rahimi, K. et al. (2016). Blood pressure lowering for prevention of cardiovascular disease and death: A systematic review and meta-analysis. *Lancet, 387*(10022), 957–967. doi:10.1016/S0140-6736(15)01225-8 PMID:26724178

European Commission Information Society. (2009). *Internet of Things Strategic Research Roadmap 2009*. Obtido de European Commission Information Society: www.internet-of-things-research.eu

Eurostat. (2008). *The Life of Women and Men in Europe: A Statistical Portrait*. Luxembourg: Eurostat.

Evans, D. (2013). *What is BYOD and why is it important?* Academic Press.

Ewer, A. K. (2014, August). Pulse oximetry screening: Do we have enough evidence now? *Lancet, 384*(9945), 725–726. doi:10.1016/S0140-6736(14)60575-4 PMID:24768154

Falchuk, B., Famolari, D., Fischer, R., Loeb, S., & Panagos, E. (2010). The mHealth stack: Technology enablers for patient-centric mobile healthcare. *International Journal of E-Health and Medical Communications, 1*(1), 1–17. doi:10.4018/jehmc.2010010101

Fan, Y. J., Yin, Y. H., Da Xu, L., Zeng, Y., & Wu, F. (2014). IoT-based smart rehabilitation system. *IEEE Transactions on Industrial Informatics, 10*(2), 1568-1577.

Fan, J., & Liu, H. (2013). Statistical analysis of big data on pharmacogenomics. *Advanced Drug Delivery Reviews, 65*(7), 987–1000. doi:10.1016/j.addr.2013.04.008 PMID:23602905

Fayyad, U., Piatetsky-Shapiro, G., & Smyth, P. (1996). From data mining to knowledge discovery in databases. *AI Magazine*, 37.

Fayyad, U., Piatetsky-Shapiro, G., Smyth, P., & Uturusamy, R. (1996). *Advances in knowledge discovery and data mining.* Cambridge, MA: The MIT Press.

Feldman, R., & Sanger, J. (2007). *The text mining handbook: advanced approaches in analyzing unstructured data.* Cambridge University Press.

Feller, E., Ramakrishnan, L., & Morin, C. (2015). Performance and energy efficiency of big data applications in cloud environments: A Hadoop case study. *Journal of Parallel and Distributed Computing, 79*, 80–89. doi:10.1016/j.jpdc.2015.01.001

Ferguson, N. D., Cook, D. J., Guyatt, G. H., Mehta, S., Hand, L., Austin, P., & Meade, M. O. et al. (2013). High-Frequency Oscillation in Early Acute Respiratory Distress Syndrome. *The New England Journal of Medicine, 368*(9), 795–805. doi:10.1056/NEJMoa1215554 PMID:23339639

Fernandes, A. (2013). *Early imagiology criteria for the screening of possible brain-death donors at the emergency room.* University of Barcelona.

Fernandes, A., Gomes, A., Ermida, D., & Vardasca, T. (2015). Imaging screening of catastrophic neurological events using a software tool: Preliminary results. *Transplantation Proceedings, 47*(4), 1001–1004. doi:10.1016/j.transproceed.2015.03.021 PMID:26036504

Fernandes, A., Perelman, J., & Mateus, C. (2010). *Health and Healthcare in Portugal: Does Gender Matter?.* Lisboa, Portugal: Instituto Nacional Ricardo Jorge.

Fernandez, F., & Pallis, G. C. (2014, November). Opportunities and challenges of the Internet of Things for Healthcare: Systems engineering perspective. In *Wireless Mobile Communication and Healthcare (Mobihealth), 2014 EAI 4th International Conference on* (pp. 263-266). IEEE.

Fernández, D. R. (2010). An agent-based architecture to ubiquitous health. In S. Mohammed & J. Fiaidhi (Eds.), *Ubiquitous health and medical informatics: The ubiquity 2.0 trend and beyond* (pp. 213–232). Hershey, PA: IGI Global. doi:10.4018/978-1-61520-777-0.ch011

Ferreira, J., Miranda, M., Abelha, A., & Machado, J. (2010). O Processo ETL em Sistemas Data Warehouse. *INForum 2010 - II Simpósio de Informática*, 757–765.

Ferreira, J., Miranda, M., Abelha, A., & Machado, J. (2010). O processo etl em sistemas data warehouse. INForum, 757-765.

Ferreira, J., Miranda, M., Abelha, A., & Machado, J. (2010). O processo ETL em sistemas data warehouse. In *INForum 2010* (pp. 757–765). II Simpósio de Informática.

Ferreira-Satler, M., Romero, F. P., Menendez-Dominguez, V. H., Zapata, A., & Prieto, M. E. (2012). Fuzzy ontologies-based user profiles applied to enhance e-learning activities. *Soft Computing*, *16*(7), 1129–1141. doi:10.1007/s00500-011-0788-y

Filkins, B. L. (2016). Privacy and security in the era of digital health: What should translational researchers know and do about it?. *Am J Transl Res.*, *8*(3), 1560–1580. PMID:27186282

Finkle, J. (2016). *J & J warns diabetic patients: Insulin pump vulnerable to hacking*. Academic Press.

Fischer, J., Neff, M., Freudenstein, D., & Bartz, D. (2004). Medical Augmented Reality based on Commercial Image Guided Surgery. *EGVE'04 Proceedings of the Tenth Eurographics Conference on Virtual Environments*, 83–86. https://doi.org/10.2312/EGVE/EGVE04/083-086

Fisher, D., DeLine, R., Czerwinski, M., & Drucker, S. (2012). Interactions with big data analytics. *Interactions, 19*(3), 50-59.

Folami, F. F. (2014). M-health technology as a transforming force for population health. In B. Adeoye & L. Tomei (Eds.), *Effects of information capitalism and globalization on teaching and learning* (pp. 256–262). Hershey, PA: IGI Global. doi:10.4018/978-1-4666-6162-2.ch021

Free, C., Phillips, G., Galli, L., Watson, L., Felix, L., Edwards, P., & Haines, A. et al. (2013). The effectiveness of mobile-health technology-based health behaviour change or disease management interventions for health care consumers: A systematic review. *PLoS Medicine*, *10*(1), e1001362. doi:10.1371/journal.pmed.1001362 PMID:23349621

Gaglani, S. M., & Topol, E. J. (2014). iMedEd: the role of mobile health technologies in medical education. *Academic Medicine: Journal of the Association of American Medical Colleges, 89*(9), 1207–9. https://doi.org/10.1097/ACM.0000000000000361

Galani, O., & Nikiforou, A. (2006). Electronic health records. In A. Lazakidou (Ed.), *Handbook of research on informatics in healthcare and biomedicine* (pp. 1–8). Hershey, PA: IGI Global. doi:10.4018/978-1-59140-982-3.ch001

Gandomi, A., & Haider, M. (2015). Beyond the hype: Big data concepts, methods, and analytics. *International Journal of Information Management*, *35*(2), 137–144. doi:10.1016/j.ijinfomgt.2014.10.007

Gao, H., & Liu, H. (2014). Data Analysis on Location-Based Social Networks. *Mobile Social Networking*, 165–194.

Gao, R., Zhao, M., Qiu, Z., Yu, Y., & Chang, C. H. (2015, June). Web-based motion detection system for health care. In *Computer and Information Science (ICIS), 2015 IEEE/ACIS 14th International Conference on* (pp. 65-70). IEEE.

Gao, W., Emaminejad, S., Nyein, H., Challa, S., Chen, K., Peck, A., & Javey, A. et al. (2016). Fully integrated wearable sensor arrays for multiplexed in situ perspiration analysis. *Nature*, *529*(7587), 509–514. doi:10.1038/nature16521 PMID:26819044

Gardner, S. R. (1998). Building the data warehouse. *Communications of the ACM*, 53.

Gartner, I. (2014). *Glossary Big data*. Academic Press.

Gartner. (2015). *Gartner says 6.4 billion connected ''things''will be in use in 2016, up 30 percent from 2015*. Retrieved June 10, 2016, from Http://www.gartner.com/newsroom/id/3165317

Gasparrini, A., Guo, Y., Hashizume, M., Lavigne, E., Zanobetti, A., Schwartz, J., & Armstrong, B. et al. (2015). Mortality risk attributable to high and low ambient temperature: A multicountry observational study. *Lancet*, *386*(9991), 369–375. doi:10.1016/S0140-6736(14)62114-0 PMID:26003380

Ge, B., Ge, S., & Minard, T. (2014). Visualizations make big data meaningful. *Communications of the ACM*, *57*(6).

Gelder, I. C. V. (2016). Rate control in atrial fibrillation. *Lancet*, *388*(10046), 818–828. doi:10.1016/S0140-6736(16)31258-2 PMID:27560277

Gentag. (2016). *NFC Skin Patches*. Retrieved August 3, 2016, from http://gentag.com/nfc-skin-patches/

Ghezzi, A., Balocco, R., & Rangone, A. (2015). A fuzzy framework assessing corporate resource management for the mobile content industry. *Technological Forecasting and Social Change*, *96*, 153–172. doi:10.1016/j.techfore.2015.01.004

Gia, T. N., Thanigaivelan, N. K., Rahmani, A. M., Westerlund, T., Liljeberg, P., & Tenhunen, H. (2014, October). Customizing 6LoWPAN networks towards Internet-of-Things based ubiquitous healthcare systems. In NORCHIP, 2014 (pp. 1-6). IEEE.

Gibson, C. J., & Abrams, K. J. (2010). Will privacy concerns derail the electronic health record? Balancing the risks and benefits. In S. Kabene (Ed.), *Healthcare and the effect of technology: Developments, challenges and advancements* (pp. 178–196). Hershey, PA: IGI Global. doi:10.4018/978-1-61520-733-6.ch011

Goldsmith, A. (2005). *Wireless communications*. Cambridge University Press. doi:10.1017/CBO9780511841224

Goletsis, Y., Exarchos, T. P., Giannakeas, N., Tsipouras, M. G., & Fotiadis, D. I. (2011). Integration of clinical and genomic data for decision support in cancer. In *Clinical technologies: Concepts, methodologies, tools and applications* (pp. 412–421). Hershey, PA: IGI Global. doi:10.4018/978-1-60960-561-2.ch212

Goligher, E. C., Ferguson, N. D., & Brochard, L. J. (2016). Clinical challenges in mechanical ventilation. *Lancet*, *387*(10030), 1856–1866. doi:10.1016/S0140-6736(16)30176-3 PMID:27203509

Gong, T., Tan, C. L., Leong, T. Y., Pang, B. C., Lim, C. T., Tian, Q., & Zhang, Z. et al. (2008). Text mining in radiology reports. *2008 Eighth IEEE International Conference on Data Mining* (pp. 815-820). IEEE. doi:10.1109/ICDM.2008.150

Gonzales, K. (2010). Medication administration errors and the pediatric population: A systematic search of the literature. *Journal of Pediatric Nursing*, *25*(6), 555–565. doi:10.1016/j.pedn.2010.04.002 PMID:21035020

Gorp, V. P., & Comuzzi, M. (2014). Lifelong personal health data and application software via virtual machines in the cloud. *IEEE Journal of Biomedical and Health Informatics*, *18*(1), 36–45. doi:10.1109/JBHI.2013.2257821 PMID:24403402

Gour, V., Sarangdevot, S. S., Tanwar, G. S., & Sharma, A. (2010). Improve Performance of Extract, Transform and Load (ETL) in Data Warehouse. *International Journal on Computer Science and Engineering*, *1*(3), 786–789.

Gowin, M., Cheney, M., Gwin, S., & Franklin Wann, T. (2015). Health and fitness app use in college students: A qualitative study. *American Journal of Health Education*, *46*(4), 223–230. doi:10.1080/19325037.2015.1044140

Goyal, S., Morita, P., Lewis, G. F., Yu, C., Seto, E., & Cafazzo, J. A. (2016). The systematic design of a behavioural mobile health application for the self-management of type 2 diabetes. *Canadian Journal of Diabetes*, *40*(1), 95–104. doi:10.1016/j.jcjd.2015.06.007 PMID:26455762

Greenhalgh, T., Potts, H., Wong, G., Bark, P., & Swinglehurst, D. (2009). Tensions and paradoxes in electronic patient record research: A systematic literature review using the meta-narrative method. *The Milbank Quarterly*, *87*(4), 729–788. doi:10.1111/j.1468-0009.2009.00578.x PMID:20021585

Gubbi, J., Buyya, R., Marusic, S., & Palaniswami, M. (2013). Internet of things (iot): A vision, architectural elements, and future directions. *Future Generation Computer Systems*, *29*(7), 1645–1660. doi:10.1016/j.future.2013.01.010

Guillemin, P., & Friess, P. (2009). *Internet of things strategic research roadmap*. The Cluster of European Research Projects. Tech. Rep.

Guimarães, T., Coimbra, C., Portela, F., Santos, F., Machado, J., & Abelha, A. (2015). Step towards Multiplatform Framework for supporting Pediatric and Neonatology Care Unit decision process. *Procedia Computer Science*, *63*, 561–568.

Gundlapalli, A. V., Reid, J. H., Root, J., & Xu, W. (2011). Regional and community health information exchange in the United States. In A. Shukla & R. Tiwari (Eds.), *Biomedical engineering and information systems: Technologies, tools and applications* (pp. 198–218). Hershey, PA: IGI Global. doi:10.4018/978-1-61692-004-3.ch011

Guo, Q., Wang, Z., Li, M., & Aghajan, H. (2005). *Intelligent health recommendation system for computer users*. Academic Press.

Gupte, M. D., Ramachandran, V., & Mutatkar, R. K. (2001). Epidemiological profile of India: Historical and contemporary perspectives. *Journal of Biosciences*, *26*(4Suppl), 437–464. doi:10.1007/BF02704746 PMID:11779959

Gürsel, G. (2016). Mobility in healthcare: M-health. In A. Panagopoulos (Ed.), *Handbook of research on next generation mobile communication systems* (pp. 485–511). Hershey, PA: IGI Global. doi:10.4018/978-1-4666-8732-5.ch019

Hahn, J., & Subramani, M. R. (2000). A framework of knowledge management systems: issues and challenges for theory and practice. *Proceedings of the twenty first international conference on Information systems*, 302-312.

Hallet, J., Soler, L., Diana, M., Mutter, D., Baumert, T. F., Habersetzer, F., … Pessaux, P. (2015). Trans-thoracic minimally invasive liver resection guided by augmented reality. *Journal of the American College of Surgeons, 220*(5), e55–e60. https://doi.org/10.1016/j.jamcollsurg.2014.12.053

Hall, J. E. (2006). *Guyton and Hall Textbook of Medical Physiology (12th ed.)*. Elsevier.

Hampshire, K., Porter, G., Owusu, S. A., Mariwah, S., Abane, A., Robson, E., & Milner, J. et al. (2015). Informal m-health: How are young people using mobile phones to bridge healthcare gaps in Sub-Saharan Africa? *Social Science & Medicine*, *142*, 90–99. doi:10.1016/j.socscimed.2015.07.033 PMID:26298645

Handel, M. J. (2011). MHealth (mobile health)-Using Apps for health and wellness. *Explore (New York, N.Y.)*, *7*(4), 256–261. doi:10.1016/j.explore.2011.04.011 PMID:21724160

Han, Q., Liang, S., & Zhang, H. (2015). Mobile cloud sensing, big data, and 5G networks make an intelligent and smart world. *IEEE Network*, *29*(2), 40–45. doi:10.1109/MNET.2015.7064901

Harrison, S., & Mort, M. (1998). Which champions, which people? Public and user involvement in health care as a technology of legitimation. *Social Policy and Administration*, *32*(1), 60–70. doi:10.1111/1467-9515.00086

Hashem, I., Yaqoob, I., Anuar, N. B., Mokhtar, S., Gani, A., & Khan, S. U. (2015). The rise of big data on cloud computing: Review and open research issues. *Information Systems*, *47*, 98–115. doi:10.1016/j.is.2014.07.006

Hassanalieragh, M., Page, A., Soyata, T., Sharma, G., Aktas, M., & Mateos, G. … Andreescu, S. (2015). Health Monitoring and Management Using Internet-of-Things (IoT) Sensing with Cloud-Based Processing: Opportunities and Challenges. *Proceedings - 2015 IEEE International Conference on Services Computing*, 285–292. doi:<ALIGNMENT.qj></ALIGNMENT>10.1109/SCC.2015.47

Hassan, M. M., Albakr, H. S., & Al-Dossari, H. (2014, November). A Cloud-Assisted Internet of Things Framework for Pervasive Healthcare in Smart City Environment. In *Proceedings of the 1st International Workshop on Emerging Multimedia Applications and Services for Smart Cities* (pp. 9-13). ACM. doi:10.1145/2661704.2661707

Hassenzahl, M., & Tractinsky, N. (2006). User experience-a research agenda. *Behaviour & Information Technology*, *25*(2), 91–97. doi:10.1080/01449290500330331

Haux, R., Winter, A., Ammenwerth, E., & Brigl, B. (2013). *Strategic information management in hospitals: an introduction to hospital information systems*. Springer Science & Business Media.

Hayhurst, C. (2015). Mining for Answers from Big Data. *Biomedical Instrumentation & Technology*, *49*(2), 84–92. doi:10.2345/0899-8205-49.2.84 PMID:25793337

Hayrinen, K., Saranto, K., & Nykanen, P. (2008). Definition, structure, content, use and impacts of electronic health records: A review of the research literature. *International Journal of Medical Informatics*, *77*(5), 291–304. doi:10.1016/j.ijmedinf.2007.09.001 PMID:17951106

Hearst, M. A. (1999). Untangling text data mining. *Proceedings of the 37th annual meeting of the Association for Computational Linguistics on Computational Linguistics*, 3-10. doi:10.3115/1034678.1034679

Heidbuchel, H., Hindricks, G., Broadhurst, P., Van Erven, L., Fernandez-Lozano, I., Rivero-Ayerza, M., & Annemans, L. et al. (2015). EuroEco (European Health Economic Trial on Home Monitoring in ICD Patients): A provider perspective in five European countries on costs and net financial impact of follow-up with or without remote monitoring. *European Heart Journal*, *36*(3), 158–169. doi:10.1093/eurheartj/ehu339 PMID:25179766

Helie, S. (2017). ScienceDirect Augmented reality: An ecological blend. *Cognitive Systems Research*, *42*, 58–72. doi:10.1016/j.cogsys.2016.11.009

Hendriks, M., & Rademakers, J. (2014). Relationships between patient activation, disease-specific knowledge and health outcomes among people with diabetes; a survey study. *BMC Health Services Research*, *14*(1), 393. doi:10.1186/1472-6963-14-393 PMID:25227734

Herford, A. S., Miller, M., Lauritano, F., Cervino, G., Signorino, F., & Maiorana, C. (2017). The use of virtual surgical planning and navigation in the treatment of orbital trauma. *Chinese Journal of Traumatology*, *20*(1), 9–13. doi:10.1016/j.cjtee.2016.11.002 PMID:28202368

Heringa, M., Floor-Schreudering, A., Tromp, P. C., Smet, P. A., & Bouvy, M. L. (2015). Nature and frequency of drug therapy alerts generated by clinical decision support in community pharmacy. *Pharmacoepidemiology and Drug Safety*, *25*(1), 82–89. doi:10.1002/pds.3915 PMID:26602064

Hernandez, J., Li, Y., Rehg, J. M., & Picard, R. W. (2014). BioGlass: Physiological parameter estimation using a head mounted wearable device. *EAI 4th International Conference on Wireless Mobile Communication and Healthcare (Mobihealth)*. doi:<ALIGNMENT.qj></ALIGNMENT>10.1109/MOBIHEALTH.2014.7015908

Hevner, A. R., & Chatterjee, S. (2004). Design Research in Information Systems. *Design Research in Information Systems, 28*, 75–105. https://doi.org/10.1007/978-1-4419-5653-8

Hevner, R., March, S. T., & Park, J. (2004). Design Science in Information Systems Research. *Management Information Systems Quarterly*, *28*(1), 75–105. https://doi.org/10.2307/25148625

Hindia, M.N., Rahman, T.A., Ojukwu, H., Hanafi, E.B., & Fattouh, A. (2016). Enabling Remote Health-Caring Utilizing IoT Concept ov er LTE-Femtocell Networks. *Lista Jornal PLoS One, 11*(5).

Hindricks, G., Taborsky, M., Glikson, M., Heinrich, U., Schumacher, B., Katz, A., & Søgaard, P. et al. (2014). Implant-based multiparameter telemonitoring of patients with heart failure (IN-TIME): A randomised controlled trial. *Lancet*, *384*(9943), 583–590. doi:10.1016/S0140-6736(14)61176-4 PMID:25131977

Hirschman, L., Park, J. C., Tsujii, J., Wong, L., & Wu, C. H. (2002). Accomplishments and challenges in literature data mining for biology. *Bioinformatics (Oxford, England)*, *18*(12), 1553–1561. doi:10.1093/bioinformatics/18.12.1553 PMID:12490438

Hočevar, B., & Jaklič, J. (2010). Assessing Benefits of Business Intelligence Systems – A Case Study. *Management, 15*(1), 87–119.

Hochron, S., & Goldberg, P. (2015). Driving physician adoption of mHeath solutions. *Healthcare Financial Management, 69*(2), 36–39. PMID:26665538

Holstiege, J., Mathes, T., & Pieper, D. (2015). Effects of computer-aided clinical decision support systems in improving antibiotic prescribing by primary care providers: A systematic review. *Journal of the American Medical Informatics Association, 22*(1), 236–242. doi:10.1136/amiajnl-2014-002886 PMID:25125688

Horsky, J., Kaufman, D., Oppenheim, M., & Patel, V. (2003). A framework for analyzing the cognitive complexity of computer-assisted clinical ordering. *Journal of Biomedical Informatics, 36*(1/2), 4–22. doi:10.1016/S1532-0464(03)00062-5 PMID:14552843

Hou, Y. Z., Ma, L. C., Zhu, R. Y., & Chen, X. L. (2016). iPhone-Assisted Augmented Reality Localization of Basal Ganglia Hypertensive Hematoma. *World Neurosurgery, 94*, 480–492. https://doi.org/10.1016/j.wneu.2016.07.047

Househ, M., Borycki, E. M., Kushniruk, A. W., & Alofaysan, S. (2012). mHealth: A passing fad or here to stay? In J. Rodrigues, I. de la Torre Díez, & B. Sainz de Abajo (Eds.), Telemedicine and e-health services, policies, and applications: Advancements and developments (pp. 151–178). Hershey, PA: IGI Global. doi:10.4018/978-1-4666-0888-7.ch007

Huang, T., Lan, L., Fang, X., An, P., Min, J., & Wang, F. (2015). Promises and Challenges of Big Data Computing in Health Sciences. *Big Data Research, 2*(1), 2–11. doi:10.1016/j.bdr.2015.02.002

Hu, H., Wen, Y., Chua, T.-S., & Li, X. (2014). Toward scalable systems for big data analytics: A technology tutorial. *IEEE Access, 2*, 652–687. doi:10.1109/ACCESS.2014.2332453

Hung, M., Conrad, J., Hon, S. D., Cheng, C., Franklin, J. D., & Tang, P. (2013). Uncovering patterns of technology use in consumer health informatics. *Wiley Interdisciplinary Reviews: Computational Statistics, 5*(6), 432–447. doi:10.1002/wics.1276 PMID:24904713

Hunt, D. L., Haynes, R. B., Hanna, S. E., & Smith, K. (1998). Effects of computer-based clinical decision support systems on physician performance and patient outcomes: A systematic review. *Journal of the American Medical Association, 280*(15), 1339–1346. doi:10.1001/jama.280.15.1339 PMID:9794315

Hussey, P. A., & Kennedy, M. A. (2016). Instantiating informatics in nursing practice for integrated patient centred holistic models of care: A discussion paper. *Journal of Advanced Nursing, 72*(5), 1030–1041. doi:10.1111/jan.12927 PMID:26890201

IEC 60601. (2015). *IEC 60601-1-11:2015 RLV Redline version.* Retrieved October 11, 2016, from https://webstore.iec.ch/publication/22261

IIPRD. (2012). *Landscape analysis - bring your own device.* IIPRD.

Ikhu-Omoregbe, N., & Azeta, A. (2012). Design and deployment of a mobile-based medical alert system. In M. Watfa (Ed.), *E-healthcare systems and wireless communications: Current and future challenges* (pp. 210–219). Hershey, PA: IGI Global. doi:10.4018/978-1-61350-123-8.ch010

Ikonen, V., & Kaasinen, E. (2008). *Ethical assessment in the design of ambiente assisted living.* Assisted Living Systems – Models, Architectures and Engineering Approaches.

IMS Institute for Healthcare Informatics. (2013). *Patient apps for improved healthcare: From novelty to mainstream.* Parsippany, NJ: IMS Institute for Healthcare Informatics.

Inmon, B. (1997, January). The data warehouse budget. *DM Review Magazine*. doi:10.1145/1651291.1651297

Inmon, W. H. (2005). *Building the data warehouse*. John Wiley & Sons.

Institute of Medicine of the National Academies. (2012). *Health IT and patient safety*. Washington, DC: The National Academies Press.

Intanagonwiwat, C., Govindan, R., Estrin, D., Heidemann, J., & Silva, F. (2003). Directed diffusion for wireless sensor networking. *Networking, 11*(1).

Irving, M. J., Tong, A., Jan, S., Cass, A., Rose, J., Chadban, S., & Howard, K. et al. (2012). Factors that influence the decision to be an organ donor: A systematic review of the qualitative literature. *Nephrology, Dialysis, Transplantation, 27*(6), 2526–2533. doi:10.1093/ndt/gfr683 PMID:22193049

Işık, Ö., Jones, M. C., & Sidorova, A. (2013). Business intelligence success: The roles of BI capabilities and decision environments. *Information & Management, 50*(1), 13–23. doi:10.1016/j.im.2012.12.001

Ivan, M., & Velicanu, M. (2015). Healthcare industry improvement with business intelligence. *Informatica Economica*, 81.

Jalote-Parmar, A. (2009). Workflow Driven Decision Support Systems: A case of an intra-operative visualization system for surgeons. TU Delft, Delft University of Technology.

Jansen, N. E., de Groot, Y. J., Bakker, J., Kuiper, M. A., Aerdts, S., & Maas, A. I. (2010). Imminent brain death: point of departure for potential heart-beating organ donor recognition. *Intensive Care*, 1488-1494.

Jara, A. J., Zamora-Izquierdo, M. A., & Skarmeta, A. F. (2013). Interconnection framework for mHealth and remote monitoring based on the Internet of Things. *IEEE Journal on Selected Areas in Communications, 31*(9), 47–65. doi:10.1109/JSAC.2013.SUP.0513005

Jasemian, Y. (2009). Patient monitoring in diverse environments. In P. Olla & J. Tan (Eds.), *Mobile health solutions for biomedical applications* (pp. 129–142). Hershey, PA: IGI Global. doi:10.4018/978-1-60566-332-6.ch007

Jaspers, M. W., Smeulers, M., Vermeulen, H., & Peute, L. W. (2011). Effects of clinical decision-support systems on practitioner performance and patient outcomes: A synthesis of high-quality systematic review findings. *Journal of the American Medical Informatics Association, 18*(3), 327–334. doi:10.1136/amiajnl-2011-000094 PMID:21422100

Jee, K., & Kim, G.-H. (2013). Potentiality of big data in the medical sector: focus on how to reshape the healthcare system. *Healthcare Informatics Research, 19*(2), 79-85.

Jha, A. K., DesRoches, C. M., Campbell, E. G., Donelan, K., Rao, S. R., Ferris, T. G., & Blumenthal, D. et al. (2009). Use of electronic health records in US hospitals. *The New England Journal of Medicine, 360*(16), 1628–1638. doi:10.1056/NEJMsa0900592 PMID:19321858

Jiang, J., Zheng, J., Zhao, C., Su, J., Guan, Y., & Yu, Q. (2016). Clinical-decision support based on medical literature: A complex network approach. *Physica A: Statistical Mechanics and Its Applications, 459*, 42–54.

Jiang, Y., Sereika, S. M., Dabbs, A. D., Handler, S. M., & Schlenk, E. A. (2016). Using mobile health technology to deliver decision support for self-monitoring after lung transplantation. *International Journal of Medical Informatics, 94*, 164–171. doi:10.1016/j.ijmedinf.2016.07.012 PMID:27573324

Jiawei, H., & Kamber, M. (2001). Data mining: Concepts and techniques. San Francisco, CA: Morgan Kaufmann.

Jinpon, P., Jaroensutasinee, M., & Jaroensutasinee, K. (2011). Business intelligence and its applications in the public healthcare system. *Walailak Journal of Science and Technology, 8*(2), 97–110.

Johnson, K., & Tashiro, J. (2011). Interprofessional care and health care complexity: Factors shaping human resources effectiveness in health information management. In S. Kabene (Ed.), *Human resources in healthcare, health informatics and healthcare systems* (pp. 250–280). Hershey, PA: IGI Global. doi:10.4018/978-1-61520-885-2.ch015

JSON. (2016). *Introducing JSON.* Retrieved September 14, 2016, from http://www.json.org/

Juzwishin, D. W. (2010). Enabling technologies and challenges for the future of ubiquitous health: The interoperability framework. In S. Mohammed & J. Fiaidhi (Eds.), *Ubiquitous health and medical informatics: The ubiquity 2.0 trend and beyond* (pp. 596–622). Hershey, PA: IGI Global. doi:10.4018/978-1-61520-777-0.ch028

Kamath, J. R., & Donahoe-Anshus, A. L. (2012). Electronic health record: Adoption, considerations and future direction. In A. Kolker & P. Story (Eds.), *Management engineering for effective healthcare delivery: Principles and applications* (pp. 309–332). Hershey, PA: IGI Global. doi:10.4018/978-1-60960-872-9.ch015

Kambatla, K., Kollias, G., Kumar, V., & Grama, A. (2014). Trends in big data analytics. *Journal of Parallel and Distributed Computing, 74*(7), 2561–2573. doi:10.1016/j.jpdc.2014.01.003

Kareem, S., & Bajwa, I. S. (2013). Virtual telemedicine and virtual telehealth: A natural language based implementation to address time constraint problem. In *Data mining: Concepts, methodologies, tools, and applications* (pp. 881–892). Hershey, PA: IGI Global. doi:10.4018/978-1-4666-2455-9.ch045

Karla, P., & Gurupur, V. (2013). C-PHIS: A Concept Map Based Knowledge Base Framework to Develop Personal Health Information Systems. *Journal of Medical Systems, 37*(5), 1–16. doi:10.1007/s10916-013-9970-3 PMID:24014254

Karlof, C., & Wagner, D. (2003). Secure routing in wireless sensor networks: Attacks and countermeasures. *Ad Hoc Networks, 1*(2), 293–315. doi:10.1016/S1570-8705(03)00008-8

Karra, V., Papathanassoglou, E. D., Lemonidou, C., Sourtzi, P., & Giannakopoulou, M. (2014). Exploration and classification of intensive care nurses' clinical decisions: A Greek perspective. *Nursing in Critical Care, 19*(2), 87–97. doi:10.1111/nicc.12018 PMID:24400657

Kasemsap, K. (2015). The role of data mining for business intelligence in knowledge management. In A. Azevedo & M. Santos (Eds.), *Integration of data mining in business intelligence systems* (pp. 12–33). Hershey, PA: IGI Global. doi:10.4018/978-1-4666-6477-7.ch002

Kasemsap, K. (2016). Multifaceted applications of data mining, business intelligence, and knowledge management. *International Journal of Social and Organizational Dynamics in IT, 5*(1), 57–69. doi:10.4018/IJSODIT.2016010104

Kasemsap, K. (2017a). Telemedicine and electronic health: Issues and implications in developing countries. In K. Moahi, K. Bwalya, & P. Sebina (Eds.), *Health information systems and the advancement of medical practice in developing countries* (pp. 149–167). Hershey, PA: IGI Global. doi:10.4018/978-1-5225-2262-1.ch009

Kasemsap, K. (2017b). Analyzing the role of health information technology in global health care. In N. Wickramasinghe (Ed.), *Handbook of research on healthcare administration and management* (pp. 287–307). Hershey, PA: IGI Global. doi:10.4018/978-1-5225-0920-2.ch017

Kasemsap, K. (2017b). Artificial intelligence: Current issues and applications. In R. Das & M. Pradhan (Eds.), *Handbook of research on manufacturing process modeling and optimization strategies* (pp. 454–474). Hershey, PA: IGI Global. doi:10.4018/978-1-5225-2440-3.ch022

Kasemsap, K. (2017c). Mastering electronic health record in global health care. In N. Wickramasinghe (Ed.), *Handbook of research on healthcare administration and management* (pp. 222–242). Hershey, PA: IGI Global. doi:10.4018/978-1-5225-0920-2.ch014

Kasemsap, K. (2017c). Robotics: Theory and applications. In M. Moore (Ed.), *Cybersecurity breaches and issues surrounding online threat protection* (pp. 311–345). Hershey, PA: IGI Global. doi:10.4018/978-1-5225-1941-6.ch013

Kasemsap, K. (2017d). The perspectives of medical errors in the health care industry. In M. Riga (Ed.), *Impact of medical errors and malpractice on health economics, quality, and patient safety* (pp. 113–143). Hershey, PA: IGI Global. doi:10.4018/978-1-5225-2337-6.ch005

Kasemsap, K. (2017e). The importance of telemedicine in global health care. In N. Wickramasinghe (Ed.), *Handbook of research on healthcare administration and management* (pp. 157–177). Hershey, PA: IGI Global. doi:10.4018/978-1-5225-0920-2.ch010

Katzenbeisser, S., & Petkovic, M. (2008). Privacy-Preserving Recommendation Systems. *The Third International Conference on Availability, Reliability and Security*, 889–895. http://doi.org/ doi:<ALIGNMENT.qj></ALIGNMENT>10.1109/ARES.2008.85

Kaushik, A., & Raman, A. (2015). The new data-driven enterprise architecture for e-healthcare: Lessons from the Indian public sector. *Government Information Quarterly*, *32*(1), 63–74. doi:10.1016/j.giq.2014.11.002

Kawamoto, K., Houlihan, C. A., Balas, E. A., & Lobach, D. F. (2005). Improving clinical practice using clinical decision support systems: A systematic review of trials to identify features critical to success. *BMJ (Clinical Research Ed.)*, 465. PMID:15767266

Kazemzadeh, R. S., Sartipi, K., & Jayaratna, P. (2012). A framework for data and mined knowledge interoperability in clinical decision support systems. In J. Tan (Ed.), *Advancing technologies and intelligence in healthcare and clinical environments breakthroughs* (pp. 84–110). Hershey, PA: IGI Global. doi:10.4018/978-1-4666-1755-1.ch006

Keim, D. A., Mansmann, F., Schneidewind, J., Thomas, J., & Ziegler, H. (2008). *Visual analytics: Scope and challenges. In Visual data mining* (pp. 76–90). Springer.

Kern, J. (2009). Standardization in health and medical informatics. In J. Tan (Ed.), *Medical informatics: Concepts, methodologies, tools, and applications* (pp. 2059–2065). Hershey, PA: IGI Global. doi:10.4018/978-1-60566-050-9.ch156

Kestle, R., & Self, R. (2013). IS Practices for SME Success Series. *IS Practices for SME Success Series, 1*(1), 1–148. https://doi.org/10.1093/itnow/bws010

Ketelhöhn, N., & Sanz, L. (2016). Healthcare management priorities in Latin America: Framework and responses. *Journal of Business Research, 69*(9), 3835–3838. doi:10.1016/j.jbusres.2016.04.008

Khajouei, R., Wierenga, P. C., Hasman, A., & Jaspers, M. W. (2011). Clinicians satisfaction with CPOE ease of use and effect on clinicians' workflow, efficiency and medication safety. *International Journal of Medical Informatics, 80*(5), 297–309. doi:10.1016/j.ijmedinf.2011.02.009 PMID:21419695

Khalid, E., Muhammad, A., Patrick, M., & Hossam, S. H. (2012). Ubiquitous health monitoring using mobile web services. *Procedia Computer Science, 10*, 332–339. doi:10.1016/j.procs.2012.06.044

Khambete, P., Athavankar, U., Doke, P., Shinde, R., Roy, D., Devkar, S., . . . Chaudhary, S. (2014). A Case Study in Participatory Service Design for Rural Healthcare System in India Using a Pattern Language. ICoRD'15 – Research Into Design Across Boundaries, 1, 3-13.

Khan, A., Ehsan, N., Mirza, E., & Sarwar, S. (2012). *Integration between customer relationship management (CRM) and data warehousing*. Procedia Technology.

Khandelwal, P., Swarnalatha, P., Bisht, N., & Prabu, S. (2015). Detection of Features to Track Objects and Segmentation Using GrabCut for Application in Marker-less Augmented Reality. *Procedia Computer Science, 58*, 698–705. https://doi.org/10.1016/j.procs.2015.08.090

Khattak, H. A., Ruta, M., Di Sciascio, E., & Sciascio, D. (2014, January). CoAP-based healthcare sensor networks: A survey. In *Proceedings of 2014 11th International Bhurban Conference on Applied Sciences & Technology (IBCAST)* (pp. 499-503). IEEE. doi:10.1109/IBCAST.2014.6778196

Khodambashi, S. (2013). Business process re-engineering application in healthcare in a relation to health information systems. *Procedia Technology*, 949-957.

Kilsdonk, E., Peute, L. W., Riezebos, R. J., Kremer, L. C., & Jaspers, M. W. M. (2016). Uncovering healthcare practitioners' information processing using the think-aloud method: From paper-based guideline to clinical decision support system. *International Journal of Medical Informatics, 86*, 10–19. doi:10.1016/j.ijmedinf.2015.11.011 PMID:26725690

Kimball, R., & Ross, M. (2002). The Data Warehouse Toolkit (2nd ed.). Robert Ipsen.

Kimball, R., & Ross, M. (2013). *The data warehouse toolkit: The definitive guide to dimensional modeling*. John Wiley & Sons.

Kim, D., & Chang, H. (2007). Key functional characteristics in designing and operating health information websites for user satisfaction: An application of the extended technology acceptance model. *International Journal of Medical Informatics, 76*(11), 790–800. doi:10.1016/j.ijmedinf.2006.09.001 PMID:17049917

Kitsiou, S. (2009). Overview and analysis of electronic health record standards. In A. Lazakidou & K. Siassiakos (Eds.), *Handbook of research on distributed medical informatics and e-health* (pp. 84–103). Hershey, PA: IGI Global. doi:10.4018/978-1-60566-002-8.ch005

Klingeberg, T., & Schilling, M. (2012). Mobile wearable device for long term monitoring of vital signs. *Computer Methods and Programs in Biomedicine, 106*(2), 89–96. doi:10.1016/j.cmpb.2011.12.009 PMID:22285459

Knott, V. E., & Weller, D. (2014). Informatics and e-health: Advancing knowledge and improving cancer care. *European Journal of Cancer Care, 23*(6), 713–715. doi:10.1111/ecc.12268 PMID:25352463

Koehler, N., Vujovic, O., & McMenamin, C. (2013). Healthcare professionals use of mobile phones and the internet in clinical practice. *Journal of Mobile Technology in Medicine, 2*(11S), 3–13. doi:10.7309/jmtm.76

Koop, C. E., Mosher, R., Kun, L., Geiling, J., Grigg, E., Long, S., & Rosen, J. et al. (2008). Future Delivery of Health Care: Cybercare. *IEEE Engineering in Medicine and Biology Magazine, 27*(6), 29–38. doi:10.1109/MEMB.2008.929888 PMID:19004693

Kopetz, H. (2011). *Real-time systems: design principles for distributed embedded applications*. Springer Science & Business Media. doi:10.1007/978-1-4419-8237-7

Koren, Y. (2008). Tutorial on recent progress in collaborative filtering. *Proceedings of the 2008 ACM Conference on Recommender Systems*, 333–334. doi:10.1145/1454008.1454067

Kotsimbos, T., Williams, T. J., & Anderson, J. P. (2012). Update on lung transplantation: Programmes, patients and prospects. *European Respiratory Review, 21*(126), 271–305. doi:10.1183/09059180.00006312 PMID:23204117

Koumpouros, Y., & Georgoulas, A. (2017). mHealth R&D activities in Europe. In I. Management Association (Ed.), Gaming and technology addiction: Breakthroughs in research and practice (pp. 758–789). Hershey, PA: IGI Global. doi:10.4018/978-1-5225-0778-9.ch034

Kovalchuk, S. V. (2015). *Personalized Clinical Decision Support with Complex Hospital-Level Modelling*. Elsevier Masson SAS.

Krämer, M., & Senner, I. (2015). A modular software architecture for processing of big geospatial data in the cloud. *Computers & Graphics*, *49*, 69–81. doi:10.1016/j.cag.2015.02.005

Kuiken, P. G. B. K. D. K. S. V. (2013). *The 'big data' revolution in healthcare*. Center for US Health System Reform Business Technology Office.

Kumar, S., Nilsen, W. J., Abernethy, A., Atienza, A., Patrick, K., Pavel, M., & Spruijt-Metz, D. et al. (2013). Mobile health technology evaluation: The mHealth evidence workshop. *American Journal of Preventive Medicine*, *45*(2), 228–236. doi:10.1016/j.amepre.2013.03.017 PMID:23867031

Kum, H.-C., Stewart, C. J., Rose, R. A., & Duncan, D. F. (2015). Using big data for evidence based governance in child welfare. *Children and Youth Services Review*, *58*, 127–136. doi:10.1016/j.childyouth.2015.09.014

Kushwaha, N., Goyal, R., Goel, P., Singla, S., & Vyas, O. P. (2014). LOD Cloud Mining for Prognosis Model (Case Study: Native App for Drug Recommender System). *Advances in Internet of Things*, *4*(3), 20–28. doi:10.4236/ait.2014.43004

Lane, J., & Schur, C. (2010). Balancing Access to Health Data and Privacy: A Review of the Issues and Approaches for the Future. *Health Services Research, 45*(5), 1456–1467. <ALIGNMENT.qj></ALIGNMENT>10.1111/j.1475-6773.2010.01141.x

Langhan, M. L., Kurtz, J. C., Schaeffer, P., Asnes, A. G., & Riera, A. (2014). Experiences with capnography in acute care settings: A mixed-methods analysis of clinical staff. *Journal of Critical Care*, *29*(6), 1035–1040. doi:10.1016/j.jcrc.2014.06.021 PMID:25129575

Lang, M., Burkle, T., Laumann, S., & Prokosch, H. U. (2008). Process mining for clinical workflows: Challenges and current limitations. *Studies in Health Technology and Informatics*, *136*, 229–334. PMID:18487736

Lan, T., Zhang, J., & Lu, Y. (2016). Transforming the blood glucose meter into a general healthcare meter for in vitro diagnostics in mobile health. *Biotechnology Advances*, *34*(3), 331–341. doi:10.1016/j.biotechadv.2016.03.002 PMID:26946282

Larose, D. T. (2014). *Discovering knowledge in data: an introduction to data mining*. John Wiley & Sons. doi:10.1002/9781118874059

Laurila, J. K., Gatica-Perez, D., Aad, I., Bornet, O., Do, T.-M.-T., Dousse, O., . . . Miettinen, M. (2012). *The mobile data challenge: Big data for mobile computing research*. Paper presented at the Pervasive Computing.

Lee, J., Han, H., Ock, M., Lee, S. I., Lee, S., & Jo, M. W. (2014). Impact of a clinical decision support system for high-alert medications on the prevention of prescription errors. *International Journal of Medical Informatics*, *83*(12), 929–940. doi:10.1016/j.ijmedinf.2014.08.006 PMID:25256067

Lee, S., & Son, I. (2011). Estimated Blood Pressure Algorithm for a Wrist-wearable Pulsimeter Using Hall Device. *Journal of the Korean Physical Society*, *58*(2), 349–352. doi:10.3938/jkps.58.349

Lee, T. (2016). Mobile healthcare computing in the cloud. In *Mobile computing and wireless networks: Concepts, methodologies, tools, and applications* (pp. 1412–1432). Hershey, PA: IGI Global. doi:10.4018/978-1-4666-8751-6.ch061

Lee, T.-Y., Tong, X., Shen, H.-W., Wong, P. C., Hagos, S., & Leung, L. R. (2013). Feature tracking and visualization of the Madden-Julian Oscillation in climate simulation. *IEEE Computer Graphics and Applications*, *33*(4), 29–37. doi:10.1109/MCG.2013.36 PMID:24808057

Lerner, R. L. (2008). *Medication errors in a neonatal intensive care unit.* Jornal de Pediatria, Sociedade Brasileira de Pediatria.

LeRouge, C., Tolentino, H., Fuller, S., & Tuma, A. (2013). Doing and understanding: Use of case studies for health informatics education and training. In S. Sarnikar, D. Bennett, & M. Gaynor (Eds.), *Cases on healthcare information technology for patient care management* (pp. 1–34). Hershey, PA: IGI Global. doi:10.4018/978-1-4666-2671-3.ch001

Liao, S. H. (2005). Expert system methodologies and applications—a decade review from 1995 to 2004. *Expert Systems with Applications, 28*(1), 93–103. doi:10.1016/j.eswa.2004.08.003

Linden, G., Smith, B., & York, J. (2003). Amazon.com recommendations: Item-to-item collaborative filtering. *IEEE Internet Computing, 7*(1), 76–80. doi:10.1109/MIC.2003.1167344

Lin, J. C.-W., Gan, W., Hong, T.-P., & Vincent, S. (2015). Efficient algorithms for mining up-to-date high-utility patterns. *Advanced Engineering Informatics, 29*(3), 648–661. doi:10.1016/j.aei.2015.06.002

Lin, W., Dou, W., Zhou, Z., & Liu, C. (2015). A cloud-based framework for Home-diagnosis service over big medical data. *Journal of Systems and Software, 102*, 192–206. doi:10.1016/j.jss.2014.05.068

Liu, Z., Jiang, B., & Heer, J. (2013). *imMens: Real-time Visual Querying of Big Data.* Paper presented at the Computer Graphics Forum. doi:10.1111/cgf.12129

Liu, G. C., Odell, J. D., Whipple, E. C., Ralston, R., Carroll, A. E., & Downs, S. M. (2015). Data visualization for truth maintenance in clinical decision support systems. *International Journal of Pediatrics and Adolescent Medicine, 2*(2), 64–69. doi:10.1016/j.ijpam.2015.06.001

Liu, Y. X. L. (2015). Characterizing RESTful Web Services Usage on Smartphones: A Tale of Native Apps and Web Apps. *Proc. - 2015 IEEE Int. Conf. Web Serv. ICWS 2015*, 337–344. doi:10.1109/ICWS.2015.53

Li, W. (2015). Clinical pathway enhanced by knowledge management technology: A critical step towards medical quality improvement. In *Healthcare administration: Concepts, methodologies, tools, and applications* (pp. 978–996). Hershey, PA: IGI Global. doi:10.4018/978-1-4666-6339-8.ch051

Logan, A. G. (2013). Transforming hypertension management using mobile health technology for telemonitoring and self-care support. *The Canadian Journal of Cardiology, 29*(5), 579–585. doi:10.1016/j.cjca.2013.02.024 PMID:23618506

López, P., Fernández, D., Jara, A. J., & Skarmeta, A. F. (2013, March). Survey of internet of things technologies for clinical environments. In *Advanced Information Networking and Applications Workshops (WAINA), 2013 27th International Conference on* (pp. 1349-1354). IEEE. doi:10.1109/WAINA.2013.255

Lovelock, C., Rinkel, G., & Rothwell, P. (2010). Time trends in outcome of subarachnoid hemorrhage population-based study and systematic review. *Neurology, 74*(19), 1494–1501. doi:10.1212/WNL.0b013e3181dd42b3 PMID:20375310

Loya, S. R., Kawamoto, K., Chatwin, C., & Huser, V. (2014). Service Oriented Architecture for Clinical Decision Support: A Systematic Review and Future Directions. *Journal of Medical Systems, 38*(12), 1–22. doi:10.1007/s10916-014-0140-z PMID:25325996

Ludwick, D. A., & Doucette, J. (2009). Adopting electronic medical records in primary care: Lessons learned from health information systems implementation experience in seven countries. *International Journal of Medical Informatics, 78*(1), 22–31. doi:10.1016/j.ijmedinf.2008.06.005 PMID:18644745

Lui, K. (2013). The health informatics professional. In *User-driven healthcare: Concepts, methodologies, tools, and applications* (pp. 120–141). Hershey, PA: IGI Global. doi:10.4018/978-1-4666-2770-3.ch007

Luís, T. (2013, November). *Business Intelligence para apoio à Gestão das Listas de Inscritos para Cirurgia em Portugal Continental*. Lisboa: Universidade Nova.

Lund, D., & Dunbrack, L. (2015). *The Healthcare Industry: Embracing BYOD for Success*. IDC Opinion.

Luukkonen, I., Toivanen, M., Mursu, A., Saranto, K., & Korpela, M. (2013). Researching an activity-driven approach to information systems development. In M. Cruz-Cunha, I. Miranda, & P. Gonçalves (Eds.), *Handbook of research on ICTs and management systems for improving efficiency in healthcare and social care* (pp. 431–450). Hershey, PA: IGI Global. doi:10.4018/978-1-4666-3990-4.ch022

Machado, J., Abelha, A., Novais, P., Neves, J., & Neves, J. (2010). Quality of service in healthcare units. *International Journal of Computer Aided Engineering and Technology*, *2*(4), 436–449. doi:10.1504/IJCAET.2010.035396

Machado, J., Alves, V., Abelha, A., & Neves, J. (2007). Ambient intelligence via multiagent systems in the medical arena. *Engineering Intelligent Systems for Electrical Engineering and Communications*, 151–157.

Mackert, M., Whitten, P., & Holtz, B. (2010). Health infonomics: Intelligent applications of information technology. In M. Pankowska (Ed.), *Infonomics for distributed business and decision-making environments: Creating information system ecology* (pp. 217–232). Hershey, PA: IGI Global. doi:10.4018/978-1-60566-890-1.ch012

MacNeil, S., & Elmqvist, N. (2013). *Visualization mosaics for multivariate visual exploration*. Paper presented at the Computer Graphics Forum.

Madakam, S., Ramaswamy, R., & Tripathi, S. (2015). Internet of Things (IoT): A literature review. *Journal of Computer and Communications, 3*(5), 164-173.

Magalhães, A. S. C. (2013). *Indicadores de Qualidade na Emergência Médica Pré-hospitalar*. Retrieved from RUN - Repositório Universidade Nova: https://run.unl.pt/bitstream/10362/15233/1/RUN%20-%20Trabalho%20Final%20CEAH%20-%20Ana%20Sofia%20Carvalho%20de%20Magalhaes.pdf

Maglogiann, D. I. (2012). Bringing IoT and Cloud Computing towards Pervasive Healthcare Charalampos. *Sixth International Conference on Innovative Mobile and InternetServices in Ubiquitous Computing*.

Mahmood, O. (2008). Application of wireless data grids for health informatics. In N. Wickramasinghe & E. Geisler (Eds.), *Encyclopedia of healthcare information systems* (pp. 61–67). Hershey, PA: IGI Global. doi:10.4018/978-1-59904-889-5.ch009

Maitrey, S., & Jha, C. (2015). MapReduce: Simplified Data Analysis of Big Data. *Procedia Computer Science*, *57*, 563–571. doi:10.1016/j.procs.2015.07.392

Majchrzak, T., Jansen, T., & Kuchen, H. (2011, March 21-25). Efficiency evaluation of open source etl tools. *SAC*, *11*, 287–294.

Maksimović, M., Vujović, V., & Perišić, B. (2015, June). A custom internet of things healthcare system. In *2015 10th Iberian Conference on Information Systems and Technologies (CISTI)* (pp. 1-6). IEEE. doi:10.1109/CISTI.2015.7170415

Manaswini, P. (2017). Status and Challenges on Adaptation for Indian Healthcare Services with Data Mining Technique. In Innovative Healthcare Systems for the 21st Century. Springer.

Mansfield-Devine, S. (2012). Interview: BYOD and the enterprise network. *Computer Fraud & Security*, *2012*(4), 14–17. doi:10.1016/S1361-3723(12)70031-3

Marchionini, G. (1989). Information-seeking strategies of novices using a full-text electronic encyclopedia. *Journal of the American Society for Information Science*, *40*(1), 54–66. doi:10.1002/(SICI)1097-4571(198901)40:1<54::AID-ASI6>3.0.CO;2-R

Marchionini, G., & Komlodi, A. (1998). Design of interfaces for information seeking. *Annual Review of Information Science & Technology*, *33*, 89–130.

March, S. T., & Hevner, A. R. (2007). Integrated Decision Support Systems: A Data Warehousing Perspective. *Decision Support Systems*, *43*(3), 1031–1043. doi:10.1016/j.dss.2005.05.029

March, S. T., & Storey, V. C. (2008). Design Science in the Information Systems discipline: An introduction to the special issue on Design Science Research. *MIS Quartly*, *32*(4), 725–730.

Marcos, M., Maldonado, J. A., Martinez-Salvador, B., Bosca, D., & Robles, M. (2013). Interoperability of clinical decision-support systems and electronic health records using archetypes: A case study in clinical trial eligibility. *Journal of Biomedical Informatics*, *46*(4), 676–689. doi:10.1016/j.jbi.2013.05.004 PMID:23707417

Marins, F., Cardoso, L., Esteves, M., Machado, J., & Abelha, A. (2017). An Agent-Based RFID Monitoring System for Healthcare. In *Advances in Intelligent Systems and Computing (AISC)* (pp. 407–416). Springer. https://doi.org/10.1007/978-3-319-56541-5_42

Marins, F., Cardoso, L., Portela, F., Santos, M., Abelha, A., & Mahado, J. (2014). Improving High Availability and Reliability of Health Interoperability Systems. In *Advances in Intelligent Systems and Computing* (Vol. 275). Springer. doi:10.1007/978-3-319-05948-8_20

Martins, M. (2011). *Processo Clínico Eletrónico - Levantamentos de Processos no Hospital da Prelada* (Master Thesis). Faculdade de Engenharia da Universidade do Porto, Portugal.

Marx, V. (2013). Biology: The big challenges of big data. *Nature*, *498*(7453), 255–260. doi:10.1038/498255a PMID:23765498

Masters, J., Madhyastha, T., & Shakouri, A. (2008). ExplaNet : A Collaborative Learning Tool and Hybrid Recommender System for Student-Authored Explanations. *Journal of Interactive Learning Research*, *19*(1), 51–74.

Matesanz, R. (2001). A decade of continuous improvement in cadaveric organ donation: The spanish model. *Nefrologia*, 59–67. PMID:11881417

Matesanz, R., Dominguez-Gil, B., Coll, E., de la Rosa, G., & Marazuela, R. (2011). Spanish experience as a leading country: What kind of measures were taken?. *Transplant International*, *24*(4), 333–343. doi:10.1111/j.1432-2277.2010.01204.x PMID:21210863

Mathers, C. D., & Loncar, D. (2006). Projections of Global Mortality and Burden of Disease from 2002 to 2030. *PLoS Medicine*, *3*(11), 2011–2030. doi:10.1371/journal.pmed.0030442 PMID:17132052

Mattern, F., & Floerkemeier, C. (2010). From the Internet of Computers to the Internet of Things. In *From active data management to event-based systems and more* (pp. 242–259). Springer Berlin Heidelberg. doi:10.1007/978-3-642-17226-7_15

Mattila, J., Koikkalainen, J., Virkki, A., Van Gils, M., & Lötjönen, J. (2012). Design and Application of a Generic Clinical Decision Support System for Multiscale Data. *IEEE Transactions on Bio-Medical Engineering*, *59*(1), 234–240. doi:10.1109/TBME.2011.2170986 PMID:21990325

Mavridou, E., Kehagias, D. D., Tzovaras, D., & Hassapis, G. (2013). Mining affective needs of automotive industry customers for building a mass-customization recommender system. *Journal of Intelligent Manufacturing*, *24*(2), 251–265. doi:10.1007/s10845-011-0579-4

Ma, Y., Wang, L., Liu, P., & Ranjan, R. (2015). Towards building a data-intensive index for big data computing–A case study of Remote Sensing data processing. *Information Sciences*, *319*, 171–188. doi:10.1016/j.ins.2014.10.006

Mayora, O., Frost, M., Arnrich, B., Gravenhorst, F., Grunerbl, A., & Muaremi, A. et al.. (2016). Mobile health systems for bipolar disorder: The relevance of non-functional requirements in MONARCA project. In *E-health and telemedicine: Concepts, methodologies, tools, and applications* (pp. 1395–1405). Hershey, PA: IGI Global. doi:10.4018/978-1-4666-8756-1.ch070

Mechael, P. (2010). Opportunities and challenges of integrating mHealth applications into rural health initiatives in Africa. In M. Cruz-Cunha, A. Tavares, & R. Simoes (Eds.), *Handbook of research on developments in e-health and telemedicine: Technological and social perspectives* (pp. 704–727). Hershey, PA: IGI Global. doi:10.4018/978-1-61520-670-4.ch034

Media, D. H. (n.d.). In this. *Update, 21*(12).

MedicineNet. (2016). *Dentition of Lifestyle disease*. Retrieved September 12, 2016, from http://www.medicinenet.com/script/main/art.asp?articlekey=38316

Medicinet. (2016). *Definition of Heart Rate*. Retrieved September 17, 2016, from http://www.medicinenet.com/script/main/art.asp?articlekey=3674

Mei, T., Yang, B., Hua, X.-S., & Li, S. (2011). Contextual Video Recommendation by Multimodal Relevance and User Feedback. *ACM Transactions on Information Systems*, *29*(2), 10. doi:10.1145/1961209.1961213

Meixner, G., & Zuehlke, D. (2012). A new paradigm for the development of future medical software systems. *ACM SIGHIT Record, 2*(1), 20–20. https://doi.org/10.1145/2180796.2180812

Mendes, E.V. (2010). As redes de atenção à saúde. Ciênc. *saúde coletiva, 15*(5), 2297-2305.

Mendes, R., & Rodrigues, P. (2010). *Main Barriers for Quality Data Collection in EHR - A Review*. Porto: Universidade do Porto.

Mettler, T., & Vimarlund, V. (2009). Understanding Business Intelligence in the Context of Healthcare. *Health Informatics Journal*, *15*(3), 254–264. doi:10.1177/1460458209337446 PMID:19713399

Miah, S. J. (2014). A demand-driven cloud-based business intelligence for healthcare decision making. In Z. Sun & J. Yearwood (Eds.), *Handbook of research on demand-driven web services: Theory, technologies, and applications* (pp. 324–339). Hershey, PA: IGI Global. doi:10.4018/978-1-4666-5884-4.ch015

Michell, V., Rosenorn-Lanng, D. J., Gulliver, S. R., & Currie, W. (Eds.). (2014). *Handbook of research on patient safety and quality care through health informatics*. Hershey, PA: IGI Global. doi:10.4018/978-1-4666-4546-2

Microsoft. (2017). *O que é Power BI?*. Retrieved April 1, 2017, retrieved from https://powerbi.microsoft.com/pt-br/what-is-power-bi/

Mikkonen, M., Va, S., Ikonen, V., & Heikkila, M. O. (2002). User and concept studies as tools in developing mobile communication services for the elderly. *Personal and Ubiquitous Computing*, *6*(2), 113–124. doi:10.1007/s007790200010

Miksch, S., & Aigner, W. (2014). A matter of time: Applying a data–users–tasks design triangle to visual analytics of time-oriented data. *Computers & Graphics*, *38*, 286–290. doi:10.1016/j.cag.2013.11.002

Miller, A., Moon, B., Anders, S., Walden, R., Brown, S., & Montella, D. (2015). Integrating computerized clinical decision support systems into clinical work: A meta-synthesis of qualitative research. *International Journal of Medical Informatics*, *84*(12), 1009–1018. doi:10.1016/j.ijmedinf.2015.09.005 PMID:26391601

Miller, B. N., Albert, I., Lam, S. K., Konstan, J. a., & Riedl, J. T. (2003). MovieLens unplugged: experiences with an occasionally connected recommender. *Proceedings of the 8th international conference on Intelligent user interfaces - IUI '03*, 263–266. doi:10.1145/604045.604094

Miller, T., Chandler, L., & Mouttapa, M. (2015). A needs assessment, development, and formative evaluation of a health promotion smartphone application for college students. *American Journal of Health Education*, *46*(4), 207–215. doi:10.1080/19325037.2015.1044138

Minutolo, A., Esposito, M., & Pietro, G. D. (2016). Design and validation of a light-weight reasoning system to support remote health monitoring applications. *Engineering Applications of Artificial Intelligence*, *41*, 232–248. doi:10.1016/j.engappai.2015.01.019

Miorandi, D., Sicari, S., De Pellegrini, F., & Chlamtac, I. (2012). Internet of things: Vision, applications and research challenges. *Ad Hoc Networks*, *10*(7), 1497–1516. doi:10.1016/j.adhoc.2012.02.016

Miranda, M., Duarte, J., Abelha, A., Machado, J., & Neves, J. (2010). Interoperability in healthcare. In *European Simulation and Modelling Conference*. Hasselt, Belgium: ESM.

Mishra, S. (2011). Social and ethical concerns of biomedical engineering research and practice. In A. Shukla & R. Tiwari (Eds.), *Biomedical engineering and information systems: Technologies, tools and applications* (pp. 54–80). Hershey, PA: IGI Global. doi:10.4018/978-1-61692-004-3.ch003

Misra, R. (2016). The benefits and challenges of using mobile-based tools in self-management and care. In A. Dwivedi (Ed.), *Reshaping medical practice and care with health information systems* (pp. 1–13). Hershey, PA: IGI Global. doi:10.4018/978-1-4666-9870-3.ch001

Mitra, S., & Padman, R. (2014). Engagement with social media platforms via mobile apps for improving quality of personal health management: A healthcare analytics case study. *Journal of Cases on Information Technology*, *16*(1), 73–89. doi:10.4018/jcit.2014010107

Miyanji, F. O., Newton, P., Samdani, A. F. A., Shah, S., Varghese, R. A., Reilly, C. W., & Mulpuri, K. (2015). The Impact of Surgical Waitlist Times on Scoliosis Surgery: The Surgeons Perspective. *The Spine Journal*, *40*(11), 823–828. doi:10.1097/BRS.0000000000000205 PMID:24430712

Moghimi, H., & Wickramasinghe, N. (2017). The development of a secure hospital messaging and communication platform. In N. Wickramasinghe (Ed.), *Handbook of research on healthcare administration and management* (pp. 243–267). Hershey, PA: IGI Global. doi:10.4018/978-1-5225-0920-2.ch015

Mohammed, J., Lung, C. H., Ocneanu, A., Thakral, A., Jones, C., & Adler, A. (2014, September). Internet of Things: Remote patient monitoring using web services and cloud computing. *Chest*, *149*(2), 576–585.

Monroe, C. M., Thompson, D. L., Bassett, D. R. Jr, Fitzhugh, E. C., & Raynor, H. A. (2015). Usability of Mobile Phones in Physical Activity–Related Research: A Systematic Review. *American Journal of Health Education*, *46*(4), 196–206. doi:10.1080/19325037.2015.1044141

Montes-Garcia, A., Alvarez-Rodriguez, J. M., Labra-Goyo, J. E., & Martinez-Merino, M. (2013). Towards a journalist-based news recommendation system : The Wesomender approach. *Expert Systems with Applications*, *40*(17), 6735–6741. doi:10.1016/j.eswa.2013.06.032

Moon, J. D., & Galea, M. P. (2017). Overview of clinical decision support systems in healthcare. In *Medical imaging: Concepts, methodologies, tools, and applications* (pp. 1501–1527). Hershey, PA: IGI Global. doi:10.4018/978-1-5225-0571-6.ch064

Morrell, T. G., & Kerschberg, L. (2012). Personal Health Explorer : A Semantic Health Recommendation System. In *Data Engineering Workshops (ICDEW), 2012 IEEE 28th International Conference on.* IEEE. doi:10.1109/ICDEW.2012.64

Morris, H., Liao, H., Padmanabhan, S., Srinivasan, S., Lau, P., Shan, J., & Wisnesky, R. (2008). Bringing Business Objects into Extract-transform-load (ETL) Technology. *IEEE International Conference on e-Business Engineering 2008*, 709–714. https://doi.org/10.1109/ICEBE.2008.72

Morrow, D. G., Conner-Garcia, T., Graumlich, J. F., Wolf, M. S., McKeever, S., Madison, A., & Kaiser, D. et al. (2012). An EMR-based tool to support collaborative planning for medication use among adults with diabetes: Design of a multi-site randomized control trial. *Contemporary Clinical Trials*, *33*(5), 1023–1032. doi:10.1016/j.cct.2012.05.010 PMID:22664648

Moscelli, G., Siciliani, L., & Tonei, V. (2016). Do Waiting Times affect Health Outcomes? Evidence from Coronary Bypass. *Social Science & Medicine*, *161*, 151–159. doi:10.1016/j.socscimed.2016.05.043 PMID:27299977

Moumtzoglou, A. S. (2016). The nexus of m-health and self-efficacy. In A. Moumtzoglou (Ed.), *M-health innovations for patient-centered care* (pp. 341–365). Hershey, PA: IGI Global. doi:10.4018/978-1-4666-9861-1.ch017

Moyer, J. E. (2013). Managing Mobile Devices in Hospitals: A Literature Review of BYOD Policies and Usage. *Journal of Hospital Librarianship*, *13*(3), 197–208. doi:10.1080/15323269.2013.798768

Muranaga, F., Kumamoto, I., & Uto, Y. (2007). Development of site data warehouse for cost analysis of DPC based on medical costs. *Methods of Information in Medicine*, *46*(6), 679–685. PMID:18066419

Murdoch, T. B., & Detsky, A. S. (2013). The inevitable application of big data to health care. *Journal of the American Medical Association*, *309*(13), 1351–1352. doi:10.1001/jama.2013.393 PMID:23549579

Murphy, J. (2010). Health science librarianship's legacy to health informatics. *Health Information and Libraries Journal*, *27*(1), 75–79. doi:10.1111/j.1471-1842.2010.00882.x PMID:20402807

Musen, M. A., Middleton, B., & Greenes, A. R. (2014). Clinical Decision-Support Systems. In *Biomedical Informatics* (pp. 643–674). Springer-Verlag London. https://doi.org/10.1001/jama.296.21.2624

MySQL. (2016). *MySQL Enterprise Edition.* Retrieved from https://www.mysql.com/products/enterprise/mysql-datasheet.en.pdf

Narasimhamurthy, A. (2017). An overview of machine learning in medical image analysis: Trends in health informatics. In *Medical imaging: Concepts, methodologies, tools, and applications* (pp. 36–58). Hershey, PA: IGI Global. doi:10.4018/978-1-5225-0571-6.ch002

Naseer, A., & Stergioulas, L. K. (2010). HealthGrids in health informatics: A taxonomy. In K. Khoumbati, Y. Dwivedi, A. Srivastava, & B. Lal (Eds.), *Handbook of research on advances in health informatics and electronic healthcare applications: Global adoption and impact of information communication technologies* (pp. 124–143). Hershey, PA: IGI Global. doi:10.4018/978-1-60566-030-1.ch008

Nassar, D. A., Othman, M., Hayajneh, J. A., & Ali, N. (2015). An integrated success model for an electronic health record: A case study of Hakeem Jordan. *Procedia Economics and Finance*, *23*, 95–103. doi:10.1016/S2212-5671(15)00526-2

Neff, G. (2013). Why big data won't cure us. *Big Data, 1*(3), 117-123.

Neves, J., Abelha, V., Vicente, H., Neves, J., & Machado, J. (2016). Length of Hospital Stay and Quality of Care. In Knowledge, Information and Creativity Support Systems (pp. 273-287). Springer International Publishing. doi:10.1007/978-3-319-27478-2_19

Ngai, E. W. T., & Yong Hu, Y. H. (2011). The application of data mining techniques in financial fraud detection: A classification framework and an academic review of literature. *Decision Support Systems, 50*(3), 559–569. doi:10.1016/j.dss.2010.08.006

Nguyen, L., Bellucci, E., & Nguyen, L. T. (2014). Electronic health records implementation: An evaluation of information system impact and contingency factors. *International Journal of Medical Informatics, 83*(11), 779–796. doi:10.1016/j.ijmedinf.2014.06.011 PMID:25085286

Nikou, S. (2015). Mobile technology and forgotten consumers: The young-elderly. *International Journal of Consumer Studies, 39*(4), 294–304. doi:10.1111/ijcs.12187

Nisha, N., Iqbal, M., Rifat, A., & Idrish, S. (2016). Mobile health services: A new paradigm for health care systems. In *E-health and telemedicine: Concepts, methodologies, tools, and applications* (pp. 1551–1567). Hershey, PA: IGI Global. doi:10.4018/978-1-4666-8756-1.ch078

Nitish Kirtiraj Shah, B. (n.d.). *Developing a decision support framework for planning and implementing Bring Your Own Device programmes in organizations, 2013–2015.* Academic Press.

Obiodu, V., & Obiodu, E. (2012). An Empirical Review of the Top 500 Medical Apps in a European Android Market. *Journal of Mobile Technology in Medicine, 1*(4), 22–37. doi:10.7309/jmtm.74

Ocano, S. G., Ramamurthy, B., & Wang, Y. (2015). Remote mobile screen (RMS): An approach for secure BYOD environments. In *2015 International Conference on Computing, Networking and Communications (ICNC)* (pp. 52–56). IEEE. https://doi.org/10.1109/ICCNC.2015.7069314

Oddershede, A. M., & Carrasco, R. A. (2008). Perception of mobile technology provision in health service. In W. Huang, Y. Wang, & J. Day (Eds.), *Global mobile commerce: Strategies, implementation and case studies* (pp. 345–364). Hershey, PA: IGI Global. doi:10.4018/978-1-59904-558-0.ch019

Odorico, J. S. (2014). Waiting List Management for Pancreas and Islet Transplantation. In A. D. Kirk, S. J. Knechtle, C. P. Larsen, J. C. Madsen, T. C. Pearson, & S. A. Webber (Eds.), *Textbook of Organ Transplantation* (1st ed.; pp. 482–488). John Wiley & Sons, Ltd. doi:10.1002/9781118873434.ch41

ODriscoll, A., Daugelaite, J., & Sleator, R. D. (2013). Big data, Hadoop and cloud computing in genomics. *Journal of Biomedical Informatics, 46*(5), 774–781. doi:10.1016/j.jbi.2013.07.001 PMID:23872175

Office of Civil Rights Department of Health and Human Services. (2003). *Summary of the HIPAA Privacy Rule.* OCR Privacy Brief. https://doi.org/10.1016/j.chroma.2005.11.119

Okuda, Y., Bryson, E. O., DeMaria, S., Jr., Jacobson, L., Quinones, J., Shen, B., & Levine, A. I. (2009). The utility of simulation in medical education: What is the evidence?. *Mount Sinai Journal of Medicine: A Journal of Translational and Personalized Medicine, 76*(4), 330–343. doi:10.1002/msj.20127

Oliveira, O. R. F. (2012). *Extração de Conhecimento nas Listas de Espera para Consulta e Cirurgia.* Universidade do Minho. Retrieved from http://repositorium.sdum.uminho.pt/handle/1822/23504

Oliveira, O. (2012). *Extração de Conhecimento nas Listas de Espera para Consulta e Cirurgia.* Braga, Portugal: Dissertação de Mestrado, Universidade do Minho.

Olla, P., & Tan, J. (2009). *Mobile health solutions for biomedical applications*. Hershey, PA: IGI Global. doi:10.4018/978-1-60566-332-6

Olszak, C., & Batko, K. (2012). Business intelligence systems. new chances and possibilities for healthcare organizations. *Informatyka Ekonomiczna*, 123-138.

OPSS Observatório Português dos Sistemas de Saúde. (2003). Saúde: que rupturas?. *Relatório de Primavera*, 1 – 124.

Oracle. (2016). *What Are RESTful Web Services?*. Retrieved September 14, 2016, from http://docs.oracle.com/javaee/6/tutorial/doc/gijqy.html

Orwat, C., Graefe, A., & Faulwasser, T. (2008). Towards pervasive computing in health care - a literature review. *BMC Medical Informatics and Decision Making*, *8*(1), 26. doi:10.1186/1472-6947-8-26 PMID:18565221

Osheroff, J. A., Teich, J. M., Middleton, B., Steen, E. B., Wright, A., & Detmer, D. E. (2007). A roadmap for national action on clinical decision support. *Journal of the American Medical Informatics Association*, *14*(2), 141–145. doi:10.1197/jamia.M2334 PMID:17213487

Osop, H., & Sahama, T. (2016). Data-driven and practice-based evidence: Design and development of efficient and effective clinical decision support system. In J. Moon & M. Galea (Eds.), *Improving health management through clinical decision support systems* (pp. 295–328). Hershey, PA: IGI Global. doi:10.4018/978-1-4666-9432-3.ch014

Pah, A., Rasmussen-Torvik, L., Goel, S., Greenland, P., & Kho, A. (2015). Big data: What is it and what does it mean for cardiovascular research and prevention policy. *Current Cardiovascular Risk Reports*, *9*(1), 1–9. doi:10.1007/s12170-014-0424-3

Paige, S. R., Stellefson, M., Chaney, B. H., & Alber, J. M. (2015). Pinterest as a resource for health information on Chronic Obstructive Pulmonary Disease (COPD): A social media content analysis. *American Journal of Health Education*, *46*(4), 241–251. doi:10.1080/19325037.2015.1044586

Palazzo, L., Sernani, P., Claudi, A., Dolcini, G., Biancucci, G., & Franco, A. F. (2013). A multi-agent architecture for health information systems. *International Workshop on Artificial Intelligence and NetMedicine*, 41.

Pang, Z. (2013). *Technologies and architectures of the internet-of-things (iot) for health and well-being*. Retrieved June 13, 2016, from http://kth.diva-portal.org/smash/get/diva2:621384/FULLTEXT01.pdf

Pang, Z., Zheng, L., Tian, J., Kao-Walter, S., Dubrova, E., & Chen, Q. (2015). Design of a terminal solution for integration of in-home health care devices and services towards the Internet-of-Things. *Enterprise Information Systems*, *9*(1), 86–116. doi:10.1080/17517575.2013.776118

Parry, D. (2012). Computerised decision support for women's health informatics. In *Machine learning: Concepts, methodologies, tools and applications* (pp. 1404–1416). Hershey, PA: IGI Global. doi:10.4018/978-1-60960-818-7.ch513

Parshutin, S., & Kirshners, A. (2013). Research on clinical decision support systems development for atrophic gastritis screening. *Expert Systems with Applications*, *40*(15), 6041–6046. doi:10.1016/j.eswa.2013.05.011

Parwekar, P., & Reddy, R. (2013). An efficient fuzzy localization approach in wireless sensor networks. *2013 IEEE International Conference* (pp. 1-6). IEEE. doi:10.1109/FUZZ-IEEE.2013.6622548

Pasupathy, K. S. (2011). Systems engineering and health informatics. In *Clinical technologies: Concepts, methodologies, tools and applications* (pp. 1684–1705). Hershey, PA: IGI Global. doi:10.4018/978-1-60960-561-2.ch606

Patterson, E. S., Zhang, J., Abbott, P., Gibbons, M. C., Lowry, Z. S., Quinn, T. M., & Brick, D. et al. (2013). Enhancing electronic health record usability in pediatric patient care: A scenario-based approach. *Joint Commission Journal on Quality and Patient Safety*, *39*(3), 129–135. doi:10.1016/S1553-7250(13)39019-9 PMID:23516763

Paul, M. J., & Dredze, M. (2011). You are what you Tweet: Analyzing Twitter for public health. *ICWSM*, *20*, 265–272.

Pautasso, C. (2009). RESTful Web service composition with BPEL for REST. *Data & Knowledge Engineering*, *68*(9), 851–866. doi:10.1016/j.datak.2009.02.016

Peffers, K., Tuunanen, T., Rothenberger, M. A., & Chatterjee, S. (2007). A Design Science Research Methodology for Information Systems Research. *Journal of Management Information Systems*, *24*(3), 45–77. doi:10.2753/MIS0742-1222240302

Peixoto, H., Machado, J., Neves, J., & Abelha, A. (2010). Semantic Interoperability and Health Records. *1st IMIA/IFIP Joint Symposium, E-Health 2010, IMIA; IFIP, E-HEALTH, IFIP Advances in Information and Communication Technology, 335.*

Peixoto, H., Santos, M., Abelha, A., & Machado, J. (2012, December). Intelligence in Interoperability with AIDA. In *International Symposium on Methodologies for Intelligent Systems* (pp. 264-273). Springer Berlin Heidelberg.

Peixoto, H., Machado, J., Neves, J., & Abelha, A. (2010). Semantic interoperability and health records. In *E-Health* (pp. 236–237). Springer Berlin Heidelberg. doi:10.1007/978-3-642-15515-4_30

Peixoto, H., Santos, M., Abelha, A., & Machado, J. (2012). Intelligence in interoperability with AIDA. *International Symposium on Methodologies for Intelligent Systems*, 264-273.

Pelargos, P. E., Nagasawa, D. T., Lagman, C., Tenn, S., Demos, J. V., Lee, S. J., … Yang, I. (2016). Utilizing virtual and augmented reality for educational and clinical enhancements in neurosurgery. *Journal of Clinical Neuroscience*. https://doi.org/10.1016/j.jocn.2016.09.002

Pereira, A., Portela, F., Santos, M. F., Abelha, A., & Machado, J. (2016). Pervasive business intelligence: A new trend in critical healthcare. *Procedia Computer Science, 98*, 362–367. doi:10.1016/j.procs.2016.09.055

Pereira, A., Portela, F., Santos, M. F., Machado, J., & Abelha, A. (2016). ScienceDirect Pervasive Business Intelligence: A new trend in Critical Healthcare. *Procedia Computer Science, 98*(98), 362–367. https://doi.org/10.1016/j.procs.2016.09.055

Pereira, P., Grilo, A., Rocha, F., Nunes, M., Casaca, A., & Chaudet, C. (2007). End-to-end reliability in wireless sensor networks: survey and research challenges. *EuroFGI Workshop on IP QoS and Traffic Control*, 67–74.

Pereira, S. R., & Paiva, P. B. (2011). A importância da Engenharia da Usabilidade para a Segurança de Sistemas Informatizados em Saúde. *Journal of Health Informatics*, *3*(3).

Perry, T. L., Tucker, T., Hudson, L. R., Gandy, W., Neftzger, A. L., & Hamar, G. B. (2008). The application of data mining techniques in health plan population management: A disease management approach. In J. Wang (Ed.), *Data warehousing and mining: Concepts, methodologies, tools, and applications* (pp. 1799–1809). Hershey, PA: IGI Global. doi:10.4018/978-1-59904-951-9.ch106

Peters, D. P., Havstad, K. M., Cushing, J., Tweedie, C., Fuentes, O., & Villanueva-Rosales, N. (2014). Harnessing the power of big data: Infusing the scientific method with machine learning to transform ecology. *Ecosphere*, *5*(6), 1–15. doi:10.1890/ES13-00359.1

Peverini, . (2000). Graphical user interface for a neonatal parenteral nutrition decision support system. *Proc. AMIA Symp.*, 650–654. PMID:11079964

Pfeiffer, P. N., Bohnert, K. M., Zivin, K., Yosef, M., Valenstein, M., Aikens, J. E., & Piette, J. D. (2015). Mobile health monitoring to characterize depression symptom trajectories in primary care. *Journal of Affective Disorders*, *174*, 281–286. doi:10.1016/j.jad.2014.11.040 PMID:25527999

Philips, Z., Ginnelly, L., Sculpher, M., Claxton, K., Golder, S., Riemsma, R., . . . Glanville, J. (2004). *Review of guidelines for good practice in decision-analytic modelling in health technology assessment*. Academic Press.

Piccini J.P., et al. (in press). Impact of remote monitoring on clinical events and associated health care utilization: A nationwide assessment. *Heart Rhythm*.

Pitsillides, A. (2006). DITIS: A collaborative virtual medical team for home healthcare of cancer patients M-Health. Springer.

Poenaru, E., & Poenaru, C. (2013, November). A structured approach of the Internet-of-Things eHealth use cases. In E-Health and Bioengineering Conference (EHB), 2013 (pp. 1-4). IEEE. doi:10.1109/EHB.2013.6707299

Pombo, N., Garcia, N., Bousson, K., & Felizardo, V. (2015). Machine learning approaches to automated medical decision support systems. In P. Vasant (Ed.), *Handbook of research on artificial intelligence techniques and algorithms* (pp. 183–203). Hershey, PA: IGI Global. doi:10.4018/978-1-4666-7258-1.ch006

Portela, F., Gago, P., Santos, M. F., Silva, A., Rua, F., Machado, J., & Neves, J. (2011). Knowledge Discovery For Pervasive And Real-Time Intelligent Knowledge Discovery for Pervasive and Real-time Intelligent Decision Support in Intensive Care Medicine. *Proceedings of KMIS 2011 – International Conference on Knowledge Management and Information Sharing*.

Portela, F., Santos, M. F., Silva, Á., Machado, J., Abelha, A., & Rua, F. (2014). Pervasive and Intelligent Decision Support in Intensive Medicine – The Complete Picture. In Lecture Notes in Computer Science (LNCS): Vol. 8649. Information Technology in Bio- and Medical Informatics (pp. 87-102). Springer.

Portela, F., Gago, P., Santos, M. F., Machado, J., Abelha, A., Silva, Á., & Rua, F. (2013). Implementing a pervasive real-time intelligent system for tracking critical events with intensive care patients. *International Journal of Healthcare Information Systems and Informatics*, *8*(4), 1–16. doi:10.4018/ijhisi.2013100101

Portela, F., Oliveira, S., Santos, M., Machado, J., & Abelha, A. (2015, December). A real-time intelligent system for tracking patient condition. In *Ambient Intelligence for Health* (pp. 91–97). Springer International Publishing. doi:10.1007/978-3-319-26508-7_9

Portela, F., Santos, M. F., Machado, J., Abelha, A., & Rua, F. (2017). Step Towards Pervasive Technology Assessment in Intensive Medicine. *International Journal of Reliable and Quality E-Healthcare*, *6*(2), 1–16. doi:10.4018/IJRQEH.2017040101

Portugal, G., Cunha, P., Valente, B., Feliciano, J., Lousinha, A., Alves, S., & Ferreira, R. C. et al. (2016). Influence of remote monitoring on long-term cardiovascular outcomes after cardioverter-defibrillator implantation. *International Journal of Cardiology*, *222*, 764–768. doi:10.1016/j.ijcard.2016.07.157 PMID:27521554

Power, B. I. (2017). *Guided Learning for Power BI*. Retrieved from https://powerbi.microsoft.com/en-us/documentation/powerbi-learning-0-0-what-is-power-bi/

Prescher, S. (2014). Wird Telemonitoring von Patienten mit chronischer Herzinsuffizienz angenommen?. *Dtsch Patienten*, *139*(16), 829–834.

Price, M. (2011). A bio-psycho-social review of usability methods and their applications in healthcare. In *Clinical technologies: Concepts, methodologies, tools and applications* (pp. 1874–1899). Hershey, PA: IGI Global. doi:10.4018/978-1-60960-561-2.ch704

Prokosch, H. U., & Ganslandt, T. (2009). Perspectives for medical informatics: Reusing the electronic medical record for clinical research. *Methods of Information in Medicine*, *48*(1), 38–44. PMID:19151882

Protti, D. (2008). A comparison of how Canada, England, and Denmark are managing their electronic health record journeys. In A. Kushniruk & E. Borycki (Eds.), *Human, social, and organizational aspects of health information systems* (pp. 203–218). Hershey, PA: IGI Global. doi:10.4018/978-1-59904-792-8.ch012

Pullen, T., & Al-Hakim, L. (2016). Shared electronic health records as innovation: An Australian case. In L. Al-Hakim, X. Wu, A. Koronios, & Y. Shou (Eds.), *Handbook of research on driving competitive advantage through sustainable, lean, and disruptive innovation* (pp. 500–533). Hershey, PA: IGI Global. doi:10.4018/978-1-5225-0135-0.ch021

Queirós, A., Silva, A. G., Ferreira, A., Caravau, H., Cerqueira, M., & Rocha, N. P. (2016). Assessing mobile applications considered medical devices. In M. Cruz-Cunha, I. Miranda, R. Martinho, & R. Rijo (Eds.), *Encyclopedia of e-health and telemedicine* (pp. 111–127). Hershey, PA: IGI Global. doi:10.4018/978-1-4666-9978-6.ch010

Raad, M. W., Sheltami, T., & Shakshuki, E. (2015). Ubiquitous Tele-health System for Elderly Patients with Alzheimers. *Procedia Computer Science*, *52*, 685–689. doi:10.1016/j.procs.2015.05.075

Raghupathi, W., & Raghupathi, V. (2014). Big Data Analytics in Healthcare: Promise and Potential. *Health Information Science and Systems, 2*, 3. https://doi.org/10.1186/2047-2501-2-3

Raghupathi, W. (2010). Designing clinical decision support systems in health care: A systemic view. In M. Hunter (Ed.), *Strategic information systems: Concepts, methodologies, tools, and applications* (pp. 652–661). Hershey, PA: IGI Global. doi:10.4018/978-1-60566-677-8.ch043

Raghupathi, W., & Raghupathi, V. (2014). Big data analytics in healthcare: Promise and potential. *Health Information Science and Systems*, *2*(1), 1. doi:10.1186/2047-2501-2-3 PMID:25825667

Rahman, R. M., & Md, F. R. (2011). Using and comparing different decision tree classification techniques for mining ICDDR,B Hospital Surveillance data. *Expert Systems with Applications*, *38*(9), 11421–11436. doi:10.1016/j.eswa.2011.03.015

Raja, U., Mitchell, T., Day, T., & Hardin, J. M. (2008). Text mining in healthcare. applications and opportunities. *Journal of Healthcare Information Management*, 52–56. PMID:19267032

Ranji, S. R., Rennke, S., & Wachter, R. M. (2014). Computerised provider order entry combined with clinical decision support systems to improve medication safety: A narrative review. *BMJ Quality & Safety*, *23*(9), 773–780. doi:10.1136/bmjqs-2013-002165 PMID:24728888

Ray, P. P. (2015, January). Internet of Things for Sports (IoTSport): An architectural framework for sports and recreational activity. In *Electrical, Electronics, Signals, Communication and Optimization (EESCO), 2015 International Conference on* (pp. 1-4). IEEE.

Rayport, J., & Heyward, A. (2011). *Envisioning the cloud: The next computing paradigm and its implication for technology policy*. Accessed May.

Redha, W., Hartwick, K., & Sikka, N. (2015). Mobile health in emergency care. In Z. Yan (Ed.), *Encyclopedia of mobile phone behavior* (pp. 825–838). Hershey, PA: IGI Global. doi:10.4018/978-1-4666-8239-9.ch068

Reed, S., Na, D., Mayo, T., Shapiro, L., Duty, B., Conklin, J., & Brown, D. (2010). Implementing and analyzing a data mart for the arlington county initiative to manage domestic violence offenders. *Proceedings of the 2010 IEEE Systems and Information Engineering Design Symposium*. doi:10.1109/SIEDS.2010.5469673

Ren, Y., Werner, R., Pazzi, N., & Boukerche, A. (2010). Monitoring patients via a secure and mobile healthcare system. *IEEE Wireless Commun.*, *17*(1), 59–65. doi:10.1109/MWC.2010.5416351

Reyes-Ortiz, J. L., Oneto, L., & Anguita, D. (2015). Big data analytics in the cloud: Spark on hadoop vs mpi/openmp on beowulf. *Procedia Computer Science*, *53*, 121–130. doi:10.1016/j.procs.2015.07.286

Rezende, S. O. (2003). *Sistemas inteligentes: fundamentos e aplicações*. Editora Manole Ltda.

Ribeiro, J., Alves, V., Silva, S., & Campos, J. (2015). *A 3D Computed Tomography Based Tool for Orthopedic Surgery Planning*. https://doi.org/10.1007/978-3-319-13407-9_8

Ricci, Rokach, Shapira, & Kantor. (2011). *Recommender systems handbook*. 10.1007/978-0-387-85820-3

Ries, N. M. (2011). Legal issues in health information and electronic health records. In *Clinical technologies: Concepts, methodologies, tools and applications* (pp. 1948–1961). Hershey, PA: IGI Global. doi:10.4018/978-1-60960-561-2.ch708

Rigby, M. (2014). The core vision of person-centred care in a modern information-based society. In I. Meyer, S. Müller, & L. Kubitschke (Eds.), *Achieving effective integrated e-care beyond the silos* (pp. 1–21). Hershey, PA: IGI Global. doi:10.4018/978-1-4666-6138-7.ch001

Rind, A., Wang, T. D., Aigner, W., Miksch, S., Wongsuphasawat, K., Plaisant, C., & Shneiderman, B. (2011). Interactive information visualization to explore and query electronic health records. *Foundations and Trends in Human-Computer Interaction*, *5*(3), 207–298. doi:10.1561/1100000039

Rivero-Rodríguez, A., Konstantinidis, S. T., Sanchez-Bocanegra, & Fernández-Luque, C. L. (2013). A Health Information Recommender System : enriching YouTube Health Videos with Medline Plus Information by the use of SnomedCT terms. *Proceedings of the 26th IEEE International Symposium on Computer-Based Medical Systems,* 257–261. doi:10.1109/CBMS.2013.6627798

Robson, B., & Baek, O. K. (2009). *The engines of Hippocrates: From the dawn of medicine to medical and pharmaceutical informatics*. Hoboken, NJ: John Wiley & Sons. doi:10.1002/9780470461808

Robson, B., & Boray, S. (2016). Data-mining to build a knowledge representation store for clinical decision support. Studies on curation and validation based on machine performance in multiple choice medical licensing examinations. *Computers in Biology and Medicine*, *73*, 71–93. doi:10.1016/j.compbiomed.2016.02.010 PMID:27089305

Röcker, C., Ziefle, M., & Holzinger, A. (2014). From computer innovation to human integration: current trends and challenges for pervasive Health Technologies. Pervasive Health, 1-17.

Rodrigues, F., Pereira, D., Nascimento, J. C., Ribeiro, J., Barros, P., Correia, R., . . . Gomes, R. (2013). *Interoperabilidade na Saúde - Onde Estamos?*. Retrieved from http://www.apdsi.pt/uploads/news/id719/Estudo_APDSI_Interoperabilidade_Sa%C3%BAde_completo.pdf

Romero, O., & Abelló, A. (2010). A framework for multidimensional design of data warehouses from ontologies. *Data & Knowledge Engineering*, *69*(11), 1138–1157. doi:10.1016/j.datak.2010.07.007

Rothman, B., Leonard, J. C., & Vigoda, M. M. (2012). Future of electronic health records: Implications for decision support. *Mount Sinai Journal of Medicine: A Journal of Translational and Personalized Medicine, 79*(6), 757–768. doi:10.1002/msj.21351

Rudge, C., Matesanz, R., Delmonico, F., & Chapman, J. (2012). International practices of organ donation. *British Journal of Anaesthesia, 108*(suppl 1), 48–55. doi:10.1093/bja/aer399 PMID:22194431

Ruiz-Fernandez, D., & Soriano-Paya, A. (2011). A distributed approach of a clinical decision support system based on cooperation. In *Clinical technologies: Concepts, methodologies, tools and applications* (pp. 1782–1799). Hershey, PA: IGI Global. doi:10.4018/978-1-60960-561-2.ch612

Ruiz, M. E., Suñol, M. M., Miguélez, J. R., Ortiz, E. S., Urroz, M. I., Camino, M. d., & Aloy, J. F. (2015). *Medication errors in a neonatal unit: One of the main adverse events. Anales de Pediatría.*

Saboor, S., Hörbst, A., & Ammenwerth, E. (2013). Modeling and automated examination of communication processes in integrated health information systems: A systematic approach. *International Journal of Knowledge-Based Organizations, 3*(1), 19–36. doi:10.4018/ijkbo.2013010102

Sagiroglu, S., & Sinanc, D. (2013). *Big data: A review.* Paper presented at the Collaboration Technologies and Systems (CTS), 2013 International Conference on. doi:10.1109/CTS.2013.6567202

Sako, Z. Z., Karpathiou, V., Adibi, S., & Wickramasinghe, N. (2017). Data accuracy considerations with mHealth. In N. Wickramasinghe (Ed.), *Handbook of research on healthcare administration and management* (pp. 1–15). Hershey, PA: IGI Global. doi:10.4018/978-1-5225-0920-2.ch001

Saleem, J. J., Russ, A. L., Justice, C. F., Hagg, H., Ebright, P. R., Woodbridge, P. A., & Doebbeling, B. N. (2009). Exploring the persistence of paper with the electronic health record. *International Journal of Medical Informatics, 78*(9), 618–628. doi:10.1016/j.ijmedinf.2009.04.001 PMID:19464231

Santos, M. Y., & Ramos, I. (2006). *Business Intelligence: Tecnologias da informação na gestão do conhecimento.* FCA-Editora de Informática.

Saranto, K., Jylhä, V., & Kinnunen, U. (2011). Are nurses prepared for engagement to evidence-based practice with new technologies? In A. Cashin & R. Cook (Eds.), *Evidence-based practice in nursing informatics: Concepts and applications* (pp. 98–112). Hershey, PA: IGI Global. doi:10.4018/978-1-60960-034-1.ch008

Sardini, E., & Serpelloni, M. (2010). Instrumented Wearable Belt for Wireless Health Monitoring. *Procedia Engineering, 5*, 580–583. doi:10.1016/j.proeng.2010.09.176

Satyanarayanan, M. (2001). Pervasive computing: Vision and challenges. *IEEE Personal Communications, 8*(4), 10-17.

Saxon, L. A., Hayes, D. L., Gilliam, F. R., Heidenreich, P. A., Day, J., Seth, M., & Boehmer, J. P. et al. (2010). Long-term outcome after ICD and CRT implantation and influence of remote device follow-up: The ALTITUDE survival study. *Circulation, 122*(23), 2359–2367. doi:10.1161/CIRCULATIONAHA.110.960633 PMID:21098452

Sayyad Shirabad, J., Wilk, S., Michalowski, W., & Farion, K. (2012). Implementing an Integrative Multi-agent Clinical Decision Support System with Open Source Software. *Journal of Medical Systems, 36*(1), 123–137. doi:10.1007/s10916-010-9452-9 PMID:20703742

Scarfo, A. (2012). New security perspectives around BYOD. In *Proceedings - 2012 7th International Conference on Broadband, Wireless Computing, Communication and Applications, BWCCA 2012* (pp. 446–451). IEEE. https://doi.org/10.1109/BWCCA.2012.79

Schmidt, B. (2006). Proof of Principle Studies. *Epilepsy Research, 68*(1), 48–52. doi:10.1016/j.eplepsyres.2005.09.019 PMID:16377153

Schmidt, H., Norman, G., & Boshuizen, H. (1990). A cognitive perspective on medical expertise: Theory and implication. *Academic Medicine, 65*(10), 611–621. doi:10.1097/00001888-199010000-00001 PMID:2261032

Schnall, R., & Iribarren, S. J. (2015). Review and analysis of existing mobile phone applications for health care–associated infection prevention. *American Journal of Infection Control*, *43*(6), 572–576. doi:10.1016/j.ajic.2015.01.021 PMID:25748924

Schnipper, J. L., Linder, J. A., Palchuk, M. B., Yu, D. T., McColgan, K. E., & Volk, L. A. et al.. (2010). Effects of documentation-based decision support on chronic disease management. *The American Journal of Managed Care*, *16*(12), SP72–SP81. PMID:21314226

Schoonen, A. J. M., Schmidt, F. J., Hasper, H., Verbrugge, D. A., Tiessen, R. G., & Lerk, C. F. (1990). Development of a potentially wearable glucose sensor for patients with diabetes mellitus : Design and in- vitro evaluation. *Biosensors & Bioelectronics*, *5*(1), 37–46. doi:10.1016/0956-5663(90)80025-9 PMID:2310541

Sebestyen, G., Hangan, A., Oniga, S., & Gál, Z. (2014, May). eHealth solutions in the context of Internet of Things. *Proc. IEEE Int. Conf. Automation, Quality and Testing, Robotics (AQTR 2014)*, 261-267. doi:10.1109/AQTR.2014.6857876

Secure Edge Networks, L. (n.d.). *7 Benefits of BYOD on Enterprise Wireless Networks*. Retrieved May 11, 2017, from http://www.securedgenetworks.com/blog/7-Benefits-of-BYOD-on-Enterprise-Wireless-Networks

Seidling, H. M., Klein, U., Schaier, M., Czock, D., Theile, D., Pruszydlo, M. G., & Haefeli, W. E. et al. (2014). What, if all alerts were specific – estimating the potential impact on drug interaction alert burden. *International Journal of Medical Informatics*, *83*(4), 285–291. doi:10.1016/j.ijmedinf.2013.12.006 PMID:24484781

Sen, J. (n.d.). Ubiquitous Computing: Applications, Challenges and Future Trends. In Embedded Systems and Wireless Technology: Theory and Practical Application. CRC Press.

Senathirajah, Y., Bakken, S., & Kaufman, D. (2014). The clinician in the driver's seat: Part 1 – A drag/drop user-composable electronic health record platform. *Journal of Biomedical Informatics*, *52*, 165–176. doi:10.1016/j.jbi.2014.09.002 PMID:25240253

Senkowski, V., & Branscum, P. (2015). How college students search the internet for weight control and weight management information: An observational study. *American Journal of Health Education*, *46*(4), 231–240. doi:10.1080/19325037.2015.1044139

Sergey, A. B., Alexandr, D. B., & Sergey, A. T. (2015). Proof of Concept Center — A Promising Tool for Innovative Development at Entrepreneurial Universities. *Procedia - Social and Behavioral Sciences*, *166*, 240–245. https://doi.org/10.1016/j.sbspro.2014.12.518

Sezgin, E., & Ozkan, S. (2013). A systematic literature review on Health Recommender Systems A Systematic Literature Review on Health Recommender Systems. *The 4th IEEE International Conference on E-Health and Bioengineering - EHB*. doi:<ALIGNMENT.qj></ALIGNMENT>10.1109/EHB.2013.6707249

Sezões, C., Oliveira, J., & Baptista, M. (2006). Business Intelligence. S.S. P. d. Inovação Ed. Porto.

Shachak, A., Hadas-Dayagi, M., Ziv, A., & Reis, S. (2009). Primary care physicians' use of an electronic medical record system: A cognitive task analysis. *Journal of General Internal Medicine*, *24*(3), 341–348. doi:10.1007/s11606-008-0892-6 PMID:19130148

Shareef, M. A., Ahmed, J. U., Kumar, V., & Kumar, U. (2015). Effect of mobile phone SMS on m-health: An analysis of consumer perceptions. In P. Thomas, M. Srihari, & S. Kaur (Eds.), *Handbook of research on cultural and economic impacts of the information society* (pp. 284–296). Hershey, PA: IGI Global. doi:10.4018/978-1-4666-8598-7.ch012

Shareef, M. A., Kumar, V., Kumar, U., & Hasin, A. A. (2013). Application of behavioral theory in predicting consumers adoption behavior. *Journal of Information Technology Research*, *6*(4), 36–54. doi:10.4018/jitr.2013100103

Sharmaa, S., & Reimer-Kirkhamb, S. (2015). Faith as social capital: Diasporic women negotiating religion in secularized healthcare services. *Womens Studies International Forum, 49*, 34–42. doi:10.1016/j.wsif.2015.01.005

Shea, S., DuMouchel, W., & Bahamonde, L. (1996). A meta-analysis of 16 randomized controlled trials to evaluate computer-based clinical reminder systems for preventive care in the ambulatory setting. *Journal of the American Medical Informatics Association, 3*(6), 399–409. doi:10.1136/jamia.1996.97084513 PMID:8930856

Shrestha, S. (2013). Clinical decision support system for diabetes prevention: An illustrative case. In S. Sarnikar, D. Bennett, & M. Gaynor (Eds.), *Cases on healthcare information technology for patient care management* (pp. 308–329). Hershey, PA: IGI Global. doi:10.4018/978-1-4666-2671-3.ch017

Shukla, A., & Tiwari, R. (2011). *Biomedical engineering and information systems: Technologies, tools and applications* (pp. 1–384). Hershey, PA: IGI Global. doi:10.4018/978-1-61692-004-3

Shukla, N., Keast, J., & Ceglarek, D. (2014). Modelling variations in hospital service delivery based on real time locating information. *Applied Mathematical Modelling, 38*(3), 878–893. doi:10.1016/j.apm.2013.07.024

Shvachko, K., Kuang, H., Radia, S., & Chansler, R. (2010). *The hadoop distributed file system.* Paper presented at the 2010 IEEE 26th symposium on mass storage systems and technologies (MSST). doi:10.1109/MSST.2010.5496972

Siau, K., & Shen, Z. (2006). Mobile healthcare informatics. *Medical Informatics and the Internet in Medicine, 31*(2), 89–99. doi:10.1080/14639230500095651 PMID:16777784

Siciliani, L., & Hurst, J. (2005). Tackling excessive waiting times for elective surgery: A comparative analysis of policies in 12 OECD countries. *Health Policy (Amsterdam), 72*(2), 201–215. doi:10.1016/j.healthpol.2004.07.003 PMID:15802155

Siddiqui, M., Islam, M. Y. U., Mufti, B. A. I., Khan, N., Farooq, M. S., Muhammad, M. G., & Kazi, A. M. et al. (2015). Assessing acceptability of hypertensive/diabetic patients towards mobile health based behavioral interventions in Pakistan: A pilot study. *International Journal of Medical Informatics, 84*(11), 950–955. doi:10.1016/j.ijmedinf.2015.08.009 PMID:26321485

Sieverink, F., Siemons, L., Braakman-Jansen, A., & Van Gemert-Pijnen, L. (2016). Internet of Things & Personalized Healthcare. *Studies in Health Technology and Informatics, 221*, 129. PMID:27071903

Silas, S., & Rajsingh, E. B. (2016). Performance analysis on algorithms for selection of desired healthcare services. *Perspectives on Science, 8*, 107–109. doi:10.1016/j.pisc.2016.04.009

Siltanen, S. (2012). Theory and applications of marker-based augmented reality. *Espoo 2012. VTT Science Series 3.* Retrieved from http://www.vtt.fi/publications/index.jsp

Silva, B. M. C., Rodrigues, J. J. P. C., de la Torre Diez, I., Lopez-Coronado, M., & Saleem, K. (2015). Mobile-health: A review of current state in 2015. *Journal of Biomedical Informatics, 56*, 265–272. doi:10.1016/j.jbi.2015.06.003 PMID:26071682

Singh, N., & Phil, M. (2012). B . Y . O . D . Genie Is Out Of the Bottle – " Devil Or Angel ". *Journal of Business Management & Social Sciences Research, 1*(3), 1–12.

Singh, N. (2012). BYOD genie is out of the bottle–"Devil or angel. *Journal of Business Management & Social Sciences Research, 1*(3), 1–12.

Skiba, D. J. (2014). The Connected Age: Big Data & Data Visualization. *Nursing Education Perspectives, 35*(4), 267–269. doi:10.5480/1536-5026-35.4.267 PMID:25158424

Skorin-Kapov, L., Dobrijevic, O., & Piplica, D. (2014). Towards evaluating the quality of experience of remote patient monitoring services: A study considering usability aspects. *International Journal of Mobile Human Computer Interaction, 6*(4), 59–89. doi:10.4018/ijmhci.2014100104

Škrobáčková, M., & Kopáčková, H. (2006). *Decision support systems or business intelligence: what can help in decision making?. Scientific papers of the University of Pardubice. Series D.* Faculty of Economics and Administration.

Sneed, W. (2011). A treatise on rural public health nursing. In *Clinical technologies: Concepts, methodologies, tools and applications* (pp. 2013–2028). Hershey, PA: IGI Global. doi:10.4018/978-1-60960-561-2.ch711

Sood, V. R., Gururajan, R., Hafeez-Baig, A., & Wickramasinghe, N. (2017). Adoption of mobile devices in the Australian healthcare: A conceptual framework approach. In N. Wickramasinghe (Ed.), *Handbook of research on healthcare administration and management* (pp. 662–685). Hershey, PA: IGI Global. doi:10.4018/978-1-5225-0920-2.ch040

Srivastava, S. K., & Ray, S. (2016). Disasters and Recommender System: Setting the Research Agenda for Developing Nations. *International Journal of Innovation, Management and Technology, 7*, 52–56. doi:10.18178/ijimt.2016.7.2.644

Stankovic, J. (2014). Research Directions for the Internet of Things. *Internet of Things Journal, 1*, 3-9.

Stavros, A., Vavoulidis, E., & Nasioutziki, M. (2016). The use of mobile health applications for quality control and accreditational purposes in a cytopathology laboratory. In A. Moumtzoglou (Ed.), *M-health innovations for patient-centered care* (pp. 262–283). Hershey, PA: IGI Global. doi:10.4018/978-1-4666-9861-1.ch013

Stolba, N., Nguyen, T. M., & Tjoa, A. M. (2010). Data warehouse facilitating evidence-based medicine. In T. Nguyen (Ed.), *Complex data warehousing and knowledge discovery for advanced retrieval development: Innovative methods and applications* (pp. 174–207). Hershey, PA: IGI Global. doi:10.4018/978-1-60566-748-5.ch008

Strachan, H., Murray, P., & Erdley, W. S. (2011). Nursing informatics history and its contributions to nursing knowledge. In A. Cashin & R. Cook (Eds.), *Evidence-based practice in nursing informatics: Concepts and applications* (pp. 78–97). Hershey, PA: IGI Global. doi:10.4018/978-1-60960-034-1.ch007

Strack, R. W., Orsini, M. M., Fearnow-Kenney, M., Herget, J., Milroy, J. J., & Wyrick, D. L. (2015). Developing a web-based tool using information and communication technologies to expand the reach and impact of Photovoice. *American Journal of Health Education, 46*(4), 192–195. doi:10.1080/19325037.2015.1044585 PMID:27642378

Stroetmann, K. A. (2013). Achieving the integrated and smart health and wellbeing paradigm: A call for policy research and action on governance and business models. *International Journal of Medical Informatics, 82*(4), e29–e37. doi:10.1016/j.ijmedinf.2012.05.008 PMID:22727880

Suchanek, F., & Weikum, G. (2013). Knowledge harvesting in the big-data era. *Proceedings of the 2013 ACM SIGMOD International Conference on Management of Data.* doi:10.1145/2463676.2463724

Sung, S.-F., Hsieh, C.-Y., Yang, Y.-H. K., Lin, H.-J., Chen, C.-H., Chen, Y.-W., & Hu, Y.-H. (2015). Developing a stroke severity index based on administrative data was feasible using data mining techniques. *Journal of Clinical Epidemiology, 68*(11), 1292–1300. doi:10.1016/j.jclinepi.2015.01.009 PMID:25700940

Swan, M. (2013). The quantified self: Fundamental disruption in big data science and biological discovery. *Big Data, 1*(2), 85-99.

Swanson, D. R., & Smalheiser, N. R. (1997). An interactive system for finding complementary literatures: A stimulus to scientific discovery. *Artificial Intelligence, 91*(2), 183–203. doi:10.1016/S0004-3702(97)00008-8

Sweeney, R.M., McAuley, D.F. (in press). Acute respiratory distress syndrome. *Lancet.*

Świątek, P., & Rucinski, A. (2013, October). IoT as a service system for eHealth. In *e-Health Networking, Applications & Services (Healthcom), 2013 IEEE 15th International Conference on* (pp. 81-84). IEEE. doi:10.1109/HealthCom.2013.6720643

Tabish, R., Ghaleb, A. M., Hussein, R., Touati, F., Mnaouer, A. B., Khriji, L., & Rasid, M. F. A. (2014, February). A 3G/WiFi-enabled 6LoWPAN-based U-healthcare system for ubiquitous real-time monitoring and data logging. In *2nd Middle East Conference on Biomedical Engineering* (pp. 277-280). IEEE doi:10.1109/MECBME.2014.6783258

Tam, N. T., & Song, I. (2016). *Big Data Visualization. In Information Science and Applications (ICISA) 2016* (pp. 399–408). Springer. doi:10.1007/978-981-10-0557-2_40

Tamposis, I., Pouliakis, A., Fezoulidis, I., & Karakitsos, P. (2017). Mobile platforms supporting health professionals: Need, technical requirements, and applications. In *Medical imaging: Concepts, methodologies, tools, and applications* (pp. 1020–1043). Hershey, PA: IGI Global. doi:10.4018/978-1-5225-0571-6.ch041

Tatarchuk, N., Shopf, J., & DeCoro, C. (2008). Advanced interactive medical visualization on the GPU. *Journal of Parallel and Distributed Computing*, *68*(10), 1319–1328. doi:10.1016/j.jpdc.2008.06.011

Technology, C. U. (2015). Pediatric Aspects of Inpatient Health Information Technology Systems. *Pediatrics, 135*(3), 756–768.

Testa, A., Coronato, A., Cinque, M., & de Pietro, G. (2016). Services and monitors for dependability assessment of mobile health monitoring systems. In *E-health and telemedicine: Concepts, methodologies, tools, and applications* (pp. 602–618). Hershey, PA: IGI Global. doi:10.4018/978-1-4666-8756-1.ch030

Thabit, H., Bally, L., & Hovorka, R. (in press). Available at a flash: a new way to check glucose. *Lancet.*

Thalhammer, T., Schrefl, M., & Mohania, M. (2001). Active data warehouses: Complementing olap with analysis rules. *Data & Knowledge Engineering*, *39*(3), 241–269. doi:10.1016/S0169-023X(01)00042-8

The Impact of BYOD on Healthcare Providers and Hospitals. (2017). Retrieved March 29, 2017, from http://mhealthintelligence.com/features/the-impact-of-byod-on-healthcare-providers-and-hospitals

Thomas, D. J. (2016). Augmented reality in surgery: The Computer-Aided Medicine revolution. *International Journal of Surgery*, *36*(October), 25. doi:10.1016/j.ijsu.2016.10.003 PMID:27741424

Thomas, J., & Kielman, J. (2009). Challenges for visual analytics. *Information Visualization*, *8*(4), 309–314. doi:10.1057/ivs.2009.26

Thorvaldsdóttir, H., Robinson, J. T., & Mesirov, J. P. (2013). Integrative Genomics Viewer (IGV): High-performance genomics data visualization and exploration. *Briefings in Bioinformatics*, *14*(2), 178–192. doi:10.1093/bib/bbs017 PMID:22517427

Timmerer, C., Ebrahimi, T., & Pereira, F. (2015). Toward a new assessment of quality. *Computer*, *48*(3), 108–110. doi:10.1109/MC.2015.89

Tin, E. E., Cummings, E., & Borycki, E. (2014). Review of the consumer perspective framework for healthcare applications. In M. Househ, E. Borycki, & A. Kushniruk (Eds.), *Social media and mobile technologies for healthcare* (pp. 1–15). Hershey, PA: IGI Global. doi:10.4018/978-1-4666-6150-9.ch001

Treurnicht, M. J., & van Dyk, L. (2012). Clinical-pull approach to telemedicine implementation policies using health informatics in the developing world. In J. Rodrigues, I. de la Torre Díez, & B. Sainz de Abajo (Eds.), *Telemedicine and e-health services, policies, and applications: Advancements and developments* (pp. 424–450). Hershey, PA: IGI Global. doi:10.4018/978-1-4666-0888-7.ch016

Trujillo, J., & Maté, A. (2012). Business Intelligence 2.0: A General Overview. *Lecture Notes in Business Information Processing, 96*, 98–116. https://doi.org/10.1007/978-3-642-27358-2_5

Tsai, C. Y., Wang, S. H., Hsu, M. H., & Li, Y. C. (2016). Do false positive alerts in naïve clinical decision support system lead to false adoption by physicians? A randomized controlled trial. *Computer Methods and Programs in Biomedicine, 132*, 82–91. doi:10.1016/j.cmpb.2016.04.011 PMID:27282230

Turban, E., Rainer, R., & Potter, R. (2005). *Introduction to information technology.* Academic Press.

Turban, E., Aronson, J., & Liang, T.-P. (2005). *Decision Support Systems and Intelligent Systems* (7th ed.). Pearson Prentice Hall.

Turban, E., Sharda, R., & Delen, D. (2011). *Decision support and business intelligence systems.* Pearson Education India.

UE. (2012). *eHealth Action Plan 2012-2020-Innovative healthcare for the 21st century.* UE.

UNICEF, WHO, & The World Bank Group. (2016). *Levels and trends in child Malnutrition.* Retrieved from http://www.who.int/nutgrowthdb/jme_brochure2016.pdf?ua=1

UNICEF. (2006). *Nutrition, survival and development.* Retrieved from https://www.unicef.org/progressforchildren/2006n4/index_undernutrition.html

Uramoto, N., Matsuzawa, H., Nagano, T., Murakami, A., Takeuchi, H., & Takeda, K. (2004). A text-mining system for knowledge discovery from biomedical documents. *IBM Systems Journal, 43*(3), 516–533. doi:10.1147/sj.433.0516

Vaishnavi, V. K., & Kuechler, W. (2015). *Design Science Research Methods and Patterns: Innovating Information and Communication Technology* (2nd ed.). CRC Press. Retrieved from https://books.google.pt/books?hl=pt-PT&lr=&id=OOE_CQAAQBAJ&oi=fnd&pg=PP1&dq=Design+science+research+methods+and+patterns:+innovating+information+and+communication+technology&ots=ZFBpZsW9gs&sig=wGD5o_q96t1Z_xZqHKYxjOOUSpo&redir_esc=y#v=onepage&q=Designsci

Vaitsis, C., Nilsson, G., & Zary, N. (2014). Visual analytics in healthcare education: Exploring novel ways to analyze and represent big data in undergraduate medical education. *PeerJ, 2*, e683. doi:10.7717/peerj.683 PMID:25469323

van der Valk, S., Myers, T., Atkinson, I., & Mohring, K. (2015, April). Sensor networks in workplaces: Correlating comfort and productivity. In *Intelligent Sensors, Sensor Networks and Information Processing (ISSNIP), 2015 IEEE Tenth International Conference on* (pp. 1-6). IEEE.

Varma, N., Piccini, J. P., Snell, J., Fischer, A., Dalal, N., & Mittal, S. (2015). Relationship between level of adherence to automatic wireless remote monitoring and survival in pacemaker and defibrillator patients. *Journal of the American College of Cardiology, 65*(24), 2601–2610. doi:10.1016/j.jacc.2015.04.033 PMID:25983008

Varshney, U. (2003). Pervasive healthcare. *IEEE Computer, 36*(12), 138–140. doi:10.1109/MC.2003.1250897

Varshney, U. (2005). Pervasive healthcare: Applications, challenges and wireless solutions. *Communications of the Association for Information Systems, 16*(1).

Varshney, U. (2007). Pervasive healthcare and wireless health monitoring. *Mobile Networks and Applications, 12*(2–3), 113–127. doi:10.1007/s11036-007-0017-1

Varshney, U. (2009). *Pervasive healthcare computing: EMR/EHR, wireless and health monitoring.* Springer Science & Business Media. doi:10.1007/978-1-4419-0215-3

Vassiliadis, P., Simitsis, A., & Baikousi, E. (2009). A taxonomy of ETL activities. In *Proceedings of the ACM twelfth international workshop on Data warehousing and OLAP* (pp. 25-32). ACM.

Vatovec, E. (2011). *Intelligent Value Chain Networks: Business Intelligence and Other ICT Tools and Technologies in Supply/Demand Chains.* Supply Chain Management - New Perspectives.

Ventola, C. L. (2014). Mobile devices and apps for health care professionals: uses and benefits. *P & T, 39*(5), 356–64. Retrieved from http://www.pubmedcentral.nih.gov/articlerender.fcgi?artid=4029126&tool=pmcentrez&rendertype=abstract

Vermesan, O., Friess, P., Guillemin, P., Gusmeroli, S., Sundmaeker, H., Bassi, A., et al. (2011). *Internet of Things: Global Technological and Societal Trends 1.* Academic Press.

Vervloet, M., Van Dijk, L., Santen-reestman, J., Van Vlijmen, B., Bouvy, M. L., & De Bakker, D. H. (2011). Improving medication adherence in diabetes type 2 patients through Real-time Medication Monitoring : A Randomised Controlled Trial to evaluate the effect of monitoring patients ' medication use combined with short message service (SMS) reminders. *BMC Health Services Research, 11*(1), 1. doi:10.1186/1472-6963-11-5 PMID:21199575

Vervloet, M., Van Dijk, L., Van Vlijmen, B., Van Wingerden, P., Bouvy, M. L., & De Bakker, D. H. (2012). SMS reminders improve adherence to oral medication in type 2 diabetes patients who are real-time electronically monitored. *International Journal of Medical Informatics, 81*(9), 594–604. doi:10.1016/j.ijmedinf.2012.05.005 PMID:22652012

Vidal-Petiot, E., et al. (in press). Cardiovascular event rates and mortality according to achieved systolic and diastolic blood pressure in patients with stable coronary artery disease: an international cohort study. *Lancet.*

Vincent, G. K., & Velkof, V. A. (2010). *The Older Population in the United States: 2010 to 2050: Population Estimates and Projections.* New York: United States Census Bureau.

Vuk, J., Anders, M. E., Mercado, C. C., Kennedy, R. L., Casella, J., & Steelman, S. C. (2015). Impact of simulation training on self-efficacy of outpatient health care providers to use electronic health records. *International Journal of Medical Informatics, 84*(6), 423–429. doi:10.1016/j.ijmedinf.2015.02.003 PMID:25746460

Walji, M. F., Kalenderian, E., Tran, D., Kookal, K. K., Nguyen, V., Tokede, O., & Stark, P. C. et al. (2013). Detection and characterization of usability problems in structured data entry interfaces in dentistry. *International Journal of Medical Informatics, 82*(2), 128–138. doi:10.1016/j.ijmedinf.2012.05.018 PMID:22749840

Walji, M. F., Taylor, D., Langabeer, J. R., & Valenza, J. A. (2009). Factors influencing implementation and outcomes of a dental electronic patient record system. *Journal of Dental Education, 73*(5), 589–600. PMID:19433534

Wang, Y., Wei, J., & Vangury, K. (2014). Bring your own device security issues and challenges. *2014 IEEE 11th Consumer Communications and Networking Conference (CCNC)*, 80–85. https://doi.org/10.1109/CCNC.2014.6866552

Wangberg, S. C., Arsand, E., & Andersson, N. (2006). Diabetes education via mobile text messaging. *Journal of Telemedicine and Telecare, 12*(S1), 55–56. doi:10.1258/135763306777978515 PMID:16884582

Wang, S. L., Chen, Y. L., Kuo, A. M. H., Chen, H. M., & Shiu, Y. S. (2016). Design and evaluation of a cloud-based mobile health information recommendation system on wireless sensor networks. *Computers & Electrical Engineering, 49*, 221–235. doi:10.1016/j.compeleceng.2015.07.017

Wang, T. D., Wongsuphasawat, K., Plaisant, C., & Shneiderman, B. (2011). Extracting insights from electronic health records: Case studies, a visual analytics process model, and design recommendations. *Journal of Medical Systems, 35*(5), 1135–1152. doi:10.1007/s10916-011-9718-x PMID:21541691

Wendel, S., Dellaert, B. G. C., Ronteltap, A., & Van Trijp, H. C. M. (2013). Consumers' intention to use health recommendation systems to receive personalized nutrition advice. *BMC Health Services Research, 13*(1), 126. doi:10.1186/1472-6963-13-126 PMID:23557363

Wen-ying, S. C., Hunt, Y. M., Beckjord, E. B., Moser, R. P., & Hesse, B. W. (2009). Social media use in the United States: Implications for health communication. *Journal of Medical Internet Research, 11*(4), e48. doi:10.2196/jmir.1249 PMID:19945947

White, J. V., Guenter, P., Jensen, G., Malone, A., & Schofield, M. (2012). Consensus statement of the Academy of Nutrition and Dietetics/American Society for Parenteral and Enteral Nutrition: Characteristics recommended for the identification and documentation of adult malnutrition (undernutrition). *Journal of the Academy of Nutrition and Dietetics, 112*(5), 730–738. doi:10.1016/j.jand.2012.03.012 PMID:22709779

Whittaker, A. A., Aufdenkamp, M., & Tinley, S. (2009). Barriers and facilitators to electronic documentation in a rural hospital. *Journal of Nursing Scholarship, 41*(3), 293–300. doi:10.1111/j.1547-5069.2009.01278.x PMID:19723278

WHO. (2016). *Global Health Observatory indicator views.* Retrieved from http://apps.who.int/gho/data/node.imr.NCD_BMI_30A?lang=en

WHO. (2017). *Body mass index - BMI.* Retrieved from http://www.euro.who.int/en/health-topics/disease-prevention/nutrition/a-healthy-lifestyle/body-mass-index-bmi

WHO. (n.d.). *Glossary.* Obtido em 01 de 2017, de World Health Organization: http://www.who.int/trade/glossary/story021/en/

Wickramasinghe, N., & Goldberg, S. (2007). The Wi-INET model for achieving m-health success. In D. Taniar (Ed.), *Encyclopedia of mobile computing and commerce* (pp. 1004–1010). Hershey, PA: IGI Global. doi:10.4018/978-1-59904-002-8.ch168

Wieder, B., & Ossimitz, M. (2015). The impact of Business Intelligence on the quality of decision making – a mediation model. *Procedia Computer Science Conference, 64*, 1163 – 1171.

Wiesner, M., & Pfeifer, D. (2014). Health recommender systems: Concepts, requirements, technical basics and challenges. *International Journal of Environmental Research and Public Health, 11*(3), 2580–2607. doi:10.3390/ijerph110302580 PMID:24595212

Wimmer, H., Yoon, V. Y., & Sugumaran, V. (2016). A multi-agent system to support evidence based medicine and clinical decision making via data sharing and data privacy. *Decision Support Systems, 88*, 51–66. doi:10.1016/j.dss.2016.05.008

Woltmann, E., Grogan-Kaylor, A., Perron, B., Georges, H., Kilbourne, A. M., & Bauer, M. S. (2012). Comparative effectiveness of collaborative chronic care models for mental health conditions across primary, specialty, and behavioral healthcare settings: Systematic review and meta-analysis. *The American Journal of Psychiatry, 169*(8), 790–804. doi:10.1176/appi.ajp.2012.11111616 PMID:22772364

Wright, H., Mathers, C., & Walton, J. (2013). Using visualization for visualization: An ecological interface design approach to inputting data. *Computers & Graphics, 37*(3), 202–213. doi:10.1016/j.cag.2013.01.013

Wu, J. (2013). *Biomedical engineering and cognitive neuroscience for healthcare: Interdisciplinary applications* (pp. 1–472). Hershey, PA: IGI Global. doi:10.4018/978-1-4666-2113-8

Wu, M., Lu, T., Ling, F., Sun, J., & Du, H. (2010). Research on the architecture of Internet of things. *3rd International Conference Advanced Computer Theory and Engineering (ICACTE)*, 484-485.

Wyber, R., Vaillancourt, S., Perry, W., Mannava, P., Folaranmi, T., & Celi, L. A. (2015). Big data in global health: Improving health in low-and middle-income countries. *Bulletin of the World Health Organization, 93*(3), 203–208. doi:10.2471/BLT.14.139022 PMID:25767300

Xia, F., Yang, L. T., Wang, L., & Vinel, A. (2012). Internet of things. *International Journal of Communication Systems*, *25*(9), 1101–1102. doi:10.1002/dac.2417

Xue, X., Li, G., Liu, L., & Liu, M. (2012). Perspectives on Internet of Things and Its Applications. In *2nd International Conference on Computer Application and System Modeling*. Atlantis Press. doi:10.2991/iccasm.2012.6

Yadav, N., Aliasgari, M., & Poellabauer, C. (2016). Mobile healthcare in an increasingly connected developing world. *International Journal of Privacy and Health Information Management*, *4*(2), 76–97. doi:10.4018/IJPHIM.2016070106

Yang, G., Xie, L., Mäntysalo, M., Zhou, X., Pang, Z., Da Xu, L., ... Zheng, L. R. (2014). A health-IoT platform based on the integration of intelligent packaging, unobtrusive bio-sensor, and intelligent medicine box. *IEEE Transactions on Industrial Informatics*, *10*(4), 2180-2191.

Yang, C. T., Liu, J. C., Liao, C. J., Wu, C. C., & Le, F. Y. (2013, December). On Construction of an Intelligent Environmental Monitoring System for Healthcare. In *2013 International Conference on Parallel and Distributed Computing, Applications and Technologies* (pp. 246-253). IEEE. doi:10.1109/PDCAT.2013.45

Yang, Y., Zhang, L., Zhen, Y., & Ji, R. (2015). Learning for visual semantic understanding in big data. *Neurocomputing*, (169): 1–4.

Yao, Q., Tian, Y., Li, P.-F., Tian, L.-L., Qian, Y.-M., & Li, J.-S. (2015). Design and development of a medical big data processing system based on hadoop. *Journal of Medical Systems*, *39*(3), 1–11. doi:10.1007/s10916-015-0220-8 PMID:25666927

Yeha, J.-Y., Wub, T.-H., & Tsaoa, C.-W. (2011). Using data mining techniques to predict hospitalization of hemodialysis patients. *Decision Support Systems*, *50*(2), 439–448. doi:10.1016/j.dss.2010.11.001

Yinong, C. (2016). Analyzing and visual programming internet of things and autonomous decentralized systems. *Simulation Modelling Practice and Theory*, *65*, 1–10. doi:10.1016/j.simpat.2016.05.002

Yoo, K. L. (2002). Issues and challenges in ubiquitous computing. *Introduction. Commun. ACM*, *45*(12), 62–65.

Young, S. D. (2015). A big data approach to HIV epidemiology and prevention. *Preventive Medicine*, *70*, 17–18. doi:10.1016/j.ypmed.2014.11.002 PMID:25449693

Yuehong, Y. I. N. (2016). The internet of things in healthcare: An overview. *Journal of Industrial Information Integration*, *1*, 3–13. doi:10.1016/j.jii.2016.03.004

Zaheer, S. (2014). Implementation of evidence-based practice and the PARIHS framework. In C. El Morr (Ed.), *Research perspectives on the role of informatics in health policy and management* (pp. 19–36). Hershey, PA: IGI Global. doi:10.4018/978-1-4666-4321-5.ch002

Zanchetti, A., Thomopoulos, C., & Parati, G. (2015). Randomized controlled trials of blood pressure lowering in hypertension: A critical reappraisal. *Circulation Research*, *116*(6), 1058–1073. doi:10.1161/CIRCRESAHA.116.303641 PMID:25767290

Zandomenighi, R. C., Mouro, D. L., Oliveira, C. A., & Martins, E. A. P. (2014). Cuidados intensivos em um serviço hospitalar de emergência: Desafios para os enfermeiros. REME rev. min. *Enferm*, *18*(2), 404–414.

Zaverucha, G. M., & Cercone, N. (2007). Web Based Health Recommender System Using Rough Sets, Survival Analysis and Rule Based Expert Systems. In *Rough Sets* (pp. 491–499). Fuzzy Sets, Data Mining and Granular Computing.

Zhang, J., & Walji, M. (2011). TURF: Toward a unified framework of EHR usability. *Journal of Biomedical Informatics*, *44*(6), 1056–1067. doi:10.1016/j.jbi.2011.08.005 PMID:21867774

Zhang, J., Wolfram, D., Wang, P., Hong, Y., & Gillis, R. (2008). Visualization of health-subject analysis based on query term co-occurrences. *Journal of the American Society for Information Science and Technology*, *59*(12), 1933–1947. doi:10.1002/asi.20911

Zhang, Y., Yu, P., & Shen, J. (2012). The benefits of introducing electronic health records in residential aged care facilities: A multiple case study. *International Journal of Medical Informatics*, *81*(10), 690–704. doi:10.1016/j.ijmedinf.2012.05.013 PMID:22749424

Zhou, X., Han, H., Chankai, I., Prestrud, A., & Brooks, A. (2006). Approaches to text mining for clinical medical records. *Proceedings of the 2006 ACM symposium on Applied computing*, 235-239. doi:10.1145/1141277.1141330

Zolfo, M. (n.d.). *How to weight BYOD benefits and risks*. Academic Press.

Zuehlke, P., Li, J., Talaei-Khoei, A., & Ray, P. (2009). *A functional specification for mobile eHealth (mHealth) systems*. Paper presented at the 11th International Conference on e-Health Networking, Applications and Services (Healthcom 2009), Sydney, Australia.

About the Contributors

José Machado is an Associate Professor with Habilitation in the Department of Informatics, Universidade do Minho. He got his PhD in Informatics, in 2002, and Habilitation in 2011. He is a researcher of the ALGORITMI research centre, in the line Computer Science and Technology (CST) and the group Knowledge and Data Engineering (KDE). He is the coordinator of the CST. His research interests span the domain of Biomedical Informatics, Electronic Health Records, Interoperability, Databases, Business Intelligence and Applied Artificial Intelligence. He is the header of the CST since 2015 and the director of the former Computer Science and Technology Center since September 2013.

António Abelha is an Assistant Professor at the Department of Informatics of the University of Minho, in Braga, Portugal. He got his PhD in 2004. He is a member of ALGORITMI research centre and co-founder of the Knowledge and Data Engineering Lab. His research interests span the domain of Knowledge and Data Engineering, Health Informatics and Artificial Intelligence. He is the author of over 150 papers in international books, journals and conference proceedings.

Manuel Filipe Santos received his Ph.D. in Computer Science (Artificial Intelligence) from the University of Minho (UMinho), Portugal, in 2000. He is associate professor with habilitation at the Department of Information Systems, UMinho, teaching undergraduate and graduate classes of Business Intelligence and Decision Support Systems. He is the head of Intelligent Data Systems group (www.algoritmi.uminho.pt) and coordinator of Healthy and Secure People thematic strand (http://algoritmi.uminho.pt/ts-healthy) of the R&D Algoritmi Centre, with the current research interests: Business Intelligence and Decision Support Systems; Data Mining and Machine Learning (Learning Classifier Systems); Grid Data Mining.

Carlos Filipe Portela went to the University of Minho in Guimarães, where he studied information system and obtained his degree in 2007 (Lic), 2009 (MSc) and 2013 (PhD). He holds a PhD in Information Systems and Technologies in 2013. He belongs to the Research Centre ALGORITMI where he is developing his post-doctoral research work in the topic "Pervasive Intelligent Decision Support Systems". His research was started in the INTCare R&D project (Intensive Medicine area) being then extended to education and public administration areas. He already has relevant indexed publications in the main research topics: Intelligent Decision Support Systems, Intelligent Systems, Pervasive Data, Business Intelligence, Data Mining and Knowledge Discovery. He has also been co-organizer of several workshops and reviewer of many indexed journals and conferences in these topics. Currently he also is an Invited Assistant Professor of the Information Systems Department, School of Engineering, University of Minho, Portugal, where he has been supervising several master students in the areas above mentioned and a Guest Lecturer in Porto Polytechnic - ESMAD. He is always in a continuing looking for opportunities to research and innovation in the society.

* * *

Victor Alves is an assistant professor in the Department of Informatics at University of Minho, Portugal, member of the Algoritmi Centre, performing his research activities within the Computer Science and Technologies (CST) R&D line in the area of biomedical engineering, particularly in medical imaging.

Gibeon Aquino holds a Ph.D in Computer Science from Federal University of Pernambuco (UFPE) in 2010, with thesis in the area of Software Engineering. He has background in Software Architecture, especially in Enterprise Information Systems and more recently in Mobile Applications. Before joining UFRN in August 2010 he worked at the Center of Studies and Advanced Systems of Recife (CESAR) as Software Architect of several systems for more than 10 years. His current research interest involve mobile and ubiquitous computing, Internet of Things and Smart Cities. He teaches undergraduate and postgraduate courses including Mobile Programming, Software Configuration Management and Software Architecture. Currently, he is the Head of Systems Division at UFRN, being responsible for the development and maintenance of important systems like SIGAA, SIPAC and SIGRH, which are used by several public organisations in Brazil.

Itamir Barroca is Professor at the Digital Metropole Institute of Federal University of Rio Grande do Norte, computer engineer with emphasis on computer systems. Master in systems and computing and expert on computer networks. He worked in the development of systems using the Java EE platform and mobile computing. Currently, he is the Director of Information Technology of Digital Metropole Institute.

Jaime Campos graduated in Informatics for Healthcare at IPCA (Instituto Politécnico do Cávado e do Ave). His academic career allowed him to acquire skills in computer engineering, health sciences and healthcare facilities' management. He took part in multiple projects related to the application of technological systems in healthcare. The MindCompanion project stands out among them and it was ranked third in the Microsoft ImagineCup idea contest nationally. Started his career as a software developer being now CTO at Peek Health S.A.

Joyram Chakraborty is a Human Factors Engineer and an Assistant Professor in the Department of Computer and Information Science at Towson University. His current work concerns the internationalization of interfaces design, cross cultural game design and the standardization of health care records. This work relies heavily upon the use of cognitive theories of decision-making. Dr. Chakraborty has conducted several usability studies into cross cultural gaming strategy to design more culturally inclusive video games. His collaborative works have been accepted in several peer reviewed journals and have also resulted in a patent with IBM Research. Dr. Chakraborty has also studied automated speech recognition (ASR) systems. This work investigated the use of cross cultural behavior patterns to establish a cognitive framework to develop learning algorithms to support data centers. He has also investigated the cognitive processes that are involved in designing, comprehending, and maintaining user interfaces for Tele-health devices in the support of Emergency Medical Technicians (EMT). Dr. Chakraborty is currently collaborating with The Johns Hopkins University School of Public Health and the Bloomberg Foundation to improve user experiences in m-heath interventions. In addition, he is currently working on an Army Research Laboratory grant to develop algorithms based on user preferences.

Inês Dias is a student of the Master degree in Biomedical Engineer with long interest in Electronic Health Records and Health Information Systems. Worked in several projects involving different areas such as Relational Databases, Applications for Clinical Management, Medical Inventory Management, Internet of People, Learning Systems and Knowledge Extraction, Multi-agent System, Data Mining, Business Intelligence, Image Processing, Operating Systems, Ontologies, Object Oriented Programming, Medical Image, Artificial Intelligence.

Marisa Esteves is currently a researcher in Algoritmi Research Centre at the University of Minho (UMinho), in Braga, Portugal, and in an Innovative Car HMI Program project resulting from the partnership between UMinho and Bosch Car Multimédia Portugal S.A. She recently concluded her Master's Degree in Biomedical Engineering at UMinho, specializing in Medical Informatics, and thereafter became a PhD student in the Doctoral Program in Biomedical Engineering at UMinho.

Bruno Fernandes was born in Guimarães, Portugal and obtained a MSc degree in Biomedical Engineering (Medical Informatics) in 2016 from the University of Minho in Braga, Portugal. His research interests include Business Intelligence, Data Mining, Decision Support Systems and Knowledge and Management Systems.

Diana Ferreira is a Biomedical Engineering student with master's degree in medical informatics and interest in eHealth, machine learning, healthcare systems, medical informatics and information technology. Programming and communication skills alongside with knowledge in various fields from computer science, physics, biology, chemistry, electronics, mechanics, and physiology.

Teresa Guarda has been scholar since 1991 and currently is teacher and investigator at the University, of Santa Elena and in University of Fuerzas Armadas of the Republic of Ecuador. She is Doctor in Technologies and Information Systems from the Minho University (Guimarães, Portugal) and M.S. in Systems and Information Technologies from the University of Coimbra (Coimbra, Portugal). She is researcher at ALGORITMI Research Centre.

José Inácio is a researcher at Algoritmi Centre, University of Minho. José is currently developing a solution and application to be used by Peek Health S.A in the future that uses Augmented Reality technologies in mobile applications for surgical assistance. He decided to embrace this project, because of his belief, passion and willingness to contribute for the development and use of technologies for medical purposes which can help not only their professionals, but mainly the patients. He has already worked in several projects such as applications for clinical use and medical inventory management, learning and knowledge extraction systems, image processing and Business Intelligence which used multiple technologies such as relational, non-relational and multidimensional databases, object oriented programming, data mining, artificial intelligence and computer vision.

Kijpokin Kasemsap received his BEng degree in Mechanical Engineering from King Mongkut's University of Technology, Thonburi, his MBA degree from Ramkhamhaeng University, and his DBA degree in Human Resource Management from Suan Sunandha Rajabhat University. Dr. Kasemsap is a Special Lecturer in the Faculty of Management Sciences, Suan Sunandha Rajabhat University, based in Bangkok, Thailand. Dr. Kasemsap is a Member of the International Economics Development and Research Center (IEDRC), the International Foundation for Research and Development (IFRD), and the International Innovative Scientific and Research Organization (IISRO). Dr. Kasemsap also serves on the International Advisory Committee (IAC) for the International Association of Academicians and Researchers (INAAR). Dr. Kasemsap is the sole author of over 250 peer-reviewed international publications and book chapters on business, education, and information technology. Dr. Kasemsap is included in the TOP 100 Professionals–2016 and in the 10th edition of 2000 Outstanding Intellectuals of the 21st Century by the International Biographical Centre, Cambridge, England.

Maria Lima received the PhD in Nursing from the Federal University of Ceará (2014). A master's degree in Nursing from the Federal University of Ceará (2011), Specialization in Nursing in Nephrology at the State University of Ceará (2009), degree in Nursing from the Federal University of Ceará (2007), incomplete degree in Chemistry from the State University of Ceará (2003). It was a lecturer at the Federal University of Piauí (UFPI) and is currently an adjunct professor of the Graduate Program in Nursing of the Federal University of Rio Grande do Norte (UFRN). It has experience in nursing, with emphasis in Medical-Surgical Nursing, acting on the following topics: health promotion, educational materials, technology, health education and emergency.

Ana Mendonça is a Biomedical Engineering student with master's specialization in Medical Informatics. Knowledge in multi-disciplinary areas such as: biology, electronics, chemistry, Medical Imaging, Databases Management or Artificial Intelligence, Healthcare systems, Machine learning.

Cristiana Neto is a student of the Master degree in Medical Informatics (Biomedical Engineer) with long interest in Electronic Health Records and Health Information Systems. Worked in several projects such as: Internet of Things: RAID technology in Healthcare, implementation of a system for the management of pharmacies and electronic prescriptions using JAVA, development of a program that deals with the information of a blood donation unit in JAVA, realization of an ontology based on a clinical protocol for chronic kidney disease and image segmentation for diabetic foot analysis. Currently working on some projects such as: development of a multiagent system that simulates the Manchester Triage system existing in the current public health services, 3D reconstruction of a knee using MRI images and Restrictions on Recipe Recommendations due to Allergies and Health Problems.

Hugo Peixoto is an IT specialist with long-held interests in eHealth, Medical Informatics and interoperability in healthcare. Programming and design ability, alongside communication skills spanning teaching, writing, and speaking, to audiences containing university students and International researchers.

João Ribeiro is a Biomedical Engineer with a Master's degree in Medical Informatics by the University of Minho in 2012. João has a passion for computer science and medicine since his childhood. In 2010, he began his master thesis which became the foundation for the development of the technology now being used by Peek Health S.A, where he is CEO, for the product PeekMed. He was also the FACE project promoter, developed at the Computer Engineering Department, University of Minho, which was a security and access control system to hospitals based on facial monitoring and recognition. His interests are related with MedTech, Medical Imaging, Technology in Health and Entrepreneurship.

Rita Reis is an Engineering and IT enthusiast with a drive to find new challenges where her creativity skills will merge with the need to connect IT and healthcare. As a problem-solving person, she uses her engineering knowledge to press for change in a non-profit organization and she acts efficiently as a web developer.

Sudipendra Roy has completed M.S. (Pharm) degree in Pharmacoinformatics from National Institute of Pharmaceutical Education & Research, Kolkata, India. Currently, he is pursuing doctoral studies in Management at Indian Institute of Management Indore, India.

Maria Santos is a student of the Informatics Master degree in Biomedical Engineer with long interest in Electronic Health Records and Health Information Systems. Previously she has worked in several projects such as "Clinical Protocols for Automatic Interpretation" or "Restrictions on Recipe Recommendations Due to Allergies and Health Problems."

Nancy Shipley is an experienced professional with a broad background in software engineering and information technology, seeking a challenging career in software application development.

Sara Silva has a master's degree in Biomedical Engineering. She is specialized in Medical Electronics. For her master's thesis, she developed a study about robotics applied to the autistic spectrum disorder. She wanted to understand how these robots could influence the learning process in children with this disorder. Four papers were published from this study, three for conferences and one for a journal. In August 2012, she also won a scholarship grant for a Summer School at the University of Bielefeld, themed: "Verbal and non-verbal communication". She began her career as a manager of software quality at a software development company for the retail sector, being now COO at Peek Health S.A.

Shashi Kant Srivastava is a doctoral participant in the Information Systems area of Indian Institute of Management (IIM) Indore. He holds a Bachelor's degree in Architecture from University of Roorkee and Masters in Ekistics (Science of Human Settlements) from Jamia Millia Islamia, New Delhi. Prior to current engagement, he worked as an Associate Professor at Apeejay Institute of Technology, Greater Noida.

Index

A

App 12-13, 55-58, 65, 116-117, 122
Appointments 69, 87, 186-187, 192-193, 195-197, 202
Augmented Reality 96-97, 99-100, 102, 104, 108

B

Big Data 14, 46-58, 65, 117, 119, 134, 189
Biomedical Engineering 153, 155, 158-159, 169
Brain Dead (BD) 128-129, 152
Bring Your Own Device (BYOD) 32, 34
Business Intelligence 54, 129, 132, 171, 173, 175-177, 183, 186-188, 192-194, 196-197, 203-206, 216
BYOD Benefits 41
BYOD SWOT Analysis 39

C

Client-Server Architecture 152
Clinical decision support 72, 86, 88, 130, 132, 153, 155-158, 169, 187, 193
Clinical Decision Support System 86, 153, 155-158, 169, 187, 193
Clinical Indicator 152
Cloud Computing 46-48, 50, 52, 55, 58, 66
Communication 1-2, 4-5, 13-14, 22-25, 28, 31-32, 55, 67-68, 70-72, 88-90, 92-93, 101, 109, 112, 120-121, 129, 153-154, 157, 188, 191, 204, 206
Computer 1, 3, 11, 14, 25-26, 34, 46-47, 50-51, 53, 66, 68, 85, 99, 104, 119, 141, 152-155, 157-158, 171, 202, 220, 222, 224
Computerized Physician Order Entry 153, 157, 169
Cranio-Encephalic Computerized Tomography (CE CT) 136, 152
Crowdsourcing 46, 66

D

Dashboard 180, 202, 210
Data 2, 4-6, 8-14, 22-25, 27-28, 31, 36, 40-42, 46-58, 65-66, 68-73, 85, 87-91, 93, 97-98, 100-101, 104, 107, 112-121, 123, 129-135, 137, 140-141, 143-147, 152-158, 170, 173-183, 187-190, 193-197, 202-203, 205-211, 215-216, 219-224, 227, 229
Data Mart 129, 189-190, 202
Data mining 134-135, 156, 194, 197, 206, 219-220, 222-224, 229
Data Warehousing 177, 187, 189-190, 203, 206, 208-209, 216
Decision Making 47, 51, 65, 71-72, 93, 132, 147, 153-159, 173, 176-177, 205, 208, 220-224
Decision Support Systems 88, 130, 132, 172, 187, 206, 209
Decision-Making Process 5, 128, 131-132, 134, 140, 174, 186-188, 190, 192-193, 195-197, 206
Diagnosis 5, 11, 34, 47-50, 54, 56, 58, 68, 98, 100, 107, 119, 129, 139, 141, 143, 147, 154-156, 158, 172, 174, 210, 220

E

Electronic Health Record (EHR) 67, 69, 72, 85, 143, 155, 169, 171-172, 183, 187, 197, 202
Electronic Medical Records (EMR) 66
ETL 134, 173, 175, 177, 179-180, 183, 187, 189-190, 195, 206-208

G

Genetic Algorithm 219, 223, 226-227, 229

H

Hadoop Distributed File System (HDFS) 52, 66
HDFS 52, 66
Health Informatics 153-159, 170
Health Management 71
Healthcare 1-6, 8-15, 22-23, 26-28, 32-34, 39-42, 46-50, 53-58, 71, 87, 117, 119, 128-133, 135, 154, 171, 173-174, 187-189, 192-193, 195, 210, 216, 219-224, 226
Hospitalization 1-2, 4-5, 204

I

Image Processing 100-101
Incremental spanning 219, 223, 225
Indicators 14, 87, 121-122, 132, 145-147, 173, 178-183, 187, 193, 195, 197, 202, 205, 207, 210-211, 215-216
Information 2, 4, 6-8, 10-14, 23-28, 31-34, 40-41, 46-48, 50-52, 54-58, 65-67, 69-73, 85, 87-88, 90-91, 93-94, 97-101, 103-104, 106, 109, 111-112, 114-122, 128-135, 137, 139-140, 143, 145-147, 153-159, 170-180, 183, 186-191, 193, 195-197, 202-206, 210, 213, 215-216, 220-221, 223-224, 227, 229
Information Technology 14, 32, 68, 85, 87, 155, 187, 193, 195, 203
Infrastructure 1-3, 5, 9-10, 13-15, 24-25, 28, 34, 52, 55, 70, 121, 133, 220
Intensive Care 3, 86-87, 129, 157, 170
Intensive Care Unit 157, 170
Internet of Things 1-2, 22-23, 31, 122, 220
Interoperability 13-14, 27, 68, 85, 87-88, 90, 92-93, 154, 173-174, 177, 205-206
Intranet 147, 202

K

Knowledge 5, 11, 24, 33, 46-51, 53-57, 72, 111-112, 116, 121, 128-131, 134-135, 137, 145-146, 153, 156-158, 170, 174, 177, 179, 186, 188, 191-193, 197, 206, 220, 223

M

MapReduce 52, 66
Medical Experts 46, 50, 53
Mobile Applications 55, 71, 96, 119
Mobile Devices in Healthcare 39-40
Mobile Health 2-4, 55, 67-73, 85
Monitoring 1-6, 8-15, 24-28, 34, 67-73, 88, 90, 113-114, 116-121, 123, 139-140, 183, 193, 204
Multidimensional Process 203

N

Neonatology 86-88, 90, 93
NoSql 52, 66
Nutrition Evaluation 203, 205, 216

O

Organ Transplantation 128, 131, 140, 145

P

Patient 1-15, 28, 34, 40, 47-50, 55-58, 67-70, 72-73, 85, 87-91, 93, 96-101, 103-104, 107, 109, 112-117, 119-122, 128-129, 135-136, 139-143, 146, 152-155, 157-159, 171-174, 178-179, 182, 187, 203-205, 208-210, 215, 220, 222
Pervasive 2, 22-24, 26, 31, 33-34, 42, 86-88, 93, 111-112, 186-187, 190, 192-193, 196-197
Pervasive Computing 2, 33-34, 86, 88
Pervasive Health Care Systems 22-23, 26, 31
Physician 6, 8-9, 11-12, 42, 69, 85, 88, 97, 100, 102, 129, 153, 157, 169, 172, 174, 213, 215
Pinterest 46-48, 54, 56-58
Plugin 202
Portal 46, 53, 56-58
Prescription 47-48, 86, 90, 116, 156-157
Proof of Concept 187, 190, 192-193, 196

Q

Queries 47, 52, 88, 91, 188, 193, 202, 209-210

R

Remote 1-6, 8-9, 12-15, 34, 66-67, 71-73, 88, 90, 97-98, 100-101, 107, 109, 219

S

Sabichão 86-88, 90-94
Smart Health and Well-being 46, 49
Social Media 46-51, 56, 58
Surgeries 97-99, 174, 178, 181, 186-187, 192-193, 195-197, 202
Surgical Planning 96, 98, 101, 103, 107-109

T

Technology 1-2, 4-5, 14-15, 23-24, 27, 32, 39, 41, 46-50, 52-58, 67-71, 73, 85, 87, 101, 109, 112, 114-117, 119-123, 131, 134, 152-158, 171, 176-177, 187-188, 193, 195, 203, 220, 223, 231
Technology-Centric 1, 3, 13
Text Mining 134-135, 137, 146-147, 152

U

Ubiquitous 22-24, 33-34, 68, 70, 86, 88, 92, 112, 154
User-Friendly 26, 93, 158, 202

V

Visual Analytics 54, 66
Visualization 9, 47-48, 52-54, 57-58, 66, 97, 100-101, 103-104, 109, 141, 144, 189, 193, 197, 207, 209

W

Waiting Lists 171-174, 183, 186-187, 192-193, 195-197
Wearable health gadgets 112, 118
Web 12, 52, 54, 87, 89-90, 92-94, 97, 100, 140-141, 186-187, 192-197, 202
Web Browser 140, 193, 202
Wireless Sensor Networks 10, 22, 25

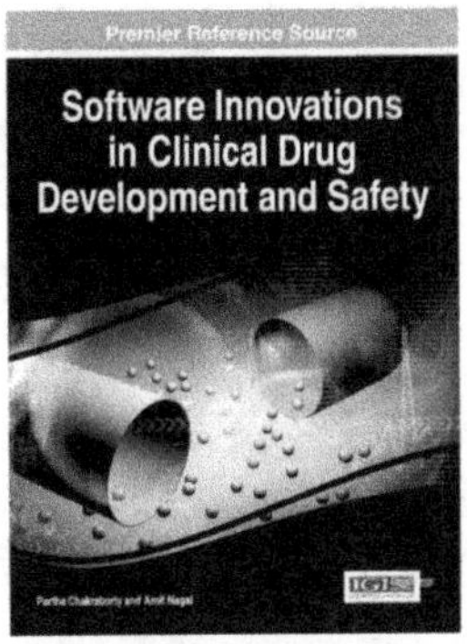
Premier Reference Source
Software Innovations in Clinical Drug Development and Safety

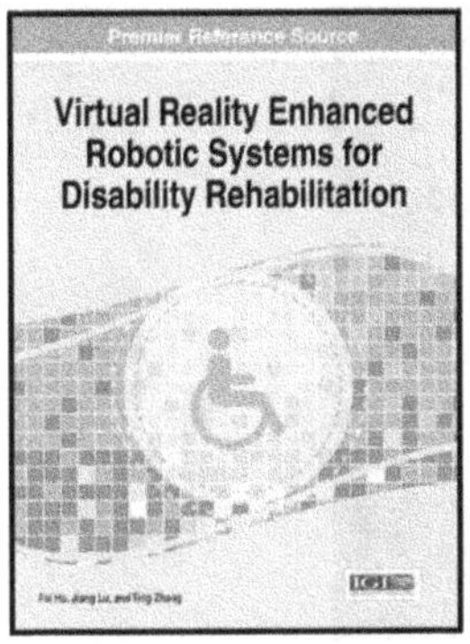
Premier Reference Source
Virtual Reality Enhanced Robotic Systems for Disability Rehabilitation

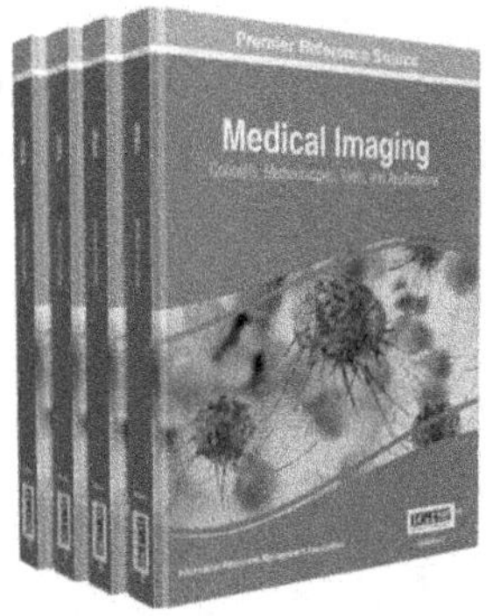
Medical Imaging

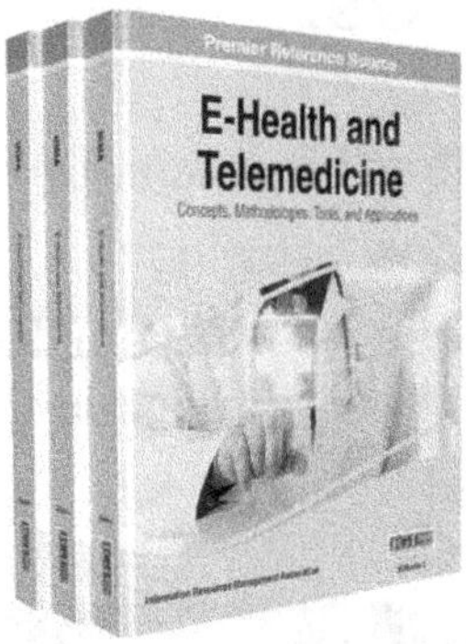
Premier Reference Source
E-Health and Telemedicine

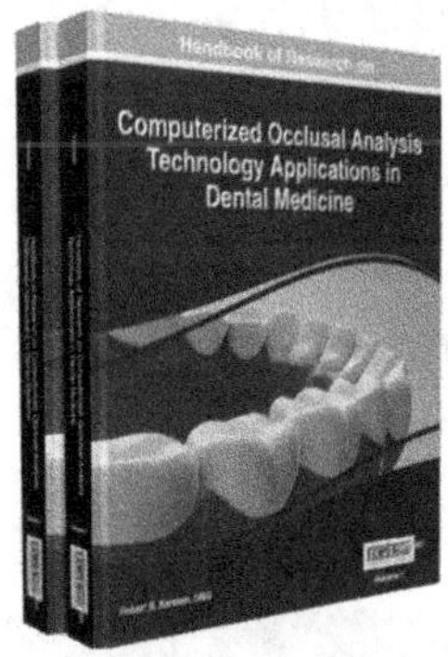
Handbook of Research on
Computerized Occlusal Analysis Technology Applications in Dental Medicine

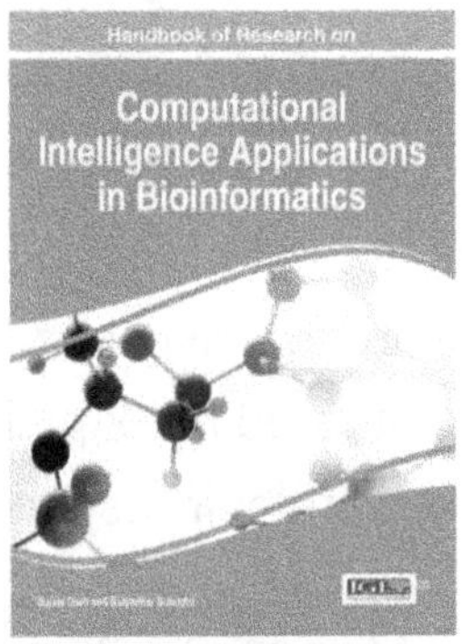
Handbook of Research on
Computational Intelligence Applications in Bioinformatics

www.ingramcontent.com/pod-product-compliance
Lightning Source LLC
LaVergne TN
LVHW062152300926
849161LV00010B/2651